The Making of the
Unborn Patient

The Making of the Unborn Patient

A Social Anatomy of Fetal Surgery

Monica J. Casper

Rutgers University Press

New Brunswick, New Jersey, and London

Library of Congress Cataloging-in-Publication Data

Casper, Monica J., 1966–
    The making of the unborn patient : a social anatomy of fetal
surgery / Monica J. Casper.
        p.   cm.
    Includes bibliographical references and index
    ISBN 0-8135-2515-2 (cloth : alk. paper). — ISBN 0-8135-2516-0
(pbk. : alk. paper)
    1. Fetus—Surgery—Social aspects.   2. Fetus—Surgery—Moral and
ethical aspects.   I. Title
RG784.C37   1998
619.8—dc21   97-39331
                                                              CIP

British Cataloging-in-Publication data for this book is available from the British Library

Manufactured in the United States of America

In memory
of my grandfather
Earl Hans Christensen
who gave me books

For my mother
Patricia A. Struck
who gave me life

For my sister
Tanya L. Casper
who gave me faith

Contents

Acknowledgments

Unlike the mythical free-floating fetus, I did not go solo for this project. I have been helped, challenged, supported, and tethered along the way by many people. Foremost, I am deeply grateful to the many informants who opened their homes and workplaces to my scrutiny. In New Zealand, Margaret Liley, Stephanie Liley, Bill Liley, Jr., Graham Liggins, Ross Howie, Florence Fraser, Pat McCarthy, and David Becroft were gracious and forthcoming. Graham Liggins provided encouraging feedback on an earlier version of Chapter 2 and valuable assistance in locating key materials while I was finishing this book. I am especially grateful to Margaret Liley for making me feel welcome on her beautiful farm in Taumarunui and for patiently answering all of my probing questions about her late husband. Peggy Lawsom of the Auckland Society for the Protection of the Unborn Child, whom I did not get a chance to meet, sent important information, including an obituary of William Liley. Val Corcoran, Kevin Townend, and Helen Hopman at National Women's Hospital provided helpful organizational and logistical support. Kevin kept me connected to the Northern Hemisphere through electronic mail, and Val was stalwart in helping me lug heavy boxes of files down from the attic of National Women's Hospital. I spent a sweltering but lovely afternoon with Karliss Adamsons in San Juan, Puerto Rico, and I deeply appreciate his interest in this project. Arsenio Comas in San Juan and Vincent Freda in New York helped bring additional aspects of the experimental work of the 1960s to life for me.

I am grateful to the clinical and administrative staff of the Fetal Treatment Unit at Capital Hospital for sharing their experiences and insights with me. I do not name them here in order to protect their identities, but I hope that they recognize their many contributions to this project. My story would have been enriched by a more thorough, less anonymous description of each explorer of this new frontier, interesting and committed people all. Those who work on and around the unborn patient may not agree with my interpretations of their livelihood, but their input has substantially shaped this project in numerous ways and I admire their passion. I owe a great debt of gratitude to the staff of the Institutional Review Board at Capital Hospital for their tireless efforts in preparing human subjects documents for me. When I invoked the Freedom of Information Act to access records, the IRB staff was gracious in what might have been an awkward situation. Thanks must also go to the patients and their families who shared their stories with me both directly and indirectly. I cannot name them but I hope they know that they are the lifeblood of fetal surgery.

My original dissertation committee—Adele Clarke, Virginia Olesen, Anselm Strauss, and Donna Haraway—shaped my thinking profoundly. Adele has been a superb mentor, colleague, and friend, and has offered much support and insight for this book. Virginia and Donna are model feminist scholars, whose work has challenged and inspired me. Anselm was influential in my emergence as a symbolic interactionist, and he is sorely missed. I owe a huge debt of gratitude to Marc Berg, Mary Sue Heilemann, Sharon Kaufman, Susan Kelly, Bill Magee, and Lynn Morgan for reading and commenting with care on the entire manuscript. Their many helpful criticisms and insights are present in the final product. Lisa Jean Moore, Linda Hogle, Debora Bone, and Mike Curtis provided feedback on earlier versions of this book, and their friendship and support through graduate school and beyond have continually revitalized me. My growth as a scholar and a person benefited enormously from a decade spent with Matt Kling, who nurtured my career and this book in their embryonic stages in more ways than one. Thanks to Barbara Koenig for helpful feedback on chapter 5 and for giving me a job when I needed one. Thanks also to the many friends and colleagues—too numerous to name—in medical sociology, science and technology studies, and feminist studies with whom I have been in conversation over the years. Finally, thanks to my colleagues in the Sociology Department at the University of California, Santa Cruz, for making me feel welcome, especially to Craig Haney for helping me get time off from teaching to write this book, to Candace West for feedback on chapter 3, and to Herman Gray for feedback on chapter 1. Vivian Christensen, my remarkable research assistant, spent her time organizing my next project while I finished this one.

My experience in publishing this book with Rutgers University Press has been remarkably painless and even fun. In large part this was due to Martha Heller, my hip, smart editor. A marvelous "midwife," Martha read everything I wrote, often more than once, and always seemed to know precisely what I was trying to say. Martha's editorial judgment was impeccable, and each chapter—indeed, the entire book—bears her savvy imprint. Thanks also to Karen Reeds who warmly brought me into the fold at Rutgers, to Betty Levin for her very helpful initial review of the manuscript, and to my agent, Ronald Goldfarb. I also received excellent feedback from Rayna Rapp and Elizabeth Knoll, each of whom reviewed the manuscript for other publishers before I signed with Rutgers.

My family is an ongoing source of comfort and encouragement. Ross Smith sustains me with his humor and love, and our busy, full life together has given me many positive things to work on besides the unborn patient. Ross contributed constructive criticism and moral support while also challenging and fueling my sociological imagination. Loving thanks to my parents, Pat and Denny Struck, for believing in me and helping me to grow, to Tanya Casper for being exactly what a big sister should be, and to Gramps, wherever he may be. I am also grateful to Derrell Struck, Dean Struck, Beth Struck, Don Wolkowitz, Sally Carlson, Don Carlson, and Ted Smith for their love, support, and interest in my work.

During this project I was generously assisted by a series of fellowships from the Graduate Division at the University of California, San Francisco, a University of California President's Research Fellowship in the Humanities, a Doctoral Dissertation Improvement Grant from the National Science Foundation (#SBR-9320173), and funding from the Social Science Division at the University of California, Santa Cruz.

Clearly, the world of the unborn is not the impenetrable
mystery that tradition claimed. The fetus is now
coming of age as a candidate for the best that modern
diagnosis and treatment can provide. He may be the
littlest patient but he is by no means the least.
—New York Academy of Sciences (1968)

Liley's needle had penetrated barriers beyond flesh and
death on its way to the heart of the womb: breached, too,
was the metaphysical barrier between the world of life
that is and the universe of life that is yet to be.
A fetus had been treated, medically, as one of us.
—David Zimmerman (1973)

Treatment of the unborn has had a long and
painstaking gestation; the date of confinement is still
questionable; and viability is still uncertain.
But there is promise that the fetus may become
a "born-again" patient.
—Michael Harrison (1991)

Who speaks for the fetus?
—Donna Haraway (1992)

The Making of the Unborn Patient

Chapter 1

Introduction
Fetal Matters

A gripping drama is unfolding in a busy urban hospital in the western United States. A young pregnant woman has recently been told that the fetus she is carrying has a fatal defect. There is a hole in its diaphragm and its abdominal organs have begun migrating up into its chest cavity, impairing lung development. Without any kind of intervention, the fetus will surely die. The woman and her husband, ardent Christians, do not believe in abortion, nor do they want their baby to die in utero or at birth, struggling for oxygen. After weeks of agonizing indecision in the face of these limited choices, the couple has learned of an experimental treatment called fetal surgery. They have traveled across the country to this imposing medical facility where the woman and her 22-week-old fetus will be operated on. The couple is nervous and frightened, but they believe that God will protect their unborn baby, and the woman herself, during the intricate and dangerous operation.

While her husband paces nervously in a nearby waiting room, the woman lies on an operating table in a hot, noisy surgical theater. Anesthetized, she is surrounded by gowned and masked medical workers and high-tech equipment. With bright lights shining on her body, the woman is transformed into a flesh-and-blood operating theater. A team of surgeons slices her abdomen, peels back its layers, and clamps it open with large silver clips. Her uterus and amniotic sac are surgically opened and the amniotic fluid is drained. The exposed fetus, the diminutive star of the show, is partially removed from the woman's uterus and placed on her abdominal wall. A small incision is made in the fetus's chest, into which is placed a monitoring device. The surgeons then slice directly into the fetal body. After almost an hour, they repair the hernia but there is not enough room in the fetus's abdominal cavity to replace the organs that the surgeons have retrieved from its chest cavity. To avoid a fetal abdominal rupture during *continued growth in the womb, the surgeons capture the fetus's organs and meticulously seal them in a small Gortex sac that is then attached to the outside of the fetus's body. When they have completed their work, the surgeons close the fetal incisions, replace the altered fetus within the amniotic sac along with saline solution, and reseal the young woman's uterus and abdomen.*

The surgery itself is successful and the woman is placed immediately on an intense regimen of antilabor medications. When she wakes up, she is in a great deal of pain and has difficulty moving, but she and her husband are deeply relieved that both she and the fetus survived the operation. Together they begin the long, slow process of recovery, while also happily anticipating their baby's birth. Sadly, the couple's relief is short-lived; their fetus dies two days later. The fetal surgeons and their obstetrician colleagues are not entirely sure what went wrong, but they will conduct an autopsy to determine the cause of death. The young couple leave the hospital several days later, devastated by their loss.

Locating Fetal Surgery

This book is about fetal surgery, a new medical treatment in which a pregnant woman's at-risk fetus is partially taken out of her uterus, operated on and, if it survives the operation, replaced in her womb for continued gestation. Although fetal surgery has existed in various forms for three decades, it is only just beginning to capture the public's imagination. People in the United States and elsewhere are far more familiar with the highly controversial debates about embryo research and fetal tissue research than they are with the making of the unborn patient. Whenever I discuss fetal surgery, whether at academic conferences or dinner parties, I am routinely met with open-mouthed awe and the now familiar question, "Can they really do that?" When I describe how some fetuses, depending upon gestational age at the time of surgery, are born without scars, jaws drop even further. What is striking in an era that heralds every new medical innovation is that so few people have heard about this rather remarkable procedure. Indeed, almost all of my wide-eyed, intent listeners tell me that fetal surgery sounds like science fiction rather than real life. Surely it is both amazing and troubling, something one sees on *Star Trek* rather than at the hospital around the corner.

This new practice both fascinates and horrifies precisely because it transgresses a number of medical and cultural boundaries. Not only does fetal surgery breach the womb in new and profoundly unsettling ways, it also performs a kind of cultural work in making us rethink some of our most cherished assumptions about life and the natural body. Fetal

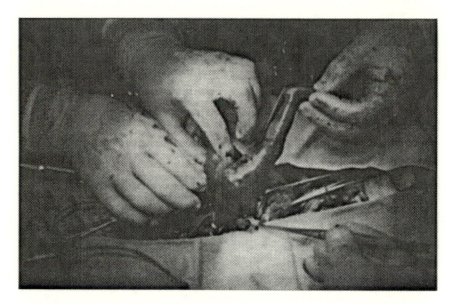

Surgeons operating on a fetus inside a woman's uterus, whose layers are peeled back to expose the unborn patient. In visual records of fetal surgery, pregnant women are routinely erased from the frame, as here. A ureterostomy is the surgical establishment of an external opening in the ureter (conducts urine from the kidney to the bladder). Source: M. R. Harrison, M. S. Golbus, and R. A. Filly. 1991. *The Unborn Patient: Prenatal Diagnosis and Treatment.* Philadelphia: W. B. Saunders Company, p. 384.

surgery challenges what we think we know about pregnancy, the autonomous fetus, maternal-fetal relationships, how and to whom health care is provided, the limits and potential of technology, and what counts as personhood at the close of the twentieth century. Like other cutting-edge medical procedures, such as cloning and genetic therapy, fetal surgery is the stuff of *Nova,* inspiring wonder and concern about our capacity to alter human destiny. But also like many other medical innovations, especially those at the beginnings and ends of human life, fetal surgery is proceeding rapidly ahead of careful reflection about what it means and without public debate about its consequences. This book offers a critical social and cultural analysis of this nascent yet significant innovation in biomedicine.

There are many overlapping stories contained within the story of fetal surgery. In this book, I "read" and interpret the stories of medical workers, pregnant women, and fetal surgery watchers of various sorts, critically weaving these together within my own ethnographic narrative. In one version of the story—certainly the most dominant in medicine and popular culture—fetal surgery is about biomedicine's heroic intervention in reproductive health over the past thirty years. In this version, brave and talented surgeons, self-sacrificing mothers, and fragile, ailing fetuses are brought together in busy operating rooms to fulfill technodreams of medical progress. Consider, for example, the enthusiastic, expansive, and uncritical terms in which the following quote portrays fetal surgery: "Treatment of the unborn patient is an exciting endeavor that is itself in its infancy. The heretofore hidden world of the fetus is coming under closer scrutiny, and the scope of medicine, both its science and humanity, has been forever broadened" (Camosy 1995, 1391). Similar versions of the fetal surgery story, laudatory and devoid of social and ethical analysis, have appeared in numerous magazine articles and newspaper accounts, on television shows such as *20/20* and *Body Human 2000*, and on radio programs such as National Public Radio's "Science Friday."

But another version of the story, one in which I am more deeply invested, extends beyond the operating room to the cultural milieus that both cradle and seep into biomedical work. In this framing, fetal surgery embodies how we think about reproduction, pregnant women, families, and most of all, those tiny dependent occupants of women's bodies—fetuses. Fetal surgery, as I shall show, is intimately connected to other social practices, like abortion politics, in which the personhood and worth of a fetus are salient. Because many women who select fetal surgery are opposed to abortion, the procedure itself is often touted as a benevolent alternative to abortion that rescues fetuses that would otherwise die either from disease or by women's hand. It is also embedded within a broader set of social phenomena that I call "fetal politics," including the crafting of a new science called fetology, controversies over fetal tissue research, the emergence of fetal rights in law and ethics, debates about and proscriptions on pregnant women's behavior, a cultural obsession with fetal images, and the relentless pursuit of new reproductive technologies. Many of these practices themselves are sites at which fetal personhood and maternal identity are constructed and contested. All these enduring, troubled relationships mark fetal surgery as a controversial practice; in part they explain why it has been something of a medical "secret" for more than a decade despite often glowing media coverage (Cadoff 1994; Kolata 1983).[1] The connections and tensions among the many different versions of the story of fetal surgery form the narrative core of this book.

Along with the emergence of this new specialty has come a new category of person whose "birth" this book charts. Like fetal surgery, this new subject has been fashioned at the intersection of an array of social, cultural, and political processes. The specialty and its often elusive client have developed in tandem, each serving as a justification for the existence of the other. Because of its single-minded focus on the fetus, fetal surgery has contributed substantially, although not without challenge, to defining the fetus as a patient in its own right with clinical (and legal) interests distinct from those of the pregnant woman in whom it is gestating (Mattingly 1992). In this sense, fetal surgery participates in the erasure of pregnant women that has occurred as fetuses continue to attract greater attention from health care providers. Despite women's own commitments to securing healthier babies, fetal surgery feeds into cultural preoccupations with maternal-fetal conflict. It fuels rather than resolves ongoing social confusion about where women end and fetuses begin. In the face of considerable cultural ambiguity about maternity and fetal life, then, some fetuses have been constructed, individually and collectively, as a shocking new object of the "clinical gaze" (Foucault 1973): the unborn patient.

Although it may provide a graphic and disturbing preview of the future of human reproduction, fetal surgery both has a rich history and is located very much in the present. Building on work done in the 1960s in New Zealand and Puerto Rico in which fetuses were treated using a variety of techniques, surgeons in California performed a successful "open" fetal surgery in 1981. Media accounts of this surgical feat characterized it as a "bold operation" and a "dramatic new enterprise," and the fetus itself was described then and subsequently as a "miracle baby."[2] Although the baby died shortly after birth, suggesting a short-lived miracle, this operation nonetheless marked the beginning of an ambitious program of clinical research on open fetal surgery. For more than fifteen years, a small number of women carrying fetuses diagnosed with life-threatening conditions have chosen experimental fetal surgery as a last chance effort to save their babies. They have eschewed other options, such as abortion, postnatal treatment, or no treatment at all, and hoped instead that high-tech intervention would salvage their otherwise doomed fetuses. They have done so within a context that celebrates progress, life at any cost, and the amazing accomplishments of modern medicine. As the pediatrician and bioethicist Perri Klass (1996, 119) has written about fetal surgery, "It is impossible not to be dazzled by the idea of what they can already do and by what they will be able to do." In clinical and popular literature, as well as in the lives of some very brave women and their families, fetal surgery is increasingly portrayed as an operation to the rescue.

Yet despite its promises and the excitement that it has generated, fetal surgery is fraught with problems on several levels. Perhaps most significantly and in contrast to many nonsurgical fetal treatments that have been more successful, this technology actually succeeds in rescuing very few fetuses. Although exact numbers are difficult to ascertain—for reasons that will become clear later—fewer than one hundred fetuses have been operated on for congenital defects and only about 35 percent have survived. While some surgical procedures have become more acceptable in routine use than others because they result in fewer fetal deaths, fetal mortality rates are as high as 80 percent for certain operations such as diaphragmatic hernia repair (Adzick and Harrison 1994). Even when surgery is successful and the fetus lives, there is no guarantee that it will survive birth or grow into a healthy child free of disabilities. Barry Kogan (1991, 399) has argued that "Fetal physicians, more than others, must be driven by the Hippocratic dictum, 'Primum, non nocare'—'In the first instance, do no harm.'" It is not clear that practitioners of fetal surgery have, in fact, remained faithful to this ethical injunction. Precisely because it has not been an unqualified success, there is considerable dissent both within medicine and among its critics about just how much a role fetal surgery should have in the future of human reproduction. But if the promise of fetal surgery currently exceeds what it can actually deliver, why has it been pursued with such zeal and why is it so beginning to capture people's imaginations?

On the surface, fetal surgery and the unborn patient exist because pregnant women and medical workers want to save babies from certain death. As an experimental procedure, the use of fetal surgery has, up until recently, been limited to fatal conditions, or those defects such as congenital diaphragmatic hernia (CDH), congenital cystic adenomatoid malformation (C-CAM), or sacrococcygeal teratoma (SCT) that would likely kill fetuses or newborns without any treatment. The prevailing logic is that these fetuses will die anyway and thus make perfect candidates for a new and uncertain treatment. The basic clinical rationale is that structural problems in a fetus's body can be diagnosed and treated early enough to prevent more serious conditions from developing. Or, as fetal surgeons Scott Adzick and Michael Harrison (1994, 901) have written, "The promise of fetal therapy is that the earliest possible intervention for a life-threatening fetal disorder may produce the best results." By nipping problems in the bud, so to speak, fetal surgeons believe that prenatal treatment can prevent a domino effect of cascading physical defects that would ultimately prove lethal. This certainly sounds pretty amazing, and it is easy to see why fetal surgery resonates so deeply with a cultural belief in the power of medicine as well as with science fiction's celebration of technical prowess.

Above and beyond clinical factors and the deceptively simple goal of "saving babies," however, there are other reasons why fetal surgery has emerged as a new medical specialty in the past thirty years. These reasons, many of which will be explored in this book, have to do with broader cultural milieus alluded to above that provide fruitful contexts for fetal surgery while also shaping its content. They include increasing medical specialization and the search for new health care markets, research trajectories within experimental medicine, the seductive allure of technology, intense cultural and political investments in human fetuses over the past few decades, reproductive and abortion politics, notions of gender and motherhood, women's own desires for healthier babies, and social discomfort with and stigmatization of disability coupled with a wide array of efforts to minimize birth defects. Fetal surgery intersects and animates all of these cultural and political fault lines that themselves form the basis of ongoing social conflicts. While fetal surgery is interesting and fascinating in its own right, examining it sociologically enables us to see the issues and practices encircling it in a different way. Like peering through a womb awash in semiotic fluid, fetal surgery acts as a cultural prism enabling a deeper analysis of the many layers of social relations, meanings, and politics that infiltrate the operating room.

As a new medical specialty, fetal surgery is embedded within the institutional and professional politics of health care in multiple ways. Because of its experimental status, fetal surgery occupies a limited and somewhat precarious place alongside other fetal therapies that are more common in advanced health care systems, including drug therapy (Schulman and Evans 1991), nutritional supplements (Harding and Charlton 1991), fetal blood sampling (Moise 1993), selective termination of a defective fetus when there is more than one fetus per pregnancy (Golbus 1991), the use of hormones to prevent respiratory distress syndrome (Liggins and Howie 1972), the use of catheters to drain fluids from malformed fetal organs (Harrison and Filly 1991), and fetoscopy and embryoscopy in which various miniature optical tools are used to diagnose and treat fetuses (Quintero et al. 1993). Beginning in the 1930s with the administration of penicillin to pregnant women to prevent syphilis in their fetuses, each of these treatments—all, for the most part, easier to perform and less risky than fetal surgery—has been an incremental step toward the making of the unborn patient. Each technical advance has rendered the womb and its contents more visible, often erasing pregnant women in the process. Indeed, obstetrical and fetal treatment practices are increasingly defined as maternal-fetal medicine (Creasy and Resnick 1994) or even abbreviated as fetal medicine (Manning 1995), underscoring the degree to which fetal health is considered paramount and maternal health issues are sidelined.

Unlike some of the more ubiquitous treatments (e.g., nutritional therapy), fetal surgery is enormously complex and requires the participation and coordination of a broad array of medical workers, each of whom brings to the table his or her own unique expertise. It is also clinically quite challenging, in part because fetuses, located inside living pregnant female bodies, are notoriously difficult to access if one wants to keep them alive. Multiple skills and tools must be deployed to find and operate on the delicate fetal patient while also struggling to avoid maternal damage. Fetal surgery attracts many different kinds of medical workers and its institutional contours are constantly reinforced through professional interaction. But fetal surgery is still evolving; its territory is not yet defined and staked out. Of the many medical specialists involved in fetal surgery, which set of workers will ultimately control fetal surgery remains to be established. There is continual jockeying for position among the various groups of medical workers, and this maneuvering has ramifications for future directions of fetal treatment. These dynamics make for some very interesting politics as medical professionals responsible for the unborn patient struggle over resources, access to "their" patients, new innovations, and a host of other issues.

Largely because of its experimental and tentative status, fetal surgery is an unusual and localized practice. There are only about fifteen centers in five or six countries pursuing invasive fetal treatments such as surgery.[3] According to one obstetrician I spoke to, there is a general consensus that many institutions are "waiting to see what happens" at one of the premier fetal treatment facilities. Capital Hospital is a major medical center in the western United States with a thriving experimental fetal surgery program, and it figures prominently in this book as a key site in the making of the unborn patient. Despite limited success and very low fetal survival rates for some operations, the Fetal Treatment Unit (FTU) at Capital Hospital has invested a great deal in fetal surgery. Medical workers there strive to propel their specialty from an experimental procedure to the standard of care for congenital defects, but they attempt to do so in the face of criticism and controversy—both within their own institution and beyond. At Capital Hospital, fetal surgery has evolved from an experimental medical innovation fraught with controversy to an established clinical research program offering a range of treatments, some deemed acceptable and others not. As a microcosm of the broader professional context, there is ongoing negotiation at Capital Hospital about whether fetal surgery should become a routine treatment. Not all medical workers, either at Capital Hospital or elsewhere, agree that operating on a fetus still in a pregnant woman's womb is a good idea. Some, in fact, think it is quite a bad idea, as we shall see.

There are other ways in which fetal surgery intersects with the politics of health care, largely having to do with money. Of the available prenatal treatment options, fetal surgery is by far the most expensive. A single operation can cost tens of thousands of dollars, and every successful fetal surgery requires at least two operations on the pregnant woman (the surgery itself and cesarean delivery).[4] Patients and their partners must often travel long distances to hospitals and pay for their own accommodations once they arrive. Federal funding of clinical trials has provided some opportunity for women of different economic brackets to choose fetal surgery, but the majority of patients are those most capable of paying for the treatment themselves and are usually (but not always) white, middle- to upper-class couples. Insurance companies are occasionally persuaded to pay for fetal surgery as a supposedly cheaper alternative to neonatal care or a lifetime of managing chronic illness or defects, eliding the fact that fetal surgery itself may result in both of these conditions. Insurance coverage would likely increase if fetal surgery were to become a routine procedure, although the widespread practice of fetal surgery may also be constrained by managed care, which rations health services on the basis of cost containment. Additional funding to offset patient costs comes from hospitals with fetal surgery programs and from nonprofit sources committed to fetal and maternal health such as the March of Dimes.

Just as significant as the actual cost of fetal surgery is the cultural work it does in detracting attention from the health care crisis in the United States. While fetal surgeons access new patients in the womb, patients outside the womb struggle to access an increasingly expensive and ineffective health care system. Daring and glamorous medical feats that make headlines can bewitch us into forgetting that many people cannot get basic health care services because they do not have any insurance or other benefits. According to the Census Bureau, in 1992 roughly 14.7 percent of the population—about 37 million Americans—was uninsured (Himmelstein and Woolhandler 1994). In 1993, that number had risen to 38.9 milion uninsured, and another 53 million people were without coverage for part of the year (Freund and McGuire 1995). Latinos are twice as likely to lack health insurance as whites, while one out of five African-Americans is uninsured. Moreover, as federal and state policies continue to dismantle the welfare state, certain groups—especially the poor, new immigrants, women, and children—have been, and will likely continue to be, severely affected by eroding public benefits. There is little doubt that the United States health care system is in big trouble.

These issues are especially relevant to reproductive health, where significant race and class disparities exist between pregnant women who have access to prenatal care (and which types of care) and those who do not (Leigh 1994). It is ironic and unfortunate that in an age of expensive high-tech medicine, many women cannot receive even basic services such as good nutrition and checkups. The California Department of Health Services estimates that almost 25 percent of all pregnant women in the United States do not receive *any* prenatal care in their first trimester, and the National Center for Health Statistics reports that 16 percent of all women giving birth receive *inadequate* prenatal care.[5]

While 87 percent of white and Asian women receive adequate care, only 74 percent of African-American women, 70 percent of Latina women, and 68 percent of Native American women receive adequate care. In addition, if the current national gap in infant mortality rates continues to widen, African-American babies will be three times as likely to die as white babies by the year 2000 (Associated Press 1994). Perhaps more important, however, across all racial and ethnic groups poverty translates into lack of access to services, including basic prenatal care *and* high-tech fetal treatments.

These figures beg a serious analysis of the politics of investing fervidly in some fetuses while ignoring others.[6] The unborn patient appears, overwhelmingly, to be white and privileged, rendering it capital-intensive in more ways than one. The costs of invasive fetal surgery, coupled with high fetal mortality rates and significant risks to pregnant women and fetuses, suggests that surgical treatment may not be the best way to ensure healthy babies and mothers.[7] Fetal surgery throws into stark relief the politics of prenatal care specifically and health care generally, raising important questions about access to health services of all kinds. Given that many women do not have access to adequate basic prenatal care, should a risky, expensive treatment like fetal surgery be considered a standard part of reproductive medicine? If so, who will have access to it? Will it be a "boutique" form of care, available only to those who can pay, or will all fetuses at high risk be eligible for treatment? Most significant, should fetal interventions be allowed to assume a more central role in prenatal care in the future if we cannot guarantee that all pregnant women will have access to basic prenatal care for themselves and their fetuses?

As a medical specialty designed to save unborn fetuses, fetal surgery also intersects with both reproductive and abortion politics, with a number of striking implications for women's health. I define reproductive politics as the multiple ways in which human reproduction, particularly as women experience it, is shaped by power, inequality, and social location. A wide range of reproductive issues—including contraception, pregnancy, childbirth, infertility, surrogacy, in vitro fertilization, abortion, infant feeding, childcare, prenatal diagnosis and care, menstruation, adoption, miscarriage, and menopause serve as critical and contested aspects of most women's lives. Reproduction is a key site of social control over women and of women's agency, both of which differ by race, ethnicity, class, and sexuality. In the United States and elsewhere, women's reproductive processes are contested and stratified at interpersonal, biomedical/scientific, cultural, economic, political, and global levels of social life (Ginsburg and Rapp 1995). The politics of reproduction may take the form of, for example, struggles for better contraception, bureaucratic hand-wringing over teenage pregnancy, battles with federal agencies over new reproductive technologies, public debates about abortion, proscriptions on pregnant women's behavior, and women's interactions with medical providers. Increasingly, reproductive politics also include the proliferation of cultural images and discourses of the fetus, technological surveillance of fetuses, and scientific and medical constructions of fetal personhood (Hartouni 1997).

Fetal surgery embodies a particular configuration of these reproductive politics, while also resonating with others such as individual women's experiences with the health care system. As a new and dubious medical procedure, fetal surgery is like many other rescue treatments but with a crucial difference. The fetus is no simple organ or body part within a woman's body; it evokes a whole set of complicated social and cultural meanings both on its own and in relation to pregnancy and women's experiences of it. Operating on fetuses has serious implications for maternal health, and pregnant women who undergo fetal surgery uniformly describe it as "a major ordeal." More than any other fetal treatment, fetal surgery requires major intrusion into a pregnant woman's body. It thus provides an unsurpassed opportunity to reconsider prenatal care in terms of women's health rather than fetal health. With this in mind, two aspects of fetal surgery stand out.

First, in almost all fetal surgery cases, there is nothing physiologically wrong with the pregnant woman choosing it. Fetal surgery is designed to benefit fetuses, especially those at great risk. Women benefit—sometimes enormously—from fetal surgery to the degree that they may end up with a living baby, invoking the social "good" of benevolent maternal sacrifice. Yet fetal surgery is not medicine for women's own good (Ehrenreich and English 1978), but rather medicine for the ostensible good of the fetus—although these may be conflated in practice. What if a woman does not accept a procedure designed to rescue her dying fetus? As ethical and legal discourses more fully embrace a doctrine recognizing "the best interests of the fetus," maternal-fetal conflict issues come into play and women's autonomy may be threatened (AAP Committee on Bioethics 1990; ACOG Committee on Ethics 1990; Knopoff 1991; Macklin 1990; Purdy 1990). In this framework, the actions and intentions of a pregnant woman are viewed as conflicting with the needs, interests, and rights of her fetus. What if a pregnant woman "refuses" the treatment her doctor recommends? Is she then culpable if her fetus dies? Will she be censured by family members? Can she be forced by the courts to undergo fetal surgery, as many women have been legally required to undergo cesarean sections on behalf of their fetuses? How is a woman's decision to undergo a risky intervention on behalf of her fetus shaped by these broader ethical, legal, and political factors?

Second, these issues are compounded by the technical difficulties of performing fetal surgery. Accessing the fetus always means somehow getting inside a pregnant woman's body, most commonly by opening the abdomen and uterus via a hysterotomy or type of cesarean section. Once a woman's uterus is surgically opened, preterm labor is an inevitable major risk; it is the most vexing problem faced during and after fetal surgery (Harrison and Longaker 1991; Jennings, MacGillivary and Harrison 1993). Fetal surgery is an extremely complicated procedure that cannot be performed quickly, safely, or on an outpatient basis. Pregnant women who choose it must undergo uterine surgery (almost always more than once), face all of the usual risks of anesthesia and major surgery including death, and take several antilabor medications for up to several weeks after surgery. In a medical specialty focused therapeutically on the fetus alone, the pregnant woman becomes, in the words of one fetal surgeon, merely "the best heart-lung machine available" for maintaining the unborn patient. Even after all of these considerable efforts, there is no guarantee that a woman who undergoes fetal surgery will have a healthy, or even living, baby in the end or that her own health will be unaffected.

These factors clearly mark fetal surgery as a women's health issue par excellence with major consequences for some women's reproductive lives. Indeed, consider the words of a representative from the March of Dimes, the nation's premier philanthropy focused on maternal and infant health and a major funder of fetal research and treatment: "Fetal surgery itself may be seen as a threat to maternal health. This causes a dilemma for us because we want to save babies without harming mothers." Balancing maternal risk and fetal health issues is a problem for many participants in this domain. Fetal surgery is especially poignant and complicated because the women who choose it are so desperate to save their babies. Like many pregnant women, these women will, in fact, do almost anything on behalf of their fetuses, and they will likely be socially rewarded for their actions. For a variety of reasons, they have selected this most intensive and invasive of fetal treatments and have willingly entered into the health care system as patients/objects solely for the sake of their fetuses. A number of feminist scholars have documented women's myriad and often painful encounters with the health care system (Fisher 1988; Lewin and Olesen 1985; Sherwin 1992; Todd 1989). Fetal surgery may be seen as an extension of some of these dynamics as the medicalization of women's bodies and experiences expands into previously uncharted territory (Riessman 1983). It is a key goal of this book to reframe fetal surgery as a women's health issue and to resituate fetal personhood within the specific bodies and social relations in and by which it is produced.

Fetal surgery is also part and parcel of other battles waged upon the terrain of women's bodies, most notably the enduring, public struggles over abortion. But the link between fetal surgery and abortion is not clear-cut, with "pro" and "con" lining up on the frontlines like black and white chess pieces. The unborn patient is imbued with many meanings, and fetal surgery has been taken up quite differently by different individual and collective participants in the abortion struggle. It is true that some reproductive rights groups are cautious and watchful, and many pro-choice organizations nervously track fetal surgery's progress. In contrast, many antiabortion groups have jumped on the fetal surgery bandwagon with zeal, energized by a new practice that so graphically and generously contributes to notions of fetal personhood. A few examples: the Fetal Treatment Unit at Capital Hospital was offered (and refused) a large sum of money by a major pro-life figure for fetal images captured during surgery, particularly an image of a tiny fetal hand extending out of the womb. The cable television show *Celebrate Life!* featured an exultant story about fetal surgery, focusing on a Christian couple's successful experience. And fetal surgery has been the subject of several positive, life-affirming articles in antiabortion newspapers.

But viewing abortion politics through the lens of fetal surgery raises many provocative questions and quandaries, and one can imagine all sorts of scenarios that confound the issues. For example, which of the following women would be more likely to choose fetal surgery if she had access to it: a 42-year-old pro-choice woman who is pregnant with what will likely be her first and only baby, or a 26-year-old, pro-life, Christian woman with two children who believes that one should let nature take its course? A 19-year-old, single, poor woman with limited social support and one healthy child, or a 35-year-old, relatively well-off, antiabortion activist who is already raising a physically disabled child? If any of these women decide against fetal surgery, what are the implications for each of them in choosing an abortion, opting for a less invasive form of treatment, or doing nothing at all? How will their choices, whatever they may be, affect their relationships with medical providers, their partners and families, and their broader social networks? And what about pro-choice activists who want to respect and honor all of women's choices, including the decision to undergo fetal surgery? Likewise, what should we make of antiabortion activists who oppose fetal surgery, as they oppose fetal tissue research, because it intervenes in human life, which they view as sacred? Which is the more "pro-life" version of medical work: surgeons who operate on fetuses in the womb in order to save their lives or surgeons who experiment on the fetus in the womb in order to advance knowledge? Does it matter—and if so, how—that both kinds of activities go on in fetal surgery and are done by many of the same practitioners?

Abortion politics also influence how medical workers view their work. Although the Fetal Treatment Unit turned down the offer from the pro-life figure, fetal surgeons and their collaborators at Capital Hospital were, at the time of my research, compiling their own history of fetal surgery. They intended to use that very meaningful image of a fetal hand extending out of the womb, along with many other compelling images, in their "insider" account celebrating the new specialty. They hoped to market their book as an objective and apolitical tale of fetal surgery. In the words of one member of the fetal surgery team, "We don't want it to be a manifesto for the right-to-life folks." But regardless of who ultimately writes it and with what intentions, it is likely that any such popular account of fetal surgery would cause quite a splash in the public domain and be used by antiabortion groups for a variety of purposes. As one fetal surgeon told me, "I'll tell you a truly interesting ethical problem. We have ten surgeons in this lab whose only focus the majority of the time is the fetus as a patient. We're all operating on fetuses, trying to do our best to protect them, yet when we're done with the operation that fetus could still be legally aborted." Obviously, the connections between fetal surgery and abortion politics are tangled, and one of the tasks of this book is to begin to unravel them.

Finally, fetal surgery intersects with another set of politics, those related to disability and bodily defects. Fixing fetuses, apparently at all costs, taps into a deep vein of cultural discomfort with birth defects, physical disabilities, and deformities of any kind that both remind us of our own vulnerability as human beings and threaten to disrupt social orders based on physiognomy. Congenital defects, the very presence of which often elicit horror, anguish, and shame, are the visceral terrain upon which fetal surgeons operate. In this sense, fetal surgery is intimately related to teratology, the branch of embryology concerned with the production, development, anatomy, and classification of malformed fetuses. In a rather evocative etymological association, teratology means quite literally the science of monsters. As Marie-Hélène Huet (1993, 108) has written, "the nineteenth century is credited with having finally created a science of monsters, or teratology . . . which first attempted to classify all monstrosities." But teratologists were not content simply to describe the laws of nature; they "also hoped to formulate new laws that would permit this recent science to compete with nature, perhaps to surpass it as well. Thus was born the adjunct science of teratogenesis, whose objective was the controlled production of monsters in the laboratory" (Huet 1993, 111). As we shall learn later, there has been a ostensibly logical progression from teratology to teratogenesis to fetal surgery, or what we might call *teratotracto*, the treatment of "monsters."

Georges Canguilhem's (1977) eloquent distinction between the normal and pathological is stunningly realized in fetal surgery, which strives to transform the "monstrous" fetus into a normal baby. These associations resonate deeply with many women's own fears of having abnormal fetuses, but they do so within a social context that fails to accommodate differences in any meaningful way. There is little social, cultural, or economic support for birthing and raising a disabled child and often much pressure to avoid babies who are believed to be a drain on the health care system. It is little wonder, then, that obdurate cultural fears of the abnormal and a hatred of difference give rise not only to snazzy medical procedures designed to fix defective babies, but also to other practices such as prenatal diagnosis and abortion that can eliminate the different before they are born. A fundamental irony is that while abortion and prenatal diagnosis are used to destroy defective fetuses, fetal surgery may transform some fetuses facing certain death into potentially disabled babies. A procedure far from perfect itself, fetal surgery may produce babies with chronic illnesses and persistent defects, making its promise seem more hollow and its connections to disability politics more salient.

Like reproductive and abortion politics, then, disability politics are vivified by fetal surgery in convoluted and troubling ways. A few puzzling questions point to some of the dilemmas this connection excites. For example, what kinds of fates might pregnant women choose for their desired but deformed fetuses if they lived in a different kind of world, one in which disability was not a measure of worth and resources were available to help all women raise all of their children, both "normal" and different? Would fetal surgery exist in such a world? If so, what would its purpose be? In a culture where disabilities do matter and often painfully so, what messages (if any) does fetal surgery send to the disabled? Is it possible for an individual woman to make an agonizing decision to save her own highly valued, at-risk fetus without striking a raw nerve among the disabled? Lastly, how might we value both women's reproductive choices and the lived experiences of the disabled while also maintaining a critical perspective on prenatal diagnosis and treatment? These questions are profound; as Rosi Braidotti (1996, 136) has argued, "We all have bodies, but not all bodies are equal: some matter more than others; some are, quite frankly, disposable." Ironically, given the current feverish and mean context of reproductive politics, this statement could apply equally to disabled bodies, to women's bodies, and to fetal bodies. Contradictions abound on the frontiers of biomedicine.

Analytical Framework

This book chronicles two intertwined historical processes as they have unfolded within a broader cultural and political context: the emergence of a new medical specialty, fetal surgery, and the social and cultural debut of a new fetal subject, the unborn patient. Following Michel Foucault's (1972) notion of archaeology, which focuses on the conditions of possibility of new forms of knowledge and new subjects, this project excavates the unborn patient from the many sedimentary layers in which it is embedded and which have molded it for thirty years. I argue that the unborn patient is not a natural phenomenon, merely reflecting the physiological, developmental, or philosophical status of the fetus. Nor is it simply technologically determined, the next step in a long series of events historically medicalizing the womb and its contents. Rather, I show that the fetal patient is a social and cultural achievement that has unfolded on the terrain of Western medicine. As a new subject, it is the product of a multitude of factors coalescing, although not always smoothly, at particular historical moments. The processes and connections that have intersected in the making of the unborn patient over the past three decades have done so largely within the fledgling world of fetal surgery, itself messy, complicated, and full of contradictions and conundrums. Both of these processes—the making of the unborn patient and the emergence of fetal surgery—demand a deeper analysis of the multiple ways in which fetuses and medicine are socially meaningful.

Culturing the Fetus

Like the oversized fetus in *2001: A Space Odyssey*, fetuses are increasingly portrayed as free-floating and larger than life. Where fetuses were once confined to anonymity and invisibility inside pregnant women's bodies, the fetus has now gone solo. Never mind that most fetuses cannot actually live outside of a woman's body. Contemporary fetal representations routinely erase women's agency and bodies.[8] In the new cultural discourse, fetuses are increasingly represented as free agents with their own needs and interests, and even their own doctors and lawyers. They are deemed worthy of protection, often from the women in whose bodies they are gestating; these representations give rise to the notions of maternal-fetal conflict that are prevalent in medicine, law, ethics, and politics. The autonomous fetus dominates political debates about abortion, appearing in Mason jars, on curbside card tables, in newsletters, and on placards at protests. Crazed young men who murder abortion providers and bomb women's health clinics, and the extremists who celebrate their actions, do so in the name of this individuated, hallowed fetus. From all indications, the autonomous fetus is a seemingly permanent fixture on the popular cultural scene and has become firmly lodged in the social imaginary. Orphan fetuses have even been sighted at that most American of institutions, the garage sale (Rojas 1994).[9]

What does it mean to culture the fetus? Usually the term culturing refers to growing a virus or other organic material in a laboratory. But it also captures the intensive activities and meanings that can congeal around a particular social object at certain historical moments. Culture includes material culture, social practices, identities, communities, language, and meanings—in short, the full range of a society's beliefs, representations, and communicative practices (Nelson, Treichler and Grossberg 1992; Rouse 1993). The private fetus, once hidden inside the womb, has now become what Rosalind Petchesky (1990) calls the "public fetus," given substance and legitimacy by a range of cultural practices. This public fetus is made to stand for, or represent, a range of interests and desires. But fetuses are not just symbols or images, empty simulacra devoid of social context. In attempting to make sense of various fetal positions (Casper 1994a), it is sociologically important to insist on the contingent, embedded, constructed, and meaningful character of who and what gets to count as a "human" or "person." Fetuses are multiply meaningful and they are fertile signifiers, but such representations are only possible in specific social, cultural, and economic relations. The potency and appeal of the fetus as an icon in the contemporary United States, and increasingly elsewhere,[10] marks it as a key player in a number of different social worlds.

Among other sites, fetuses are cultured in the following places: women's bodies, families, communities, popular images, magazines, discourses, institutions, political arenas, laboratories, operating rooms, and so on. Yet while new practices contribute to the making of new fetal identities, some of these practices are accorded greater legitimacy because of their particular social and cultural locations. In medical and scientific domains where human fetuses are key objects of work, such as in fetal tissue research or fetal surgery, culturing the fetus resonates in multiple, powerful ways. In these worlds, fetal status is often defined in naturalistic and biological terms (Grobstein 1988; Morowitz and Trefil 1992). Because science and medicine are considered important and authoritative sites of the production of knowledge, definitions of life created in these domains are propagated and subsequently represented in other worlds as "truth" or reality (Franklin 1991). Contemporary abortion debates are thus framed around static biological definitions of personhood and life, embodied in the compelling image of the tiny homunculus. Consider, for example, that the landmark Supreme Court decision *Roe v. Wade*, itself a social and political achievement, was based on scientific markers of trimesters in pregnancy (and physicians' assessment of them) rather than on a woman's right to privacy or choice. In this respect, the making of the unborn patient through fetal surgery has the potential to reshape the way we think about fetuses in the United States and in other nations where such operations have been attempted.

In contrast to these biological views, an alternate framework rests on the assumption that there is no "natural" meaning of the fetus outside of social and cultural claims. Contexts shape fetal ontologies, providing a locus for analysis of social practices that give rise to different versions of "the fetus." History and context matter in how meanings are attributed to individual and public fetuses (Casper 1994b; Morgan 1996).[11] Fetal subjectivities, like other social categories, are produced within social interactions rather than being endowed by nature—although materiality may be significant as we shall see. Analysis of fetal practices should begin with a recognition that fetuses are socially, culturally, and politically constructed. The analytic task then is to determine *how* and *under what conditions* these configurations occur. Understanding how and why fetuses have come to matter so much requires a rejection of the monolithic, naturalized, ahistorical fetus, and a resituating of actual fetuses, fetal meanings, and fetal subjectivities within the contexts of their origin. One important element of the context of fetal surgery is medical work, through which the unborn patient and fetal personhood are produced.

Medical Work and Its Objects

From the outset, this project was envisioned as an ethnography designed to build theory from the ground up. As I began observing fetal surgery, interviewing people, and attending staff meetings, medical work itself emerged as the heart of the dynamics in which I was interested. In part, this is because I came to see the making of the unborn patient and the emergence of fetal surgery as affiliated processes, both richly shaped by culture and politics. My initial research persuaded me that it is in the actual work involved in operating on a human fetus (and by implication the pregnant woman in whom it is gestating) that culture and politics reveal themselves most provocatively. The word "making" in my title is important because it highlights all of the work—both the nitty-gritty medical activities and tasks and the overlapping cultural and political work—that has been central to crafting the unborn patient out of specific fetal bodies. Wendy Simonds (1996:13) has argued that "abortion work cannot be an ordinary job in a culture that casts abortion as a deeply contested moral issue," and the same may be said of the work of fetal surgery, an exploratory enterprise carried out on a highly charged political terrain.

Drawing on George Herbert Mead's (1934) notion of social objects, I developed the concept of work object to explain certain interactions and activities among the many different actors involved in fetal surgery. A social object is defined according to the meanings it has for the actors for whom it is an object. In my framing, a work object is any material entity around which people make meaning and organize their work practices. In fetal surgery, work objects include both fetuses and pregnant women— almost always at the same time but with very different meanings and consequences. By focusing on how (and which) fetuses are worked on, I was able to examine all of the complicated meanings associated with this work. I found that constructions of the fetus vary depending upon who cares about it, who is attributing meaning, what the work goals are, and material contingencies such as fetal death. Moreover, the fetal work object is not simply a focus of medical work; its material and symbolic properties matter as well; they link fetal practices in medicine to other domains where human fetuses are salient, such as fetal tissue research or abortion politics (Casper 1994a). Culturing the fetal work object means recognizing how fetuses themselves, or rather fetal bodies, comprise the symbolic and pedestrian traffic between different social worlds.

There are a number of advantages to focusing on work objects. The first is in rendering a complicated and controversial subject manageable. It is all too easy to get lost in the cultural mystique and political hysteria surrounding "the fetus," and indeed many academic studies portray the fetus as a symbol without really understanding or explaining the specific social relations that underlie this construction. Grounding an analysis in work practices rescues the fetus from the lofty, abstract plane in which it floats as a monolithic, transcendant creature, and resituates it as multiple, embodied fetuses within everyday life, medical work, and women's experiences—all of which are accessible to ethnography. This approach allows for an analysis of the concrete actions, interactions, and relations that have gone into the making of the unborn patient in late twentieth-century biomedicine. Focusing on work also shows how politics and cultural meanings are woven into the fabric of clinical decisions, and are themselves in turn shaped by clinical practices. I analyze how fetuses and pregnant women become objects of medical work, how these material work objects have contributed to the emergence of a new specialty, what meanings have congealed around work objects, what kinds of investments are made in work objects, who claims to speak for work objects, and how meanings of reproductive phenomena are generated and shaped by emergent work practices. In other words, this book examines all of the fascinating, risky, and consequential work of making fetuses into unborn patients and fetal surgery into a new specialty.

The Politics of Engagement

On more occasions than I can remember during this project, I have been asked why I chose to study fetal surgery. I have also been asked, and attempt to answer in this book, what fetal surgery has to do with gender and women's health; what fetal surgery has to do with abortion politics; and how I could possibly stand to watch surgeons cutting open pregnant women. All of these questions point to obvious and highly problematic connections between me, a pro-choice feminist scholar with deep and public commitments to women's health, and my topic. There are some who will critique my story for not being "objective" enough. But this precisely misses the point of my argument: no work—not the work of fetal surgery, certainly not the work of a sociologist—occurs *outside* particular contexts. In the current political moment in which an entire nation is frantically and often painfully obsessed with fetuses, abortion, family values, and changing gender roles, it makes perfect sense that this highly contested topic and I would engage *each other.* There is something about the topic of fetuses that immediately implicates me as a political actor, subjective as well as objective, and it is not simply a question of research "problem choice" as Max Weber (1949) argued. Were I studying the social organization of the insurance industry, would I be asked quite so frequently about my own politics? Probably not.

Like many feminist scholars interested in women's health and reproduction, I have also been a participant in abortion politics and reproductive rights activities. In many ways, and often quite profoundly, my activism has shaped my intellectual work. In college during the 1980s—at the same time that I was discovering sociology and feminist theory—I staffed telephone lines at Planned Parenthood, campaigned for the ill-fated but pro-choice presidential candidacy of Michael Dukakis, and helped write position papers for local reproductive rights groups. When I moved to a different state and began graduate school in 1990, I joined the board of directors of a local advocacy organization focused on reproductive health issues so that I could remain connected to, or "grounded" in, the real world of women's health activism. I continue to work with women's health groups. Throughout this period, abortion rights have been further eroded and abortion providers (as well as women who seek abortions) are more than ever at risk. Abortion politics have become increasingly centered around fetuses, often erasing women as agents or, even worse, portraying women as selfish strumpets so blinded by our own desires as to be incapable of making informed moral decisions. Where once a coat hanger symbolized the dangers of abortion for women, the iconography is now dominated by fetal body parts displayed graphically or by helpless, free-floating fetuses resembling out-of-control balloons at a Macy's parade.

As a sociologist *and* a women's health activist, I am captivated by the fetus as a cultural icon, a political symbol, an object of desire (including my own), a social debutante, and a medical patient. I first discovered fetal surgery in 1991 in a file called "Fetal Rights" at the office of the advocacy group on whose board I served. The file contained a yellowed newspaper clipping heralding an operation performed in the mid-1980s, describing fetal surgery in rather vivid terms. I was finishing up my first year of graduate school and had begun thinking about potential dissertation topics. Certain that I would investigate some aspect of reproductive health, I was trying on different ideas every day. I was fascinated by the "new" reproductive technologies, but felt that they had already received ample and insightful attention from feminist scholars. I remember vividly that resounding *ping!* of satisfaction I felt as I read with growing fascination about operating on fetuses in utero. I knew that I had found my dissertation topic in fetal surgery. It was compelling, sociologically interesting, visually exciting, and germane to all of the areas in which I worked: medical sociology, science and technology studies, cultural and feminist studies, and women's health. Moreover, I guessed that nobody else was studying fetal surgery; indeed, I had never even heard of it and I was immersed in the relevant literature. With the words of my mentors echoing in my head, I decided to "study the unstudied" (Strauss 1967), and I have been engaged with this topic ever since.

My research methods and data sources were varied, reflecting what many social scientists are usefully calling *multisite ethnography*. This expansive methodological approach enabled me to draw on a range of rich sources at different sites to access information and to attain more robust conclusions about my data. Between November 1991 and December 1994, I formally interviewed twenty-four informants in the United States, New Zealand, and Puerto Rico, including fetal surgeons, pediatricians, sonographers, obstetricians, social workers, fetal physiologists, nurses, laboratory coordinators, and a limited number of patients and their families. I informally interviewed more than thirty others, including neonatologists, geneticists, genetics counselors, other specialists, administrative staff, and activists. I attended clinical staff meetings, Ob/Gyn Grand Rounds, and brown-bag lunch presentations at Capital Hospital, and I observed four surgical operations on human fetuses

performed there. I also attended scientific and clinical meetings elsewhere, such as a conference on fetal research and treatment sponsored
by the Institute of Medicine in 1993.

I investigated several nonhuman sources, as well, including historical records and archives, biomedical literature, and popular cultural representations. In New Zealand I analyzed the papers of the late Dr.
William Liley. These were not formally archived, but rather "collected"
alongside ancient medical equipment in the dark, dingy attic of National
Women's Hospital in Auckland. The papers included correspondence,
clinical notes, laboratory records and reports, hospital protocols, patient
records, unpublished and published articles, copies of lectures and presentations, and reprints of articles on specific topics. At Capital Hospital
I reviewed nonconfidential records, such as memos, correspondence,
and copies of grant proposals relevant to the historical development of
the specialty. I also invoked the Freedom of Information Act there to investigate confidential documents related to the human subjects approval
process covering a five-year period from 1990 to 1994. These documents
included correspondence, research protocols, patient data (with identifying information concealed prior to my viewing), supporting documenta-
tion (e.g., tables of data), and informed consent documents.

In terms of clinical and scientific literature, I read and analyzed literally hundreds of articles from a variety of journals and textbooks. *The
Unborn Patient*, the major text in fetal surgery containing a wealth of scientific and clinical data, was an insightful and provocative companion
throughout my research. Among the popular cultural representations I
analyzed were *New York Times* science writer Gina Kolata's (1990) hagio-
graphic but detailed account of fetal surgery, as well as an array of videos
including those made by the Fetal Treatment Unit at Capital Hospital, a
March of Dimes commercial containing clips of an operation, and seg-
ments of *20/20, Celebrate Life!* and *Body Human 2000* that featured fetal
surgery, often in venerating terms. All of these sources, which I investigated during the period from 1991 to 1997, provided key insights into
popular cultural meanings of fetuses. All data were analyzed using modified grounded theory (Glaser and Strauss 1967).

Throughout this research and across most of the ethnographic sites
I studied, a consistent theme in the data has been political and professional controversy and conflict. While I expected to find evidence of
broader political strife, I did not seek out the theme of professional conflict. But its emergence in my fieldwork was not surprising. After all, fetal surgery is about fetuses and women's bodies, which are among the
most contested biological objects in the twentieth century and likely will
be in the twenty-first century. It is also, by extension, about abortion politics and the history of research on human fetuses, invoking deep emo-

tions and tensions. Fetal surgery turned out to be political both inside and outside of medicine. It was no accident that I first stumbled across this topic in the files of a reproductive rights organization, nor is it coincidence that abortion was a compelling and troubling issue for many of the people I interviewed for this project. Again and again, I was reminded that the history of fetal surgery as a form of medical work has been inextricably caught up with the history of American and international reproductive and abortion politics. These connections significantly shaped not only my analysis, but also my engagement with this topic and my relationships with all of the people I studied who care about the fetal patient. My own commitment to reframing fetal surgery as a women's health issue is as much about the cultural and political implications of this practice as it is about the clinical implications.

My desire to engage fetal surgery certainly matched that of the women and men who have built this incipient specialty. But my sociological insistence on process—on the *making of* the unborn patient—has often run counter to prevailing clinical, scientific, and ethical assertions that "the fetus" is natural, ahistorical, and static. Moreover, my interest in learning everything possible about fetal surgery far exceeded medical workers' willingness or ability to recount their work. My commitment to reframing fetal surgery as a women's health issue greatly diverged from predominant clinical framings of the specialty as a pediatric issue. My heartfelt desire to talk to pregnant women was squelched on many occasions by medical workers who serve as gatekeepers to "their" patients. And my feminist, democratic tendency toward open dialogue and free information was often thwarted by clinical tendencies toward secrecy and nondisclosure. Many of my repeated requests for additional data (e.g., clarification of outcome statistics, fetal mortality rates, or exactly how many surgeries have been performed at various institutions) were denied or ignored. In fact, difficulties in obtaining what I saw as essential data prompted me to invoke the Freedom of Information Act to gain access to records and documents at Capital Hospital. I quickly learned that I needed to tread with great care and some boldness on this highly contested terrain.

Rather than reviewing in detail all of the specific problems I encountered in this research, many of which I have written about elsewhere (Casper 1997), I shall briefly describe a troubling incident that convinced me of the starkly political nature of this topic. Early in my research I interviewed a woman who had undergone fetal surgery at Capital Hospital and, who, along with her husband, was very active in antiabortion politics. As this couple requested during our interview, I later sent them some of my work including an earlier (unpublished) version of chapter 4. They were very upset by my critical perspective on fetal surgery and by the internal conflict I described occurring in the Fetal Treatment Unit. Because they are outspoken proponents of fetal surgery and also potential donors to Capital Hospital, they were able to convince fetal surgeons to severely curtail my access to the research site, especially to other patients and their families. Despite my diplomatic but persistent requests for access to other patients and their families—and despite their own initial enthusiasm about my project—the surgeons refused (often by simply ignoring me) to allow me to interview other patients. Of course, this only made me question more strongly medical workers' motivations for not letting patients talk to me. It struck me that surgeons seemed reluctant to grant me access to their patients because they believed that my research might threaten their own access to patients. A key informant at Capital Hospital later told me that surgeons were afraid my work might end up "cited in the *New York Times*." Ironically, although fetal surgeons and other medical workers have often called for social and ethical analysis of their work, they squirmed uncomfortably under the sociological lens when it was directed at them. Yet this is understandable, especially if one takes the deeply controversial nature and contexts of their work into account.

I learned through close encounters with those who care about the unborn patient that the research process itself (my own and theirs) could be a rich source of data in explaining some of the politics shaping fetal surgery. I discovered that the people who practice fetal surgery (medical workers), those who "consume" it (patients), and those of us who study it are all deeply embedded in this controversial world. We are not insulated from the political currents that run through fetal surgery because these currents are generated within a broader social circuitry of which we are also a part. The occasional shock reminds us of what is at stake in making connections between the medical work that goes on in an operating room and the cultural and political context in which this work takes place. For fetal surgeons, whose work exists precariously at the borders of several different worlds, to speak of abortion in a public context may be to risk losing their livelihood. There is a danger in making visible the cultural filaments that connect the operating room to the world around it; some groups have much to lose as the myth of "the natural fetus" is unraveled. It is a danger of which medical workers and sociologists alike are gravely aware: it may reduce funding for our work; it may deliver incendiary surprises in our mailboxes. I grew to appreciate that some of the problems I encountered in the field had a great deal to do with the political contexts in which we all "operate."

Donna Haraway (1997, 190) has described ethnography as "a method of being at risk in the face of the practices and discourses into which one inquires." Despite the risks involved in studying the brave new world of fetal surgery, it would be extremely difficult (as well as disingenuous) to cloak myself in an old-fashioned version of scientific objectivity. As the eminent natural historian and essayist Stephen Jay Gould (1996/1981, 36) has argued, "Impartiality (even if desirable) is unattainable by human beings with inevitable backgrounds, beliefs, and desires," a sentiment undergirding most social and cultural studies of science and medicine as well as most feminist methodologies. I care too much about the issues raised by fetal surgery and the unborn patient to assume a polite, reasonable distance, and instead embrace a politics of engagement that recognizes my own immersion in the worlds I study. I have been moved and transformed by this research in multiple ways, and fetal surgery is something I shall continue to think and talk about long after this book is published. My politics and intellectual assumptions have been shaken time and again, precisely because fetal surgery evokes persistent debates about fetuses, abortion, women's roles, the health care system, and rescue technologies. I have explicitly *not* created a study of fetal surgery that might, as Haraway (1997, 190) puts it, "stand a good chance of floating off screen into an empyrean and academic never-never land."

In writing a book that is unashamedly politically engaged, my work is in dialogue with other feminist scholars of reproduction who have begun creatively to theorize the fetus, insisting that women remain clearly inside the analytical frame. This analytical approach is an important development in reproductive studies; it marks feminist commitment to reclaiming the intellectual and political terrain upon which fetal politics are carried out. Scholarly questions about fetal subjectivity may well power the political debates about the future of human reproduction. My work is informed by the contributions of the many brave feminist scholars who labor in this area—with their own complicated and diverse political engagements—including Barbara Duden (1993a; 1993b), Sarah Franklin (1991; 1993), Donna Haraway (1992; 1997), Valerie Hartouni (1992; 1994; 1997), Linda Layne (1990; 1996), Lynn Morgan (1989; 1996), Rayna Rapp (1990; 1993a; 1995), Barbara Katz Rothman (1986; 1989), Janelle Taylor (1993), Irma van der Ploeg (1994), and others. All of this work, including mine, focuses on the many ways in which "fetal matters" on the final frontier of reproductive medicine.

To Boldly Go

The story of fetal surgery is far more complicated than I ever imagined, and I have thought long and hard about how to tell it both honestly and passionately. Foremost, I have wanted to tell an engaging sociological story about a controversial new medical procedure while also linking it to the "big picture" (Park 1952) of culture, politics, and social relations. But I have also wanted to make clear that fetal surgery and the unborn patient embody a number of hidden meanings and consequences that too few people have been talking about. In reading this book, one should think about each chapter as a site, or as a set of overlapping sites, within which the unborn patient has been made and fetal surgery has emerged as a new specialty. These sites—whether geographical, institutional, discursive, or textual—have all performed and hosted certain kinds of medical, cultural, and political work. All the sites are connected through the interwoven threads of fetal surgery and the unborn patient as they have been mutually and jointly constructed, but each site is also interesting on its own terms.

Chapter 2, "Breaching the Womb: A History of the Unborn Patient," explores early fetal surgery efforts and the debut of the fetal patient in the 1960s. This chapter touches on several themes that appear later in the book such as constructions of maternal-fetal conflict, the fetal work object, reproductive politics, and fetal personhood. Drawing on research conducted in New Zealand, Puerto Rico, and key United States locations, I follow the work of the late William Liley, Karliss Adamsons, Vincent Freda, and their many colleagues and collaborators. As with contemporary fetal surgery practices, historical efforts were undergirded by the cultural politics of abortion as shaped by specific national contexts, and these contexts are also discussed. Throughout the chapter, I describe technical and social practices that established the solid foundation upon which later practices were built.

Because fetal surgery is an innovative medical specialty, it is shaped by a variety of diverse practices utilizing different research and treatment sites. Chapter 3, "A Hybrid Practice: Traffic Between the Laboratory and the Operating Room," analyzes this unique institutional position, focusing on the complex hybrid nature of the specialty. Fetal surgery has been shaped not only by the clinical work of medical practitioners, but also by the intersections of basic scientific research and technical innovations in medicine. Building on both historical and contemporary data, this chapter explores fetal physiology, diagnostic technologies, animal experimentation, and fetal wound healing research as these practices have shaped (and been affected by) fetal surgery. In different yet interrelated ways, each of these practices has enhanced access to the fetus as a work object and legitimated the emerging specialty, thereby facilitating the making of the unborn patient.

Chapter 4, "Working On (and Around) the Unborn Patient: Negotiating Social Order in a Fetal Treatment Unit," is based on data collected at Capital Hospital and examines the institutional framework of contemporary fetal surgery. I focus specifically on the work done by medical practitioners in this field, extending my argument concerning hybridization introduced in chapter 3 to examine the interdisciplinary nature of fetal surgery today. Using the concept of work objects, the specialty of fetal surgery is presented as a dynamic, diverse, and contested domain in which actors must negotiate social order in the face of conflicting perspectives, agendas, and work practices. I show that the fetus is defined as the primary work object in fetal surgery around which commitments and practices are organized. These processes are illustrated through an analysis of several areas where negotiation and dissent occur in fetal surgery, including definitions of work objects, factors in patient selection, and definitions of a fetal disease and its treatment.

Chapter 5, "Clinical Trials in Fetal Surgery: Making, Protecting, and Contesting Human Subjects," explores the many social and ethical dilemmas involved in research on human subjects in the state-of-the-art clinical practices of fetal surgery. Again drawing on fieldwork at Capital Hospital, I analyze interactions between the fetal surgery team and the Institutional Review Board (IRB) charged with implementing guidelines to protect human subjects. This chapter presents a sociology of the human subjects approval process, offering insight into how it has shaped and delimited fetal surgery. I examine efforts to establish human subjects protection as a key organizational and textual site of ongoing negotiations at which the unborn patient is made and challenged. I focus specifically on ambiguity in definitions of "human," distinctions among innovations, experiments and standard of care in fetal surgery, the manufacture of informed consent, and the politics of accounting. Throughout, the chapter is attentive to the concrete practices through which ethical decisions are made regarding the acceptability of biomedicine.

In chapter 6, "Heroic Moms and Maternal Environments: Pregnant Women on the Final Frontier," I describe the experiences of women who undergo fetal surgery on behalf of their fetuses. All too often in clinical and cultural representations of fetal surgery, pregnant women are erased or relegated to the role of passive hosts for the patient deemed most important: the fetus. Here, countering the maternal-fetal conflict paradigm—which suggests that women and their fetuses are distinct (and even unequal) entities—I define pregnant women as engaged participants who are very much connected to and responsible for their fetuses. I analyze the activities that pregnant women participate in as they attempt to save their ailing babies, focusing on their choices and politics in fetal surgery, the organizational and emotional commitments they make, and their assumption of health risks. This chapter shows that the women are not simply fetal containers; rather, they are "talking wombs" who often present challenges to the medical workers for whom they are objects of risky clinical and technical work. Employing a women's health perspective, I describe the very real physical consequences of operating on women only for the sake of their fetuses. There are, as I show, signficant tensions stemming from the physical challenges of performing an operation in which the fetal patient is located inside a living, breathing woman's body. This chapter ultimately raises a host of questions related to reproductive politics, such as: Whose needs are being met in fetal surgery? To whom are physicians accountable?

Chapter 7, "Beyond the Operating Room," presents conclusions and implications of this research. I return to some of the major issues and questions raised in the introduction, including the relationship between medical work and reproductive politics. I also examine the fate of the unborn patient in different contexts, focusing on some of the consequences of social, cultural, and political constructions of fetuses. In addition, where earlier portions of the book address the making of the unborn patient, here I discuss what it would mean to *unmake* fetal patienthood and personhood. I preview the fate of fetal surgery, including predictions by key participants in the field and a description of technologies that are presented as alternatives to surgery. Also in this final chapter I more fully explore fetal surgery as a women's health issue and propose feminist interventions. I do not present a litany of reasons why we should do away with fetal surgery; instead I ask what needs to be in place—socially, clinically, politically, economically, ethically—in order to make fetal surgery accountable to the women who select it.

The limited scope of fetal surgery means that it is very difficult to discuss who is doing it and where without violating participants' anonymity. While I use real names in chapter 2 in order to represent historical events and actors, accurately, in the remainder of the book I use either pseudonyms or no names at all (substituting occupational descriptors) to protect the identities of all my informants. I have collected a variety of data at many sites, but most of my ethnographic observations and interviews were done at Capital Hospital. Most readers, especially those outside of medical worlds, will be unfamiliar with the scenes I describe in chapters 4, 5, and 6. But "insiders" to fetal surgery, or to reproductive medicine more generally, may well recognize certain key players, including themselves, their patients, and their colleagues. This is unavoidable, although I have taken great precautions to protect the identities of my informants. Ironically, although I offered it explicitly, very few of the medical workers, and none of the fetal surgeons and obstetricians, requested anonymity when they signed consent forms agreeing to be interviewed. However, I myself chose to mask the identities of *all* personnel and patients connected with Capital Hospital as well as the identity of the institution itself. In some cases I have changed an informant's gender or specific occupation, while in others I have melded more than one actual person into a single character. I have also changed certain details about patients, such as which part of the country they are from or how many children they have. My goal is protection rather than duplicity, and these author-imposed personality changes do not affect my core argument.

It is also important to point out that my story centers on fetal surgery's growth and emergence at certain sites in the 1960s and 1970s and at Capital Hospital in the 1980s and early 1990s based on data collected over a six-year period. Certainly it is possible that if I did this ethnography of fetal surgery today, I might well tell some different stories. One of the fetal surgeons told me early on in my research, "You'd better hurry! You're trying to do a project on a very dynamic field right now. If you don't finish it in a year, it will be old stuff." Indeed, after a few informants read earlier versions of chapters in this book, they told me that some of the most difficult conflicts had been ironed out, illustrating the phenomenon long recognized by medical sociologists that conflicts and mistakes may be normalized over time. Also, specialties may become more or less institutionalized, medical workers may move between institutions, new technologies may be added, and the contours of specialties themselves may change (Bucher 1962; Bucher and Strauss 1961). In short, some of the practices and dynamics that I describe here regarding the work of fetal surgery may strike some insiders as obvious and outdated. This is one of the few pitfalls of studying an emerging, controversial practice.

However, I argue that the skeleton of my argument remains largely the same: most of the cleavages discussed in this book are deep and fetal surgery is still quite contested. Fetal surgery is not by any means "old stuff," especially in terms of its social and political consequences. It is medicine without boundaries, cowboy surgery on what is considered, at least for now, the final frontier. We do not know what fetal surgery or procedures following in its footsteps (such as prenatal gene therapy and fetoscopy) will look like in the next century. But the social and ethical issues raised by fetal surgery and its technokin transcend the sterile confines of the operating room. This book examines many complex issues and weighty concerns through the lens of fetal surgery, offering a fresh look at some persistent questions. It points to what is unique, consequential, scary, and exhilarating about fetal surgery and the making of the unborn patient.

Chapter 2

Breaching the Womb
A History of the Unborn Patient

New York City, 1964

The 1960s, alive with social change on many fronts, were a watershed decade in fetal diagnosis and treatment. In 1964, three major figures in the history of fetal surgery spent a fruitful year together at Columbia University in New York City. Continuing work in which each of them was already engaged, Vincent Freda, Karliss Adamsons, and William Liley pursued an international collaborative enterprise with consequences that continue to reverberate. The work they accomplished, and the connections they established with each other, were vital to the making of the unborn patient. Their combined efforts led to ideas and innovations that have shaped reproductive and fetal medicine for thirty years.

Vincent Freda was a young obstetrician working in Rh research at Columbia University. Although trained in clinical obstetrics, he was keenly interested in immunology and blood and forged ties with others in these fields. Building on fetal physiological research and advances in immunology of previous decades, Freda pursued the vexing problem of Rh disease, hoping to eradicate it. Concurrently with a group of researchers from Liverpool, in the early 1960s Freda and his colleagues developed anti-D immunoprophylaxis, the Rh "vaccine," which drastically reduced the number of fetal and neonatal deaths from Rh hemolytic disease.

Karliss Adamsons, another young obstetrician, also worked at Columbia during this time. Born in Switzerland, Adamsons received his medical training in Germany, did a brief stint at Harvard, and then fulfilled a five-year residency at Columbia. During the last years of his residency, he became interested in fetal physiological problems related to cerebral palsy. He began traveling regularly to Puerto Rico to collaborate with William Mendel, who managed a large primate colony in San Juan and was conducting neurological research on monkeys. One of the striking findings of this work was how "tolerant" the monkey fetus was of surgical intrusion. After finishing his residency in 1961, Adamsons spent several months continuing this primate research, returning to New York regularly to participate in the Rh efforts. It was during this period that he and Freda, building on the monkey experiments, attempted open fetal surgery in human patients, with mixed short-term results but significant historical impact.

William Liley, on the heels of his remarkable success pioneering intrauterine transfusion for Rh disease in fetuses, moved his family from New Zealand to New York City in 1964. Liley brought with him not only an understanding of the mechanisms of intrauterine transfusion, but also a wealth of knowledge about Rh disease based on years of research and clinical care at National Women's Hospital in Auckland. Where Freda's scientific research was aimed at finding a way to *prevent* Rh disease, the transfusion efforts developed by Liley were designed to *treat* fetuses. It is for this seminal work, treating fetuses still in the womb, that Liley is considered the "father" of fetal surgery.

In 1964, then, Columbia University was a "hotbed" of fetal research and treatment, a busy urban teaching hospital where the unborn patient was enthusiastically championed. Gathered in this one place, Freda, Adamsons, and Liley merged their talents, ideas, and ambitions into the joint enterprise of crafting the fetal patient. They compared notes, shared trade secrets, and struggled to make collective sense of this new practice—not yet a specialty—that they were forging. They brought with them to this enterprise a host of experiences, skills, and interests developed at other places (indeed, in other nations) and with other colleagues. It is these different sites and practices, whose trajectory eventually converged in New York City, to which I now turn.

Rh Disease and the History of Fetal Surgery

Although many diseases and defects led to fetal and neonatal deaths in the first half of this century, hemolytic (blood) disease resulting from Rh incompatibility was especially important in the origins of fetal treatment.[1] Understanding fetal surgery at present requires looking back through time to the Rh research of the 1960s. The Rhesus factor, named after the monkeys on which this research was done, is a thin coating of chemicals that surrounds the red blood cell. About 85 percent of people have this coating, and their blood is called Rh-positive. Those with only a partial coating or with no coating on their red blood cells are called Rh-negative. People with Rh-negative blood cannot tolerate Rh-positive blood, an immunological condition with ramifications both in transfusions and in pregnancy.

During pregnancy, problems typically arise when a woman is Rh-negative and her fetus is Rh-positive, although other blood combinations can also be dangerous. In Rh disease, the woman's Rh-negative blood destroys the Rh-positive fetal blood, which is perceived as a threat, by creating antibodies against it. When this happens, and the antibodies begin to filter across the placenta to the fetus, the fetal bloodstream begins producing red blood cells at an accelerated rate to replace the blood cells destroyed by the maternal antibodies. Because red blood cell production is increased, the cells are only partly formed; these are called *erythroblasts* to distinguish them from normal or fully formed red blood cells, which are called *erythrocytes*. This process eventually leads to anemia, jaundice, erythroblastosis (too many erythroblasts in the blood), and often death of fetuses or newborns (called "blue babies" for their unhealthy pallor at birth).

Rh disease has been of interest to researchers not only because of its unique properties, but precisely because it occurs in the context of pregnancy and can shed light on how immunology works. The human body under normal circumstances manufactures biochemical substances called *antibodies* to fight foreign invaders, such as viruses or bacteria, called *antigens*. One of the most interesting physiological features of pregnancy is that a pregnant woman and her fetus exist in a state of *parabiosis* despite their genetic difference. That is, as Liley (1980, 1) argued, "Mother and baby are inevitably immunological foreigners because the baby inherits exactly half his tissue compatibility and blood group genes from his father." Yet the pregnant woman's body does not usually reject the fetus as a foreign invader; a woman's normal biological defense systems are "on hold" during pregnancy. The fetal intruder is protected from expulsion by the *trophoblast*, a thin layer of tissue forming the outer surface of the placenta and separating the pregnant woman's bloodstream from that of her fetus. The trophoblast, however, is a permeable membrane and antibodies can pass from the pregnant woman to her fetus, often with benefits to fetal and neonatal health. For example, babies who have never been exposed to measles or chickenpox enter the world with the temporary protection of their mothers' antibodies against these diseases circulating through their bloodstream. The trophoblast and its osmotic properties become a problem only when the antibodies a fetus receives from its mother across the placenta are dangerous, as in Rh disease.

Prevention and treatment of Rh disease in fetuses was a major medical and scientific goal in the first half of the twentieth century. But before this disease could be either prevented or cured, researchers first had to establish its pathology and course. As Zimmerman (1973) argues in his lively history of Rh disease, in the 1930s there was not one disease but rather several different conditions based on similar symptoms: hydrops, jaundice, anemia, and erythroblastosis. (In the fetus, hydrops refers to the abnormal accumulation of serous fluid in fetal tissues and signifies the terminal phase of hemolytic disease.) Diagnosing the individual conditions was relatively easy; putting a name on the larger disease thought to be responsible was more difficult. Eventually, through combined research in immunology, pathology, and serology, these four disorders came to be associated with a new disease: hemolytic or Rh disease. The classification of these symptoms into the condition called Rh disease was closely interwoven with scientific efforts to discover a prevention and cure. That is, as researchers worked together to unlock the secrets of Rh disease, they collectively created a common language to talk about their object of pursuit. In doing so, they participated in the biomedical construction of a new affliction called Rh disease.

In populations of European descent, approximately one in 200 pregnancies is considered to be complicated by Rhesus disease. Prior to World War II, most Rh-negative women had little hope of delivering a healthy baby. Once a woman produced antibodies in response to Rh incompatibility in one pregnancy (whether or not it came to term), they were present for life and subsequent pregnancies were at increased risk for hemolytic disease. Liley illustrated this Rh sensitization in a letter to a colleague, "Once you have them, there's nothing we can do about them. Antibodies have long memories." The persistence of Rh disease meant that physicians embraced a multistrategy prevention scheme: taking careful histories of a woman's previous blood transfusions, identifying blood type (A, B, O) and Rh-factors for all pregnant patients, screening patients for antibodies, and determining the husband or partner's Rh factor. Liley once summarized management of hemolytic disease as such: "Reassure everybody, trust nobody, and hope for the best . . . but prepare for the worst. There is little margin for error."[2]

Following the relatively grim decades of the 1930s to the 1960s, during which large numbers of fetuses and "blue babies" died, several medical treatments were developed to treat Rh-affected babies, ultimately rendering the disease much less threatening to prenatal and infant mortality. First, with the development of more sophisticated blood banking procedures in the 1930s and 1940s, and better methods for screening antenatal patients, it became possible to avoid transfusing mismatched blood into pregnant women. Second, the innovation of exchange transfusion, also called therapeutic plasma exchange, enabled pediatricians to treat babies born with conditions such as anemia caused by hemolytic disease.[3] Third, the development of anti-D immunoprophylaxis in New

York by Freda and his colleagues and in Liverpool in the mid-1960s, and its widespread use internationally after 1968, drastically reduced the number of pregnancies affected by Rh disease. This "vaccine," still in wide use as Rhogam, is given to Rh-negative women *after* their first pregnancies. The drug effectively inhibits antibody production by "lending" a woman antibodies before her body has a chance to produce them, thus preventing the development of a permanent immunity to fetal antigens that may be present in subsequent pregnancies. In other words, the Rh vaccine performs an immunological sleight of hand.

Such efforts were lifesaving for infants and of huge benefit to the pregnant women who cared deeply about their babies. But these techniques were limited either to *preventing* Rh disease in subsequent pregnancies or to treating pregnant women and fragile *newborns* with multiple blood transfusions. None of these innovations focused directly on the *fetus* at risk or already suffering from Rh disease. What medical researchers envisioned was a technique that would enable them to transfuse fetuses while still in the womb. This would involve passing needles into the fetus through a pregnant woman's body—without opening the uterus, a procedure which at that time seemed far too dangerous. When such a technique was eventually developed through a wide range of collaborative work, it made headlines and became instrumental in defining the fetus as a patient in its own right. Pioneered by Liley and his colleagues, intrauterine (literally, "within the womb") transfusion for Rh disease captured both the popular and clinical imaginations by breaching a hitherto uncrossed therapeutic and moral boundary. As news of this breathtaking achievement spread across the globe in 1963, the "unborn patient" became a new clinical and social entity. Let us now journey to one of the most important sites where the fetal patient originated.

Making the Unborn Patient in Aotearoa, "the Land of the Long White Cloud"

On the islands of New Zealand, one feels an almost primal connection to the landscape of these small volcanic jewels in the South Pacific. The Maori who settled New Zealand's northern island long before the *pakeha*, or Europeans, had a word for their beautiful and lush homeland surrounded by blue-green sea: *whenua*. This same word also refers to the placenta, the membranous organ inside a pregnant woman's uterus that nurtures the growing fetus. Given the rich and evocative meanings of *whenua*, it seems fitting that fetal surgery began in New Zealand. This exquisite island nation ably plays the part of paradise in the origin story of the unborn patient. Unsurprisingly, the *pakeha* whose work facilitated the construction of the fetal patient shared with the Maori a deep and

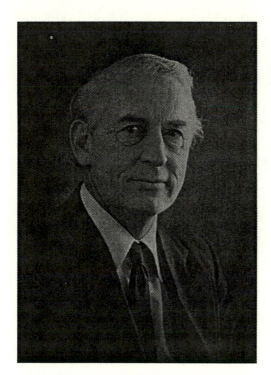

A. William Liley, the "father" of fetal surgery, c. 1975. Reprinted with permission of Graham C. Liggins.

abiding connection to their homeland. It is the unique fusion of work with culture, technology, and geography that culminated in the social debut of the unborn patient.

The Significance of Place

Albert William Liley, called "Bill" by almost everyone who knew him, was born in 1929 into a working-class Catholic family in Auckland.[4] As a child he was fascinated by New Zealand's landscape, joining the Auckland Botanical Society and planting a native forest in his family's backyard. Drawn to the natural world, he might have pursued either forestry or science. But his family physician suggested a career in medicine, and Liley responded with enthusiasm. After placing first in New Zealand's national scholarship competition in 1947, he began college at Auckland University the following year. He studied medicine at university and then went on to New Zealand's only medical school at that time, the University of Otago in Dunedin on the South Island. After graduating from medical school in 1954 with degrees in both medicine and surgery, he became interested in scientific research and was recruited by Nobelist John Eccles at Australian National University in Canberra. There he studied neurophysiology and received a Ph.D. degree in 1956.

Although fascinated by the intellectual demands of neurophysiology,

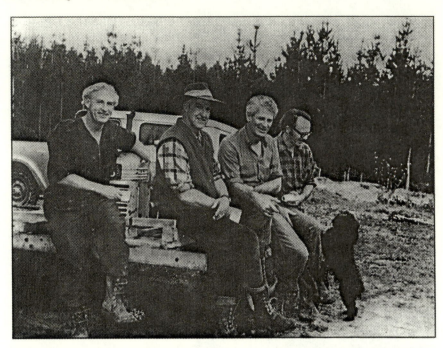

The Stoney Creek Forest Partners, c. 1975. From left, surgeon/foresters Bill
Liley, Herb Green, John Groome, Mont Liggins, and mascot, Louis I. In the mid-
1960s, they purchased 450 acres of rugged land around Kaukapakapa which is
now a thriving pine forest. "All the handiwork of men more used to dealing with
the human fetus than with pinus radiata seedlings," as one contemporary put it.
Reprinted with permission of Graham C. Liggins.

Liley also felt that scientific research was too esoteric. He wanted to
work with people and, more important, he wanted to work in New
Zealand. He had married a fellow medical student, Margaret Hunt,
shortly after graduating, and they purchased some rugged land in the
center of the North Island near Taumarunui, in the hill country. Liley felt
a deep connection to New Zealand and spent much of his spare time on
forestry and farming.[5] A contemporary of Liley's recounted that "his
weekend pursuits led to one patient complaining that she felt gorse
prickles in his hands when he examined her!" (McCarthy 1983, 5). (A fetal surgeon at Capital Hospital remembers meeting Liley once and notic-
ing how "rugged" his hands were: "They were definitely the hands of
someone who worked outside, and not really the hands of a surgeon.") In
short, Liley worried that a successful career as a research scientist would
pull him away from his beloved home, prompting a renewed interest in
medicine.

Liley was well-trained as a research scientist, but he realized that he needed clinical training for a medical career. In 1957, shortly after returning to New Zealand, he began a research fellowship in obstetrics at the University of Auckland's Postgraduate School of Obstetrics and Gynecology. Liley was the first permanent research fellow at the school, which had been created just a few years earlier in 1951.[6] Originally situated in a wide green park at the base of an extinct volcano, the school eventually became the hub of obstetrical research and training in New Zealand and attracted some of the finest scientists in the South Pacific. Ross Howie, who began as a pediatric resident in 1962 and worked closely with Liley, described it as "a good place to work. The department, under the leadership of D.G. Bonham from 1963, was not beholden to the `publish or perish mode' of most academic settings." Research was, according to Howie, cooperative and friendly, with very little competition among "talented people of ability and ideas." He pointed out that the school also benefited from readily available research materials: at that time there were 60 million sheep in New Zealand as compared to 3.5 million people.

The Postgraduate School was developed in conjunction with National Women's Hospital, within which it was, and still is, housed. The hospital was established by Parliament to provide every woman in New Zealand with free access to health care. As with any teaching hospital, this arrangement provided a steady stream of human subjects for clinical research and offered a capable group of providers versed in the most up-to-the-minute techniques. In 1964 the hospital moved to a new location near the base of One Tree Hill, the site of a Maori *pa*, or fortified village, with breathtaking vistas of the Auckland region. It sits at the end of Claude Road, in a residential neighborhood of colorful frame houses with tidy gardens. The building in which the Postgraduate School is located represents 1960s functional architecture at its zenith, and the small birds darting in and out of the open-air cafeteria add a welcome touch of whimsy to the otherwise austere setting.

As a national medical center, National Women's Hospital has, since its inception, provided health care services for women from all over New Zealand as well as from nearby areas of the South Pacific. The patient population historically has been highly ethnically and culturally diverse, including European, Polynesian, Melanesian, and Maori women. Collaborative work on Rh disease and the development of intrauterine transfusion unfolded within this rather unique institutional and geopolitical context. For example, in the 1960s and 1970s as news of Liley's work spread, women came from as far away as the United States, Spain, and India and from as near as neighboring Fiji for medical management of their pregnancies. Clearly, National Women's Hospital occupied a central role in obstetrics during that era, making it an ideal site for research on fetal interventions and the unborn patient. It was in this "exciting research climate," as Ross Howie depicted it, that Liley and his colleagues began experimenting with the technique of intrauterine transfusion.

"Peacekeeping on the Maternofetal Frontier": Intrauterine Transfusion and the Unborn Patient[7]

Although Liley is widely considered the "father" of fetology for his role in developing prenatal transfusion, there were a number of other people involved in this enterprise as well.[7] As Ross Howie pointed out, the working environment of the Postgraduate School was cooperative and encompassed a range of activities geared toward prevention and eradication of Rh disease. In addition to Howie, a pediatrician, other members of the Rh team included Florence Fraser, an obstetrician and Liley's "right arm"; Herb Green, deputy head of the department and an active clinical researcher; Graham Liggins, an obstetrician with expertise in fetal physiology; Sally Kinnock, a researcher and the Rh Committee secretary; Neal Patterson, an obstetrician; and others representing pediatrics, obstetrics, radiology, and blood banking. The Rh program undertaken at National Women's Hospital in the early 1960s mobilized this diverse group of medical workers who brought to their collective task a range of skills, interests, and commitments.

This cooperative spirit was manifest in the Rh Committee, a microcosm of the social organization of fetal treatment at that time. Cooperation was required by the clinical demands of caring for pregnant women at risk for hemolytic disease. The women who came to National Women's Hospital for evaluation and treatment were often seen by several different specialists, ranging from obstetricians caring for the women to pediatricians who would treat surviving newborns upon birth. The Rh Committee was set up to provide some cohesion to this group of practitioners and to add a degree of organization and coordination to patients' trajectories through the health care system. According to Florence Fraser, "The Rh Committee started because we had a specialized team here for managing hemolytic disease. The Committee consisted of pediatricians, obstetricians, plus the Rhesus team, and the blood bank.[8] So the decisions, even in dire emergencies, were made with consultation if there was time. And I think this led to a safer and better outcome, because forewarned you're forearmed. I think because we involved anyone that might be interested, a team of people, we didn't have any major ethical problems."[9]

Liley researched Rh disease within this collaborative climate, beginning with prenatal diagnosis (Liley 1960; 1961; 1963; 1965a). Soon after joining the faculty of the Postgraduate School, he eagerly set about selecting an area of clinical research. Graham Liggins remembers Liley wanting an area "that was both important and about which something might be done. So he identified hemolytic disease as fitting those criteria, and set about systematically to do something about it. And clearly the first step was to go and make a diagnosis of hemolytic disease and its severity." Liley was fascinated by amniotic fluid, in part because, in his view, "it belongs primarily to the fetus. It is the only part of the conceptus which can be sampled reliably with relative impunity and, if necessary, repeatedly. Tests on the amniotic fluid are tests on the fetus and his environment" (Liley 1972a, 199). Drawing on the prior efforts of Bevis (1952; 1956), Liley began using the technique of amniocentesis in pregnant women with Rh-impaired fetuses as a way to assess the course of the disease.

Amniocentesis required technical precision. Locating the sac without harming the fetus in this pre-ultrasound era was both challenging and risky.[10] After the woman emptied her bladder, Liley would attempt to locate an accessible fetal body part—the limbs, for example—in order to establish the position of the amniotic sac. He would next apply a local anesthetic to the woman's abdomen and insert a sharp lumbar puncture needle through it and into the sac, avoiding both the placenta and the fetus if possible. About ten milliliters of amniotic fluid would be removed, centrifuged, and then analyzed. In many cases of Rh disease, the fluid would become more yellow and was thus easily discernible by the naked eye, but often spectrophotometric analysis would be used. This technique involved measuring the intensity of light of a known wavelength transmitted by a solution, allowing a quantitative assessment of the amount of material in the amniotic fluid. These measurements were plotted on a logarithmic scale against wavelength on a linear scale, resulting in "peaks" of pigmentation corresponding to the level of severity of Rh disease. In some cases, amniocentesis was insufficient. For those cases requiring a more delicate assessment, Liley would inject dye into the amniotic sac that would then be swallowed by the fetus. He used radiography (X rays) to assess fetal condition, and the resulting film would show structural problems not visible with amniocentesis. In his view (Liley 1965a, 732), "amniography as an adjunct to amniocentesis" was useful in the management of Rh disease.

Amniocentesis and amniography indicated the level of anemia, or abnormally low red blood cells, in fetuses, allowing an assessment of "the condition and prognosis of the individual baby" (Liley 1963, 238). Used in this way, the techniques enabled physicians to decide in which pregnancies to induce labor to prevent stillbirths and to avoid severely anemic neonates.[11] Early treatment efforts, then, were an extension of diagnosis and focused on ascertaining when to leave low-risk fetuses in utero and when to deliver others prematurely with minimum risk. As Liley (1963, 242) put it, "the practical implications of these observations is that if all Rhesus-sensitized women are subjected to amniocentesis some time between twenty-nine and thirty-two weeks, a group may be defined in whom the fetal condition is already critical, with very premature delivery a matter of urgency and desperation." After incorporating amniocentesis into the Rh work at National Women's Hospital, "the erythroblastosis perinatal mortality was reduced from the 22–25 percent prevailing before 1958 to less than 9 percent by 1962" (Liley 1965c, 837). For most fetuses at risk for Rh disease, prenatal diagnosis and early delivery were sufficiently efficacious.

Yet, as Liley (1963, 242) wrote, "[Amniocentesis] is not a panacea but a diagnostic procedure. Discovery is not synonymous with salvage." There was one group of fetuses for which early prenatal diagnosis and selective induction were insufficient. Liley (1965c, 837) identified these fetuses as being the "third grade of severity, with very large pigment peaks portending fetal death or hydrops before 34 weeks gestation. For such patients conventional treatment has little to offer since gross immaturity and severe anemia or hydrops makes very premature induction a desperate and disappointing exercise." The Rh team wondered what to do about these severely affected fetuses. The possibility of using amniocentesis to identify at-risk fetuses prompted Liley to consider treatments beyond conventional therapy. He wrote, "It was very frustrating to have to put a diagnosis on a baby which was virtually a sentence of death and then sit back and watch the baby die" (1971b, 303). About this time, two events occurred that dramatically affected the course of fetal therapy and promised to alleviate Liley's frustrations.

First, during amniocentesis Liley accidentally punctured a distended fetal abdomen, with striking consequences: "Instead of getting deep yellow, cloudy amniotic fluid, I got brilliant, golden, clear fluid which was obviously ascitic fluid; this windfall was easily confirmed by injection of contrast medium. Now this had not been intended, and initially it was rather disconcerting, but it did not appear to disturb the fetus—who was a write-off anyway. However, it occurred to me that if we could needle the fetal peritoneum without even trying then perhaps we could do it deliberately and put it to some good use" (Liley 1971b, 303). Liley considered the possibility of using this route for transfusion, yet wondered if the fetus would absorb blood cells rapidly enough to offset anemia. Graham Liggins had also recently accidentally invaded the peritoneal cavity in a pregnancy where there was no amniotic fluid. In this case Liggins was injecting contrast medium before doing an amniogram; when the medium missed its intended mark, the amniotic fluid, it instead "gave a lovely picture of the fetal peritoneal cavity." As Liley and Liggins were about to embark on a project to determine the feasibility of peritoneal transfusion in treating fetuses, a second event occurred influencing this line of work.

A young English geneticist, whose name has long since been forgotten, stopped in Auckland on her way home from Nigeria, where she had been working on sickle-cell disease in African children (Green 1985; Liley 1971b). Liley recalled that "with her she had some beautiful blood slides from neonates and infants, homozygous for HbS [sickle cell], who had been given normal cells intraperitoneally. There were floods of normal cells in their peripheral blood, and this was good enough evidence for us that cells could be taken up from the peritoneum in massive quantity and at a relatively rapid rate. We therefore went directly to the fetus" (1971b, 303). Ironically, this technique established in a very different context—the hands-on treatment of sickle-cell anemia in an undeveloped nation—turned out to be the key to developing a procedure that revolutionized fetal medicine. The young doctor's contribution to the development of intrauterine transfusions cannot be overestimated, even if her name is, unfortunately, no longer part of the historical record—a fate shared by many women in science. As Liggins put it, "When the English lady came along, of course, Bill got the idea of putting blood into the peritoneal cavity."

The goal of fetal transfusion for Rh disease was to "tide over to a more viable maturity the baby severely affected by hemolytic disease in the second or early third trimester" (Liley 1965c, 70). In other words, transfusions could be performed in fetuses too young to survive premature delivery but that would likely die in utero if left untreated. It is important to emphasize that despite the severity of hemolytic disease, the scope of fetal transfusion for Rh-affected fetuses was quite limited. Of the approximately one in 200 pregnancies complicated by Rh sensitization, about 90 percent could be managed by more conventional methods.[12] At most, "only one in 2,000 pregnancies may require transfusion of the fetus to help protect it from intrauterine death or gross prematurity. Thus, for the whole of New Zealand the procedure need be carried out only about 30 times in a year" (Greenet al. 1964:7). For this very small number of fetuses, however, transfusions were potentially lifesaving.

Liley's first successful transfusion was performed in September 1963 on a male fetus at thirty-two weeks' gestation, followed by a second transfusion ten days later and an induced delivery at just under thirty-five weeks. It was the fourth pregnancy for the woman, identified in records and news accounts as Mrs. E. McLeod. Hospital records show that her first pregnancy had been successful, the second ended with intrauterine death, and the third resulted in stillborn twins. The fetus in question was severely affected by hemolytic disease and would likely

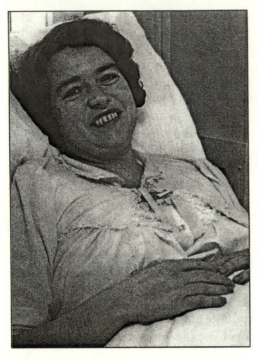

Mrs. E. McLeod after undergoing intrauterine transfusion on behalf of her fetus at National Women's Hospital, Auckland, September 1963. Source: *New Zealand Herald,* Wilson and Horton Ltd., Auckland.

have died within a week of diagnosis had treatment not been performed. Prior to this landmark procedure, which resulted in a baby named Grant Liley McLeod, Liley had attempted three unsuccessful transfusions in fetuses that died. All three efforts failed for technical reasons. Having weathered a process of trial and error, Liley realized that not only were multiple transfusions necessary to treat fetuses in utero, but that some babies would likely need to be transfused again after birth. With the McLeod fetus, Liley put this hard-won knowledge to the test—with astonishing results.

The use of new technologies to treat a fetus in the womb was greeted with excitement and wonder. Some of the headlines describing this and subsequent operations in 1963 are indicative of the absolute novelty of this procedure: "Transfusions Save Life in Fetal Anemia!" "How Unborn Baby was Transfused," "Pre-Birth Transfusion Overcomes Rh Incompatibility," "Transfusions of Blood Aid Unborn Babies," "New Technique Means Life for Baby Girl," "Blood Transfusion Before Birth," and "Unborn Babe Given Transfusion." Echoing this awestruck media coverage a decade later, Zimmerman (1973, 233) described Liley's achievements in poetic, heroic terms: "Liley's needle had penetrated barriers beyond flesh and death on its way to the heart of the womb: breached, too, was the metaphysical barrier between the world of life that is and the universe of life that is yet to be. A fetus had been treated, medically, as one of us.

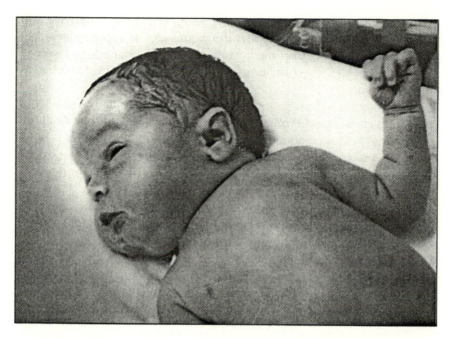

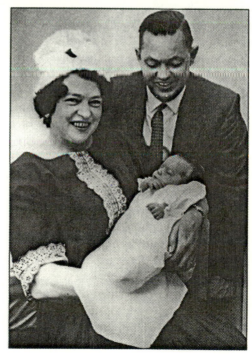

(*Above*) Grant Liley McLeod, the first success of fetal surgery, at National Women's Hospital, Auckland, September 1963. Source: *New Zealand Herald*, Wilson and Horton Ltd., Auckland.

(*Right*) A happy McLeod family on their way home from National Women's Hospital, September 1963. Source: *New Zealand Herald*, Wilson and Horton Ltd., Auckland.

Shattered, too, had been the barrier of medical custom. Prudence and caution had insisted until then that the womb and its contents were beyond the boundary of direct medical intervention." Man and technology had ushered in the era of the unborn patient, and the world responded with amazement.

Breaching the womb brought renown to Liley especially, but also to his colleagues, National Women's Hospital, Auckland, and New Zealand. As one surgeon exalted about the first successful transfusion, "It is most rewarding and encouraging to find an Auckland medical case so extensively reported. For years New Zealand has been relying on gaining medical information elsewhere. This means the turning of the tide."[13] But like most new medical procedures, intrauterine transfusions were challenging, particularly in the initial period before the technical wrinkles were ironed out in practice and many fetuses died. Much of this work took place prior to the development of ultrasound, which has made assessment of fetal position much easier to determine. In the first year during which fetal transfusions were performed at National Women's Hospital, there were sixteen cases involving twenty-two transfusions. The success rate was low: six surviving fetuses or a survival rate of 37.5 percent (Green at al. 1964). In 1969 the survival rate had risen slightly to 39.5 percent, based on 167 pregnancies, 328 fetal transfusions, and 60 survivors (Liley 1969). These numbers reflected the experimental status of this new technology: because it was an innovation in clinical research combining investigation and treatment, its problems were worked out along the way.

And there were many problems, some more challenging than others. One of the most frustrating aspects of this practice for the physicians was actually finding and penetrating the fetus with the needle. Both amniograms and hands-on examinations were used to ascertain fetal position; often, pregnant women themselves were shifted around to provide physicians with better access to fetuses. The consequences of missing the peritoneal cavity could be quite severe for both the woman and her fetus, including puncturing other fetal body parts or rupturing the amniotic sac. According to Liggins (1966a, 617), fetal movement also created problems: "as the fetus explores the roomy confines of the amnion in its efforts to evade the intruding needle, it becomes a very elusive target." Florence Fraser confirmed the technical difficulties of this work: "If the fetus wasn't in a good position, we would put a second needle in, then a third or fourth. There were very few patients where we gave up. Usually the very little ones were the very difficult ones. Sometimes between 18 and 22 weeks you can't hit your target. It's like trying to catch a golf ball in a bucket of water."[14]

Yet, despite such technical challenges, the temptation to use the

(Right) Headline from *New Zealand Herald*, September 25, 1963.

(Below) Headline from *New Zealand Herald*, September 24, 1963.

BABY MAKES HEADLINES OVER WORLD

Case a Tribute To Doctors

Grant McLeod, of Hastings, who owes his life to Auckland doctors who successfully gave him blood transfusions before birth at Auckland's National Women's Hospital, could be the first New Zealand baby to receive headlines in many parts of the world.

The fact that the operation was unique in medical history was responsible for the unprecedented publicity.

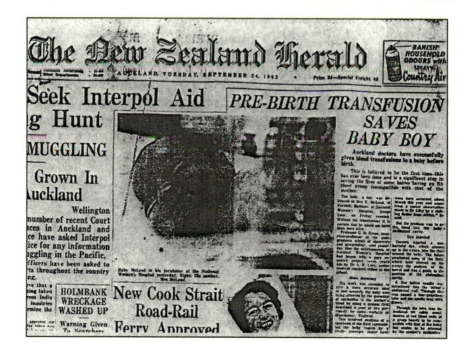

The New Zealand Herald

AUCKLAND, TUESDAY, SEPTEMBER 24, 1963

Seek Interpol Aid

g Hunt

MUGGLING

Grown In Auckland

Wellington
number of recent Court
aces in Auckland and
ce have asked Interpol
ice for any information
uggling in the Pacific.
fficers have been asked to
ts throughout the country
ng.
ve that a
ing taken
rom India
inquiries
rmine the

HOLMBANK
WRECKAGE
WASHED UP

Warning Given
To Searchers

PRE-BIRTH TRANSFUSION SAVES BABY BOY

Auckland doctors have successfully given blood transfusions to a baby before birth.

This is believed to be the first time this has ever been done and is a significant step in saving the lives of some babies having an Rh blood group incompatible with that of the mother.

Baby McLeod in his incubator at the National Women's Hospital yesterday. Right: his mother, Mrs McLeod.

New Cook Strait Road-Rail Ferry Approved

technique in fetuses at lesser risk for Rh disease was compelling. Liley (1965c:842) wrote, "if the procedure can benefit babies at 100 percent risk, it should also benefit babies at only 50 or 30 percent risk." But he also preached caution: "what is necessary is more important than what is possible, and extreme measures are best reserved for extreme situations . . . there is little justification for exposing the fetus and mother gratuitously to the risk of unnecessary transfusions when a much less complete restoration will suffice" (1965c, 841–42). His comments offered an early awareness of how fetal treatment might affect both fetuses and pregnant women. Possible maternal risks of the procedure, which required intervening in the woman's body, included "increased maternal [Rh] sensitization by placento-maternal leak, hemolytic reaction from massive feto-maternal transfusion, accidental hemorrhage, hemoperitoneum, and infection" (Liley 1964, 148). Then, as now, operating on fetuses had enormous implications for women's health. But, although Liley and others acknowledged maternal risks, clinical experiments on fetuses continued apace.

The work of transfusing Rh fetuses, highly technical in nature, was also social and involved a great deal of interaction with patients and their families. Because pregnant women came to National Women's Hospital from all over New Zealand, as well as from other countries, they often required additional support beyond clinical care. Liley, Fraser, and others who worked on the Rh team often developed close, long-term relationships with their patients. Fraser told me, "I used to spend a terrific amount of time with the mothers. We tried to keep their lives as normal as possible, as much as you can in a hospital. If they wanted to talk, both of us would make time to just sit down and talk to them, and I think that's why Bill and I both ended up with a lot of friends. You know, I still at Christmas time get fantastic little bulletins about patients." An important component of this work was providing psychosocial support for the pregnant women. Fraser described this aspect: "Your social and psychological support are terribly important, because you've got to have a peaceful calm. We did a lot of social working on the job, and to me that was part of the job. And Bill felt the same way. For both of us, our day here started with a trip to the wards to see all the patients. I couldn't start the day without knowing they were all okay and happy, and that junior [the fetus] was happy."

In addition to working with patients, Liley and Fraser also interacted with colleagues from all over New Zealand who referred patients or wrote asking for information and treatment advice. These inquiries illustrate the degree to which National Women's Hospital was an epicenter of Rh diagnosis and treatment during the 1960s and 1970s, with

Liley positioned as the expert in residence. The correspondence is testament to the routine consulting, disseminating, and negotiating work that constituted reproductive medicine. In one humorous letter Liley wrote, "In this situation it would have saved a lot of time and paper if you and I had sat down—preferably over a bottle of whiskey—and decided what to do ourselves. I appreciate that this might sound a little arrogant but by the time you have answered the same query from obstetricians in a dozen towns in New Zealand it gets a little boring." To a colleague in the South Island who had inquired about a particular case, he responded, "Mrs. P's story is interesting but by no means novel to us, at least in terms of development of antibodies after immunoprophylaxis in a previous pregnancy." And to a Fijian physician he was gently discouraging: "Your lady does not sound the most auspicious clinical prospect particularly as her husband is very likely to be homozygous. On the other hand if she is happy to attempt another pregnancy we will certainly be happy to try and help her."

Physicians were not the only people seeking advice and counsel from the increasingly popular Liley. One of the offshoots of Liley's renown was the massive amount of correspondence he received from women all over the world asking for information about Rh disease.[15] For example, in 1966, a woman from Savannah, Georgia, sent a poignant letter typed on pale blue stationery:

> I know you are a very important man so I won't take up much of your time. I got your name and address thru reader's digest. In the April addition there was an article named "Conquest of Death before Birth." . . . One year ago today they burried my baby. I carried my child nine months to the day. The week before she was born they ran an RH test on me. The Doctors said there wasn't enough RH Composits for it to be a blue baby. . . . When they tried to transfuse my childs blood she would destroy it before they could get a pint into her body. She lived twelve hours and then died. . . . My little girl who is three is very lonesome and I would like to have more children. I am so afraid that I couldn't take the chance of losing another child. . . . Do you think the reaction would show up again if I were to get Pregnant? Please help me with this.

Another sad story came from a woman in Ohio, who wrote in 1974:

> In my mind you are the highest medical authority on "life before birth" and I have read many of your articles. . . . My husband and I have the RH problem and just one month ago lost our 3rd child at 26 weeks gestation. . . . We have been advised that the possibility of producing a living child is now entirely out of the question—in other words, no hope. . . . At 26 I am finding the diagnosis of "no more children, ever" a terribly difficult burden and I guess I just wonder if you concur with the "verdict."

The woman's letter also revealed some of the connections between fetal surgery and abortion politics. In closing, she wrote, "Thank you for your tremendous fight and support of all the unborn. I am a Birthright office Chairman and we regard you and your work so highly!"

A voluminous set of letters from a man in Sri Lanka concerned his wife's pregnancy and related Rh problems. Spanning almost two years, these letters chronicle the pregnancy, birth, and death of the baby, and confronted the issue of whether the couple should travel to Auckland or to the United States or Great Britain for care in subsequent pregnancies. Liley responded that the decision might be affected by the fact that "as you probably already know, medical care does tend to be disproportionately expensive in the United States in comparison with most places in the world." Liley's correspondence is filled with letters such as these, as well as copies of his detailed and thoughtful responses. If the sheer magnitude and content of his correspondence is any indication, Liley's fame did not prevent him from treating each inquiry with concern—although he did often resort to standardized language when conveying technical information.

Transfusion work—both in and out of the operating room—kept the Rh team busy for several years. With the introduction of the Rh vaccine for hemolytic disease in the 1970s, some researchers expected that fetal transfusions would taper off or that hemolytic disease would be vanquished (Zimmerman 1973). But this was not the case. Liley believed that Rh disease was persistent and likely to remain a significant problem for at least some group of women. Fraser recalled Liley's response to the vaccine: "Everyone here, when anti-D came, said of course this is going to end hemolytic disease, and Bill said, No it's not. He said it would cut out the mild ones, but it would take an almighty blast to get the trigger happy ones, as he used to call them. There would still be a hard core of tough cases, and this is what it's turned out to be." Liley and his colleagues in Auckland believed that intrauterine transfusion technology would always have a place—albeit a limited one—in the management of fetuses at high risk for Rh disease. He wrote, "Clearly this is a somewhat long term and ambitious campaign and in this context it is both naive and arrogant to speak of 'the conquest of hemolytic disease.'"[16]

More than any of his equally devoted colleagues, innovations in prenatal treatment secured for Liley a place in the annals of medical history, as well as in the hearts of New Zealanders.[17] His work on Rh disease and the development of intrauterine transfusion technology sparked what one observer called a "revolution" in the making of the unborn patient. By breaching the womb with needles and catheters and by directly treating fetuses surgically, Liley and his colleagues expanded the scope of reproductive medicine and redefined obstetrical care. Most important, these events brought the fetus under the purview of modern medicine as a distinct patient available for treatment. Yet just as intrauterine transfusion technology was making international headlines, another chapter in the making of the unborn patient was being written. Graham Liggins and Ross Howie were quietly demonstrating that fetal treatment was not limited to the "invasive" approach in which fetuses were directly penetrated. As Liggins told me, "Surgical *and* medical intervention began in National Women's Hospital." Both forms of treatment have had far-reaching consequences for fetal medicine.

A Nonsurgical Approach: Corticosteroids and the Unborn Patient

While Liley's work emphasized direct, intrauterine treatment of fetuses using needles to breach the womb, Liggins and Howie focused on nonsurgical aspects of fetal treatment. Building on animal experiments, they administered corticosteroids (a steroid produced by the adrenal cortex) to pregnant women to facilitate lung growth in fetuses, a technique still in wide use. Considering the context in which this research unfolded, its concurrent development with surgical advances in fetal treatment is not at all surprising. As with surgical treatment, National Women's Hospital provided a fertile setting for the development and emergence of nonsurgical treatments. Liley's work with fetal transfusions depended to some degree on a solid understanding of principles of fetal physiology, which Liggins had spent years researching in animals and attempting to elucidate.[18] Liggins reminisced, "Bill and I worked very closely together. I did a lot of fetal transfusions, and Bill was away for a year [at Columbia in 1964] and I looked after the whole thing. We were also really close friends, shared not only our work interests but also our extramural interests. There was certainly a cross-fertilization." Liggins was interested in technical aspects of fetal transfusions, including the development of impaling techniques used to better grasp fetuses during diagnosis and treatment. Moreover, patients admitted to National Women's Hospital for care by the Rh team were often delivered prematurely to avoid hydrops, the usually fatal stage of Rh disease, and thus provided Liggins and Howie with a steady supply of research subjects.

Liggins had long been interested in the physiological mechanisms responsible for the onset of labor, conducting most of his research in sheep.[19] In a series of remarkable animal experiments he claimed to demonstrate that it was the fetus, not the mother, that controlled the time of onset of labor (Dawes 1989). During the course of that work, he discovered that by destroying the fetal pituitary gland, birth could be postponed or avoided while the fetus continued to grow. He recalled, "What I'd done was remove the pituitary in the fetal sheep, and allow the pregnancy to continue without the gland, and the pregnancy would go on forever. Conversely, if you infuse into the fetus the hormone ACTH, which is a pituitary hormone that drives the adrenal, or cortisol, which is an adrenal hormone in the placenta, the animals deliver prematurely. And the lungs of the babies, even though they died quickly, had retained air. So we were noting this effect and I realized that the cortisol or the ACTH was accelerating the development of the fetal lungs. Ross Howie and I then pursued this in lambs about to deliver prematurely." From his research on labor, Liggins stumbled (fortuitously, in his view) across the key to fetal lung development.

Following a trial in which 43 sheep were given cortisol and other hormones (Liggins 1969), which showed that corticosteroids administered prenatally stimulate lung development in the sheep fetus, Liggins and Howie conducted their first clinical trial in humans. Moving from experimental research in sheep to clinical care in humans required some modifications in the procedure. With sheep, fetuses were infused directly with cortisol using self-retaining catheters. In humans, however, the placenta is much more permeable; this meant that injecting pregnant women with the hormones could be "a feasible means of subjecting the human fetus to high levels of glucocorticoid activity" (Liggins and Howie 1972, 516). In other words, treatment entailed direct intervention in the pregnant woman but not in the fetus itself, which would be affected through placental transfer. This innovation had significant clinical implications for premature babies born with immature lungs who might subsequently succumb to respiratory distress syndrome. Corticosteroids promised to alleviate this problem in the fetal stage, resulting in healthier babies and higher survival rates. And, the fetus itself did not have to be directly treated.

From this experimental work carried out in the late 1960s and early 1970s, corticosteroid treatment has since become a routine practice in obstetrics. The trajectory of corticosteroid treatment was quite different from that of intrauterine transfusions, primarily because it was an easier technology to use. National Women's Hospital had become a singular center for Rh transfusion treatment because it was a difficult procedure and most other institutions were not yet prepared to do it. This was not the case with corticosteroid treatment, a much less invasive technology for the fetus and a somewhat less invasive technology for the pregnant women. Liggins stated, "Women didn't have to travel to Auckland. It was such a simple treatment anybody could do it. What happened initially is a number of centers set up similar controlled trials, and within quite a short time, say three or four years, a half dozen or more comparative studies were done." Thus, nonsurgical fetal treatment was able to be exported to other medical centers to a degree that fetal transfusion was not. Liggins told me, "Our test results have stood the test of time, and this has become standard treatment throughout the world. Probably hundreds of thousands of babies have survived who might not have survived."

It is ironic that intrauterine transfusions, which saved at most thirty fetuses per year in New Zealand, captured the world's imagination, while corticosteroid treatment, which has become standard care and has saved many more babies across the globe, did not. Both forms of treatment were based on the same body of experimental research, used many of the same techniques, were performed by many of the same practitioners on some of the same patients, and occurred within a single institution, National Women's Hospital. This distinction in public reception and the historical record indicates that although there has been tremendous clinical interest in all aspects of fetal treatment, it is viscerally breaching the womb that both fascinates and compels a wider audience. Giving hormones to a pregnant woman that are then passed to her fetus through the placenta was not nearly so exciting as the drama of penetrating the uterus and its contents with needles and catheters, fully *intervening* in pregnancy and fetal life. This was indeed revolutionary medicine, and in more ways than one. Once the Pandora's box was surgically opened, the unborn patient began to be sighted elsewhere—most significantly in Puerto Rico and New York City.

"A Bona Fide Patient": Open Fetal Surgery in Puerto Rico and New York

Despite the extraordinary success and allure of intrauterine transfusions, there were a number of clinical problems identified with this new approach to fetal treatment (Adamsons 1966; Adamsons et al. 1965). Everyone agreed that locating the peritoneal cavity of the fetus was often quite difficult. On many occasions, the "blind" needling technique pioneered by Liggins and used by the Rh team in transfusions resulted in injury to fetal organs. Even if the peritoneal cavity was adequately penetrated with needles and catheters, absorption of injected red blood cells was not always successful. Repeated punctures were often necessary because of the decay of the donor cells and expansion of the intravascular compartment of the fetus. If the fetus survived, exchange transfusions were almost always required after birth. Thus, although Liley's *closed* intrauterine transfusion method was lifesaving in many circumstances and avoided the problems associated with surgically opening the uterus,

Adamsons (1966, 204) argued that "large variations in salvage rate exist[ed]" with this technique. In an attempt to increase survival rates and expand treatment to an older group of fetuses, Adamsons, Freda, and others began pursuing *open* fetal surgery for exchange transfusions in Rh cases in New York and Puerto Rico. Open surgery promised enhanced visibility of and access to the fetus at risk for Rh disease, bringing the unborn patient more clearly within the scope of the clinical gaze.

Colonialism, Science, and Medicine

In order to understand the concurrent emergence of open fetal surgery in New York and Puerto Rico, it is first necessary to situate Puerto Rico as a U.S. colony. Throughout the nineteenth and twentieth centuries, there has been considerable political, economic, cultural, scientific, and human migratory traffic between the United States, especially New York and other urban centers, and the small, beautiful Caribbean island, which historically has been viewed as "a strategic outpost" for U.S. interests (Ramirez de Arellano and Seipp 1983). Puerto Rico was ceded to the United States in 1898 as a spoil of the Spanish-American War, and subsequently suffered from the "imperialism of neglect" by a country that did not know what to do with its newest geographic prize. Predominantly Catholic with an economy supported by coffee, sugar, and tobacco, Puerto Rico soon began to appeal to certain U.S. constituents who advocated for a greater stateside role in the island's affairs. It became known in the 1950s as the "TVA of the tropics" (Ramirez de Arellano and Seipp 1983), amenable to innovative social and economic policies designed to enhance the welfare of its inhabitants and bolster the island's economy. Currently a self-governing protectorate of the United States, Puerto Rico struggles for autonomy within a geopolitical context shaped by its history as a colony.

It is within this colonial context that the relationship between Puerto Rico and research institutions such as Columbia University developed and flourished. Puerto Rico as a colonial possession has been "studied and restudied" (Ramirez de Arellano and Seipp 1983), serving as a natural laboratory for research of all kinds on both human and nonhuman primates. Health issues, including reproduction, have been central to U.S.–Puerto Rican relations, beginning in the 1930s and 1940s with scientific interest in tropical diseases and one of the earliest programs of surgical sterilization for contraceptive purposes. For example, Haraway (1989) traced the relationship between Columbia University and the School of Tropical Medicine at the University of Puerto Rico as a partnership shaped by a convergence of interests in reproductive physiology, naturalistic behavior studies, and infectious diseases. The affiliates instituted a trial birth control clinic in 1935 and began a large-scale, island-wide birth control program shortly thereafter. The contraceptive pill, invented by Gregory Pincus, was tested on Puerto Rican women in the mid-1950s (Oudshoorn 1994; Clarke 1998). Puerto Rico was chosen for several reasons: Pincus and his colleagues knew they could not carry out a trial in the United States because of contraception laws; the nearby island was both crowded and impoverished, providing a "natural" rationale for limiting its population; and many Puerto Rican women were poor and illiterate and thus not in a position to resist being used as human guinea pigs for reproductive research (Oudshoorn 1994). (On the other hand, many women may well have welcomed an opportunity to have fewer children.)

One other factor has made Puerto Rico attractive to researchers historically: availability of research materials (Clarke 1987). A primate colony called Cayo Santiago was established in 1939 by the School of Tropical Medicine. Located off the southeast coast of Puerto Rico on a thirty-seven-acre island, the colony was originally stocked with more than four hundred Rhesus monkeys, fourteen gibbons, and three macaques transported from India (Rawlins and Kessler 1986). In 1951, control of the colony passed to the School of Medicine, which struggled to maintain it adequately as the island was ecologically incapable of sustaining the food requirements of its alien inhabitants. Upon visiting the island, one researcher wrote, "The colony appeared in lamentable condition. There was evidence of malnutrition, cannibalism, and the island was infested with rats, which would beat the monkeys in a struggle for coconuts. The delivery of food from the shore was irregular and inadequate and there was evidence of water shortage" (Rawlins and Kessler 1986). During this period, many monkeys attempted, mostly unsuccessfully, to escape the island by swimming to the mainland. An influx of NIH money in the 1950s provided necessary resources and rejuvenated a tenuous research program (Backman 1982), paving the way for a research boom in the 1960s.[20]

Puerto Rico, then, in concert with key locations in the United States, has long been an important site for certain types of scientific and medical work. Because Puerto Rico has been configured as a "natural laboratory," it has often been possible for scientists to engage in research that might be precluded by institutional barriers present on the mainland. The contraceptive pill trials offer an excellent example of this. A more "relaxed" investigative climate rendered Puerto Rico a fruitful setting for the emergence of open fetal surgery and drew fetal researchers southward from the gritty hustle of New York City. The development of open fetal surgical techniques resulted from a confluence of traffic, both human and nonhuman, between the metropolis and the Caribbean colony.

Monkeys, Medical Work, and the Unborn Patient

Karliss Adamsons had long been interested in obstetrical techniques relating to problems of the fetus. While a resident in 1958–59 he worked
with the renowned fetal physiologist Dawes (with whom Liggins had
also worked at Oxford), where he spent a productive year studying fetal
breathing in sheep. There he confirmed that sheep are able to tolerate
surgical intrusion into the womb because the junction between the placenta and fetus is very unstable in sheep, unlike in primates where
placenta and fetus are closely linked. On the basis of their research in
sheep, both Dawes and Adamsons were invited to Puerto Rico to work
with Rhesus monkeys in a small laboratory run by William Mendel located on the medical campus of the university and supplied with Rhesus
monkeys from Cayo Santiago. Adamsons and Dawes began experiments
in which monkey fetuses were lifted out of the uterus and exposed to
cooler air in order to study neonatal asphyxia and resuscitation. They
were encouraged by their results that they could open the uterus and not
be faced with irreparable problems, such as immediate fetal demise, although premature labor was still a concern. Adamsons (1966, 204)
wrote, "it could be shown that even in the monkey, complete removal of
the fetus and its subsequent replacement to the uterine cavity is compat-
ible with fetal survival, and even repeated exposures of the fetus during
the course of the development are feasible."

In the meantime, Vincent Freda was busily investigating Rh disease
at Columbia, where he was on the obstetrics faculty. This work subsequently led to the development of the Rh vaccine. Freda was quite interested in pursuing additional avenues of fetal treatment and had conducted
some animal experimentation using techniques to locate the placenta
and uterus for penetration with needles. As a practicing obstetrician,
Freda was familiar with the physiology of pregnancy and already had extensive experience with procedures such as cesarean section. When
Adamsons returned to Columbia from Puerto Rico in 1962, he became
very interested in Freda's Rh work. After hearing of Liley's work the following year and using his techniques in their own practices, Adamsons
and Freda had begun thinking about performing catheterizations and
transfusions with open surgical techniques; that is, cutting open a pregnant woman's uterus to access her fetus. Adamsons told Freda about his
research in Puerto Rico and how "tolerant" the monkey fetuses had been
of intrusion. This, coupled with Freda's technical expertise in maternal
patients, persuaded the team that they should, as Adamsons told me,
"find a willing patient and proceed apace."

Shortly after deciding on this trailblazing course, Freda located a
suitable patient, a 33-year-old woman in the fourth month of her

eleventh pregnancy, whose fetus was at grave risk and, according to Adamsons, "in dire need of a transfusion." On the basis of amniocentesis, Adamsons and Freda predicted that the fetus would probably die within two and a half weeks. Adamsons remembers being "surprised when the mother readily agreed, but also nervous and anxious." It is not clear how eager the woman was to participate or exactly what she was told about the procedure, but given the highly experimental nature of what they were attempting, Adamsons and Freda had good reason to be worried. The operation lasted three hours, and both the pregnant woman and her fetus appeared to tolerate it well. Adamsons remembers, "We were ecstatic. We felt that the next step was going to Stockholm to win the Nobel Prize." This excitement was short-lived, however. The patient went into labor just two days after surgery and, after premature vaginal delivery, her baby died of immaturity and incomplete expansion of the lungs. It is not clear from the published literature, or Adamsons's and Freda's recollections, how much the intervention itself had to do with the baby's death. Although the baby died, Adamsons and Freda considered the procedure a major success because it provided valuable information about open surgical techniques. Yet despite their claims that the procedure was successful, the pregnant woman whose baby died most likely did not view it as such.[21]

Despite the specter of fetal demise and maternal risk, Freda and Adamsons (1964) argued that there were several advantages to open surgical exchange transfusion. These included introducing the greatest volume of fresh Rh-negative blood into the fetal circulation, ensuring the broadest protection for the fetus for the longest period of time, and obviating the need for repeated "blind" needling attempts and possible fetal damage. They identified the two largest disadvantages as technical difficulties in carrying out the procedure with minimal trauma to the pregnant woman and her fetus, and the possibility of premature labor following the operation. As Adamsons knew from his monkey research, the physiological tendency in primates once the uterus is opened is onset of labor. Fetal death might be prevented, but at what cost to the pregnant woman or her fetus? In this initial surgical case, as in subsequent cases in New York, Puerto Rico, and elsewhere, premature labor has indeed proven to be a recalcitrant problem in open fetal surgery. At the time, however, these problems did not prevent Adamsons and Freda from applying for and receiving a grant from the National Institutes of Health for their experiments.

Columbia Presbyterian was an ideal place to pursue this work, as the patient population was steady, diverse, and large, with about twenty patients per month referred for Rh problems. At that time, before the widespread routinization of Liley's technique in clinical practice, Columbia was the only place in the world outside New Zealand where intrauterine transfusions were being done. According to Adamsons, however, there were differences in the patient population that suggested a different therapeutic trajectory. In New Zealand, Liley was treating patients at early gestational ages, allowing for greater absorption of blood into the fetal peritoneal cavity. In New York, many patients were classified as "already too far advanced" for intraperitoneal transfusions. Adamsons claims, "We had no other choice but to do open surgery for transfusions!" Of course, choice is contextual, and Adamsons and Freda were instrumental in defining a need for fetal surgery. Yet however ripe the conditions for the emergence of this work, Adamsons and Freda had poor success with open transfusions. There was not a single surviving fetus in the first few years of their work, beginning with their initial attempt in 1963.

In 1964, while visiting Columbia, Liley engaged with Adamsons and Freda in considerable exchange of information and collaboration. The latter researchers were interested in learning more about Liley's closed intraperitoneal transfusion technique, and Liley was curious about their forays into open surgery. Adamsons remembers Liley fondly, remarking that "he was a nice person and we got along well." Freda talked about his work with Liley that year in positive terms, stating that they had spent a lot of time discussing animal research and obstetrical techniques in humans. Yet despite this spirit of collaboration, there were major differences among the three men. According to Florence Fraser, Liley was "very scathing of Adamsons' work on open transfusions." Open surgery was never pursued at National Women's Hospital in Auckland because of concerns about maternal and fetal risk. Indeed, Liley (1968, 55–56) wrote that "[the] isolated success using hysterotomy to implant intraperitoneal catheters does little to redeem the consistent failures of Freda and associates." It is interesting to speculate, given Liley's views on open surgery, about some of the discussions these colleagues may have had in 1964. Neither Adamsons nor Freda could remember exact conversations, but both men recall a period of lively and productive debate.

After 1964 the working relationship between Adamsons and Freda began to sour. They had, at this point, attempted open fetal surgery in a handful of patients, with mixed success. Many fetuses died right away, while some lingered a bit longer; the team never achieved neonatal survival after experimental open fetal surgery. Eventually, the NIH grant expired as well. Freda told me that he had not wanted to publicize the research on open surgery because of its controversial nature and limited success; he remarked, "I wanted to keep it quiet until we got more pieces under our belt." He reportedly turned down an interview request from *Time* magazine, and was both surprised and furious to discover an article in that magazine the following month with, in his words, "Adamsons all

over it. As if Adamsons had done the surgeries or provided the patients."
Freda became angry with Adamsons for publicizing their research and
for taking sole credit for the surgery. He told me that he had been "the
main surgeon," with colleagues Albert Plentl and Adamsons assisting.
Freda retaliated by denying Adamsons access to obstetrical patients at
Columbia Presbyterian—an action both men confirmed in interviews.
This incident marked the end of their collaboration and prefigured the
intense professional conflicts that continue to pervade fetal surgery.

Freda stayed at Columbia and continued to work on Rh disease. In
1994 he told me that he had done more than five hundred closed operations and, after Adamsons left, he did nineteen additional open surgical
operations with some success. (I could not verify this in the published literature. In fact, Freda told me that he "did not write more papers" because he was "preoccupied with inventing Rhogam and running the Rh
clinic.") Adamsons left Columbia shortly after the altercation to work at
Mount Sinai and then to chair the Department of Obstetrics and Gynecology at Brown University. During this period, he began collaborating
with a team of physicians in Puerto Rico who were interested in open fetal surgery. He recounts a case involving a woman in San Juan with a
poor history of Rh treatment and a grossly hydropic fetus. Using open
surgical techniques, Adamsons and his colleagues injected red blood
cells directly into the fetus's bone marrow, administered the hormone
thyroxin to accelerate fetal growth and development, and successfully
delivered a live baby three weeks later. This operation marked the beginning of extensive collaboration between Adamsons and his colleagues in
Puerto Rico, which continued long-distance until Adamsons relocated
there permanently in 1976 as chair of obstetrics and gynecology at the
University of Puerto Rico.

The Puerto Rico team, prior to Adamsons's arrival, had made an important contribution to the field by performing the first successful open
surgery for transfusion. In 1965, building on the efforts of Liley,
Adamsons, and Freda, as well as a substantial body of monkey experiments, Stanley Asensio, Juan Figueroa, and others (Asensio et al. 1966)
performed an open intrauterine exchange transfusion on a 26-year-old
woman with Rh complications. The operation itself went relatively
smoothly. Twenty days later, the woman delivered a "living female infant
in good condition" (1966, 1130). The baby was named Miracle by her exhausted but relieved mother. Buoyed by this success, Asensio et al. (1966,
1133) wrote, "This procedure might be the safest and the one that can
provide the most definite treatment for the severely affected erythroblas-
totic fetuses." Even Liley (1968, 56) was impressed, stating a few years
later that "Asensio's single success remains the only convincing rescue by
intrauterine exchange transfusion." Remarkably, despite their achieve-

ments and the possibility of fame, Asensio and his team did not pursue open surgery beyond their first successful effort. Arsenio Comas, who was a young resident on the team, told me that this work had seemed "too experimental" to become a viable clinical procedure.

Like Liley's technique, open fetal surgery for Rh disease profoundly influenced the development of fetal medicine (Michejda and Pringle 1986a). The act of slicing open the womb and exposing the fetus for direct treatment was nothing short of amazing. In Adamsons's view, the significance of fetal surgery was in defining the fetus as "a bona fide patient, as much a patient as the mother is, available for diagnosis and treatment. There is nothing more convincing than opening the uterus, taking the fetus out, and putting it back." This facet of the making of the unborn patient thus served an important legitimating function. Adamsons told me that "breaking down barriers of the fetus as a patient makes other procedures, both diagnostic and therapeutic, more acceptable." Open fetal surgery was so graphically shocking that every other technique looked tame by comparison. Legitimacy, however, can work in both directions. Adamsons also remarked that "once the field was opened with amniocentesis and other techniques, people couldn't argue against invading the womb. People had to accept that the uterus was no longer a sanctuary." In other words, constructing the fetus as a patient through open fetal surgery served to legitimate other, less invasive fetal treatments, whose acceptance and use in turn made it possible to continue to breach the womb. All of these practices, but especially open fetal surgery, helped bring the womb and its contents—now conceptualized as the unborn patient—within the jurisdiction of medicine.

In sum, open fetal surgery enjoyed a brief but intense wave of interest in the mid-1960s that had subsided by the end of that decade. Following the New York and Puerto Rico experiments, open fetal surgery was abandoned until the early 1980s for a number of reasons. First, the technique of intraperitoneal transfusion was claimed to be both effective and safe enough that open surgery for Rh disease was viewed as both too invasive and too risky for both the woman and her fetus. According to Maria Michejda and Kevin Pringle (1986b, 8), "If the group in Auckland, New Zealand, had not been so outstandingly successful in the development of percutaneous fetal transfusions, then fetal surgery would have had to have developed to a point where major fetal surgery could have been routine by this time." Another explanation for this lag is that preventive measures such as the Rh vaccine drastically reduced the incidence of hemolytic disease, which prior to ultrasound was one of the only conditions amenable to diagnosis by amniocentesis (Michejda and Pringle 1986a). Once Rh disease became more manageable and until new conditions became diagnosable, physicians had no reason to pursue open surgical treatment. A third important reason stemmed from ethical, political, and professional opposition to this innovative and risky technology. As Adamsons told me, "there was hostility by older practitioners and scientists to notions of intervening." Thus fetal surgery was also shaped by controversy and ongoing "illegitimate" associations. In the 1960s, the making of the unborn patient was deeply connected to other politically charged issues, especially abortion, rendering fetal surgery itself a contested terrain.

Forbidden Frontier: Reproductive Politics and the Unborn Patient

Just as the present context of fetal surgery is shaped by political controversy, so too have politics permeated the historical emergence of the fetus as a patient. In New Zealand, New York, and Puerto Rico, these connections have included the changing face of reproductive politics, abortion politics, and general discomfort with fetal research in both humans and animals. By innovating new technologies and breathing life into a new medical specialty, medical workers both actively and unwittingly became embedded in broader social and political arenas of debate. Some, most notably Liley, relished their roles as scientific authorities on the fetus, while others struggled to avoid controversy and position their work as legitimate science. Clarke (1990, 18) has argued that the reproductive sciences have long been marked by controversy because it is an arena where "the politics of science confronts the politics of moral change." Operating on fetuses threatens moral order on two major fronts: it is "brave new worlds" research capable of altering human destiny, and it is associated with abortion, which is itself so highly contested. Understanding historical associations between reproductive politics and fetal surgery fleshes out our picture of this emergent specialty, while also previewing some of the issues that remain contentious today. For three decades, the making of the unborn patient has been shadowed by concerns about intervening at the beginning of human life.

"A Legacy of Life": Liley, Abortion, and Fetal Personhood

Of the many people involved in the making of the unborn patient during the 1960s and 1970s, Liley was the most passionate and articulate about abortion and fetal personhood.[22] He was deeply interested in fetal life and devoted much of his career to describing and illuminating the world of the fetus, with major linkages to and consequences for the international antiabortion movement. A colleague in the antiabortion movement once described him as "a giant among men who has dedicated his life to the tiniest human."[23] His clinical work was an integral part of a broader fascination with and commitment to fetuses, or "unborn children" in his preferred terminology. While he labored to bring fetuses under modern medicine's gaze as a new category of patient, he struggled simultaneously to foster social and cultural respect for fetal personhood. He was ardently opposed to abortion, basing his position on what he termed the "medical realities of achieving the pro-life ideal" (Liley 1979). Liley saw his mission extending beyond the clinical domain into the political sphere, both participating in antiabortion politics and serving as a "scientific" spokesman for the fetus. In what became an oft-cited quote in the antiabortion movement in New Zealand, he (Liley 1971d, 12) remarked that "it is a bitter irony that just when the fetus achieves some medical status and importance there should be pressure to make him a social non-entity."

Displaying shades of biological determinism, Liley drew upon his clinical work to propagate notions of the "natural" fetal patient, a status he then used to legitimate fetal personhood in a variety of cultural settings. Beginning with his Rh work, Liley saw himself primarily as a physician to the fetus—which he viewed as the most important work object. For example, he (1971d, 13) wrote, "We can now diagnose and treat a number of fetal maladies, and the list is growing. . . . The fetus can be sick and need diagnosis and treatment like any other patient." In an antiabortion newsletter, he (Liley n.d.-a) elaborated the issue as such: "This is the fetus we look after in modern obstetrics, the same baby we are caring for before and after birth. . . . This is also the fetus whose existence and identity must be so callously ignored or energetically denied by advocates of abortion." An important aspect of making the unborn patient, and consequently fetal personhood, was elucidating key physiological characteristics of fetal development and behavior that seemed to support this emergent status.

Yet in order to establish fetal patienthood, the fetus needed first to be framed as a distinct individual, separable and separate from the pregnant woman in whose body it resided. Reverberating with echoes of Liggins and Howie's (1972) research on the fetus's definitive role in onset of labor, Liley presented the fetus not only as a distinct patient, but as *actively* in charge of pregnancy. For example, in a paper originally presented in 1975 (Liley 1983, 6; emphasis added), he wrote, "Our new human has in hand even grander designs and undertakings than simply his own internal organization and development. He also develops his own life-support system, his placenta, and his own confines. . . . But even the organization of his own confines does not exhaust the list of achievements of our new individual. His own welfare is too important to permit leaving anything to the chance cooperation of others, and therefore *he must organize his mother to make her body a suitable home.*" Among the ways in which Liley claimed fetuses accomplished this were by producing hormones to prevent menstrual shedding of the endometrium, taking over the endometrium, manufacturing hormones necessary for pregnancy, preventing immunological rejection by the host mother, and determining the duration and onset of pregnancy. In short, according to Liley (1983, 8), "the fetus is a young human, dynamic, plastic, resilient, in command of his own environment and destiny with a tenacious purpose."

These fetal representations formed the core of Liley's (1972b, 105) classic article, "The Fetus as a Personality," in which he presented "a day in the life of a fetus."[24] He suggested: "we may not all live to grow old but we were each once a fetus ourselves. As such we had some engaging qualities which unfortunately we lost as we grew older. . . . Is it too much to ask therefore that perhaps we should accord . . . to fetal personality and behavior, rudimentary as they may appear by adult standards, the same consideration and respect?" Contradicting earlier premodern conceptions of the fetus as a passive tabula rasa in the uterus, Liley constructed it as "very much in command of the pregnancy" (1972b, 100). His account of fetal personhood is replete with action verbs: the fetus "guarantees" the success of pregnancy, "induces" changes in maternal physiology, "determines" the duration of pregnancy, "decides" which way "he" will present in labor, "learns" and "responds" to stimuli, and so on. The pregnant woman in this account is reduced to a "suitable host," "the space and shape available to [the fetus]," "the walls of the fetal world," "a pregnant uterus," and "a plastic, reactive structure."

Liley's representations of fetal individuality and agency are significant in terms of establishing historical foundations of the paradigm of maternal-fetal conflict that undergirds contemporary practices. In much of this literature, as illustrated in the above examples, pregnant women are relegated to the status of maternal environments or hosts for the developing, active fetus. Liley (1983, 6) wrote, "Women speak of *their* waters breaking and *their* membranes rupturing, but such expressions are so much nonsense—these structures belong to the fetus." He (Liley 1971d, 12) later asserted that "at no stage can we subscribe to the view that the fetus is a mere appendage of the mother. . . . The early embryo stops mother's periods and induces all manner of changes in maternal physiology to make his mother a suitable host. . . . It is argued that the fetus is incapable of independent existence. However, the fetus can outlive his mother, and dead women have been delivered of live babies. Independent existence is a relative concept." It is quite obvious here whose existence is seen to matter in Liley's framework, and whose is not.

In a rather remarkable display of deeply gendered cultural assumptions, Liley (1983, 7) also wrote,

This relationship between a baby and his mother is clearly much more than simple biological parasitism. The term parasite, so frequently applied to the fetus, is often used, not in the limited biological sense, but with the sociological overtone of describing someone who takes all and contributes nothing. Neither sense is applicable to the fetus. True, he is parasitic on mother for his nutritional requirements. In the same sense many wives could be said to be parasitic on their husband's income; but just as wives would indignantly maintain that they contribute much to a home and a marriage to justify their keep, and that really what is involved is a division of labor, so also does the fetus justify his keep by organizing and maintaining his pregnancy. Such a relationship is more accurately described as parabiosis or symbiosis, and physiologically there is no question who guarantees its success.

The notion of separate entities with distinct interests extended beyond physiological matters into the political realm. Liley often discussed abortion, which he clearly despised, in terms that exalted fetal rights and privileges while trivializing women's own concerns and needs: "We have the rather perverse situation nowadays where the perfectly healthy are clamouring for their abortions on the grounds of the inconvenience [their pregnancies] represent to them. . . . It's not continuation of the pregnancy which represents any threat whatsoever to anyone; it is the life of the child which represents a threat to somebody's convenience" (Liley 1979, 54). Twenty years later, these same cultural judgments about women's autonomy and choice dominate the discourse of the antiabortion movement. Then as now, abortion itself was portrayed by some as a maternal-fetal conflict in which a woman's own "selfish" needs and interests were believed to constitute a serious risk to her fetus, perhaps more serious even than Rh disease which could at least now be treated.

Liley's clinical work and his antiabortion activism were mutually reinforcing in another important way. He became quite distressed that certain procedures he had developed to save fetal lives were subsequently used in abortion practices. Specifically, he was upset that amniocentesis, a "life-saving diagnostic tool" in his view, was "next misapplied to detect handicapped unborn so they could be destroyed—a 'search and destroy mission'" (McCarthy 1983, 5).[25] But he was especially disturbed by the application of techniques he developed for transfusions in administering solution for saline abortions. He (Liley 1971a, 3) wrote, "A living fetus may be dismembered, poisoned or ejected to die from exposure but this must be called 'terminating a pregnancy,' not exterminating a fetus. The subterfuges necessary to maintain this approach are well seen in my own hospital where the needles used for the infusion of hypertonic saline, 7" Tuohy needles or trochars and cannulae, are the needles we originally developed for fetal transfusion." Liley was clearly bitter at this perceived "misappropriation" of fetal technologies for other than lifesaving purposes. Beyond the politico-moral question, there is also a question of professional control; some of Liley's anxiety may have stemmed from losing his position as the authority on Tuohy needles and their use.

Liley's views on abortion were shaped by collaboration with his wife, Margaret, with whom he shared a political perspective. An obstetrician and pediatrician, and a publicly acclaimed mother of six children, Margaret was considered an expert on pregnancy and fetal life. In the 1960s and 1970s, she was director of the Antenatal Clinic at National Women's Hospital, where she was responsible for patient education and instituted a number of innovative procedures, such as allowing newborn babies to remain with their mothers to facilitate bonding.[26] She coauthored two well-received books on pregnancy (Liley and Day 1966; Day and Liley 1968), and enjoyed a reputation throughout New Zealand as an obstetrical authority. Yet despite her own considerable accomplishments, Margaret Liley's renown rested on her relationship with her husband, an all-too-common position for wives of famous men.[27] For example, in the introduction to Margaret's first book, Virginia Apgar (Liley and Day 1966, viii) wrote: "Her understanding of life before birth is enhanced by a working alliance with her husband, Dr. A. William Liley, a world-renowned obstetrician who developed the daring procedure of intra-uterine transfusions for infants threatened by Rh complications."

But Margaret also wrote about fetal development and personhood, raising the possibility that both Lileys originated ideas that are usually attributed only to Bill Liley. In *Modern Motherhood*, Margaret situated pregnancy and fetal life within the context of new techniques in medicine that focus on the fetus. She (Liley and Day 1966, xiii) wrote, "Among the many fascinating discoveries that we see among our babies, I think the most important is that each baby is an individual. It is separate and distinct from every other individual, in fact, much earlier than anyone suspected." Throughout the text, she (1966, 23) refers to the fetus as "active, lively [and] independent," a "tiny Tom Thumb of a human being [who] dominates his environment." An entire chapter is devoted to "The Fetus as an Individual," and is rife with phrases similar to Bill Liley's notions of the fetus as a personality. The "unborn baby" is described as distinct and separate from the mother, with needs of "his" own: "Fetology holds many secret parcels. . . . There will be greater awareness that it is the baby who conducts the orchestra in pregnancy, and that we should be able to predict his condition more accurately by studying the ways in which he is affecting his host's body" (1966, 213).

In addition to drawing on the same cultural repository of ideas about fetal life, Margaret also shared Bill Liley's sentiment that abortion was wrong. During our visit together in 1994, she told me that she firmly believed fetuses were individual personalities and that abortion destroyed "unique human lives." She showed me a series of chalk tracings that she and her husband had made on the basis of fetal X rays. Apparently, Bill Liley had saved hundreds of fetal X rays discarded by radiologists who no longer needed them for diagnostic purposes. The chalk tracings, in bright colors on dark construction paper and resembling a child's crude artistic efforts, were used by Margaret in educational presentations about pregnancy and fetal life. While tracing the drawings with her fingers as a sort of radiant fascination danced across her face, she remarked that both she and Liley loved the images because they showed the fetus as "active and moving." She contrasted their chalk images with the famous photographic representations in *A Child Is Born* (Nilsson 1990), telling me that "because those images were based on dead fetuses, they were static and lifeless. These are pictures of *living* fetuses." Yet although she and her husband shared the belief that the fetus was a human being worthy of medical treatment and protection, Margaret Liley did not share the public spotlight of Bill Liley's antiabortion activities.

In large part, the emergence of antiabortion sentiment during this period was a reaction to developments in New Zealand's abortion law, which was becoming increasingly liberalized.[28] As a British commonwealth, New Zealand's law was historically similar to Britain's, which prohibited abortions in most cases. In 1967, in both Britain and New Zealand an act was passed allowing abortion for the mental and physical health of the pregnant woman. Some doctors began liberalizing their practices in response, and abortion clinics were established in urban areas. Pat McCarthy, an antiabortion activist and editor of *Humanity,* told me that shortly after the 1967 act was passed, "a private abortion clinic was set up in Auckland, and it was fairly clear that abortions were being performed without too much regard for the law. The law was being interpreted fairly broadly. The doctor who was performing abortions at that clinic, Dr. James Woolnough, was prosecuted. He stood trial three times but was acquitted. Abortion was a tremendously political issue at that time." In 1976, the government set up the Royal Commission on Contraception, Sterilization, and Abortion, which after a year of deliberations further liberalized abortion law.[29]

Witnessing these events, as well as the creation of the pro-choice Abortion Law Reform Association in the late 1960s, prompted Liley, along with Dr. Patrick Dunn and Leo Manning, to form the Society for the Protection of the Unborn Child (SPUC) in 1970.[30] They were joined by some of Liley's colleagues at National Women's Hospital, including Harvey Carey, Herb Green, and Ross Howie. In describing how SPUC was founded, Howie recalls that "Liley focused on the rights of the fetus, and we agreed that you can't bump off the fetus or unborn to solve social problems." According to SPUC literature, the society is "a humanitarian organization, formed out of concern at the increasing disrespect for the value of human life. [It] is involved in various programs to educate the public regarding the humanity of the Unborn Child and the fundamental value of all human life, assist the mother and child, and lobby for protective legislation."[31] Pat McCarthy told me that SPUC's mission has always been "respect for life across the board" including resistance to euthanasia at all ages, even though the organization's name evokes only abortion. When the abortion issue was more acutely politically charged in 1970, SPUC claimed a membership of about 50,000.[32]

As the first president of SPUC, a position he held for many years, Liley was far more than a figurehead. He had by that time fashioned himself into a national and international activist for fetal rights. According to McCarthy (1983, 5), "he campaigned throughout the country and far beyond for recognition of the unborn child as a human being with inalienable human rights." Yet his activism was not limited to SPUC activities. In many instances, he spoke or gave testimony as a scientific and medical expert on the fetus. Liley was seemingly always willing to speak on behalf of fetuses, often at a moment's notice. McCarthy (1983, 5) relates a story of Liley being in the middle of a surgical operation when a call came in from the United States; "five hours later he was on a plane to give evidence before a district federal court in Rhode Island." In testimony before the U.S. Senate Judiciary Subcommittee on a proposed constitutional amendment to protect fetal life, Liley took great pains to establish his professional credentials. He remarked, "I am a registered medical practitioner in New Zealand. . . . Clinically I have worked as a fetal pediatrician for most of the last seventeen years. . . . In 1963, I developed a method by which Rh babies beyond the aid of conventional therapy could be given transfusions in utero."[33] His "expert" status offered Liley legitimacy in his role as spokesman for the fetus, enabling him to move comfortably and quite visibly between his clinical work and political activities.

Liley's position on abortion often posed difficulties at National Women's Hospital, particularly for colleagues who did not fully share his views. Florence Fraser, for one, did accept the premise of fetal personhood: "I became very aware of the fetus as an individual early on. As far as I was concerned, fetuses do have personalities and I encouraged [the mothers] to think of their babies as personalities. They've always been personalities to me, they've always been people from a very early stage. I guess it was Bill's influence right at the beginning of my obstetrics career, you know, he sowed the seed." But the pragmatic Fraser, whose obstetrical training in Britain had included abortion procedures, disagreed with Liley about the morality of abortion. She told me, "Bill didn't like abortions at all but I had done abortions in Britain. In those days, here in New Zealand, you didn't get many abortions done because the law had not been liberalized at all. I've never been as rigid as Bill was about abortion because of the women, but he wasn't even keen on sterilization. And we did have a few words about that." Graham Liggins, with whom Liley shared so many interests, was also not involved in abortion politics. When I asked him if he had a role in the antiabortion group Liley formed, he replied, "No, no. I have always steered well clear of any political position."

Despite resistance from some of his colleagues, Liley continued to advocate for fetal rights until his death in 1983. The fetus was, in his view, "small, naked, nameless, and voiceless. He has no one except sympathetic adults to speak up for him and defend him—and equally no one except callous adults to condemn and attack him."[34] Yet the tension between his convictions and their public reception (and their reception closer to home) often put Liley under a great deal of stress. Reid (1973, 8) reported that Liley's "deep study of fetal medicine . . . has created a moral conviction that he must educate the public about his findings on the status of the fetus and a certainty that it must have social and legal protections. Results? . . . A load of responsibility that gives his face an unusually greyish tinge for a comparatively young man." A number of informants remarked that toward the end of his life, Liley seemed particularly "worn down" and "depressed." Many suspected that stress engendered by his dual roles as both medical practitioner and political activist contributed to his death by suicide on June 15, 1983.[35]

It is both ironic and tragic that Liley, who had claimed such deep and abiding respect for life, would take his own. Given the public pro-life stance he maintained for years, Liley's suicide was greeted with shock and disbelief by his family, friends, colleagues, former patients, the antiabortion movement, and the media.[36] Reaction to his death provided a fitting elegy for the fetophilic work to which he dedicated his life, as news accounts often stressed his political activities in equal measure to his medical contributions. For example, a colleague in the anti-abortion movement remarked, "It won't be for his professional achievements that we remember Bill so well—rather for his humanness, his magnanimity and good humor. . . . It was as though this great man, filled with care and compassion for the tiniest humans (the unborn) extended that warmth and care to all. . . . He had a unique and facile ability to present the unborn as a living individual, unique and precious."[37] John Willke, at that time president of the U.S. National Right to Life Committee, wrote to Margaret, "We were shocked to receive the news of Bill's death. He was such a good guy, so firm and consistent in his values and so vitally important to all of us in our struggle to save babies." Margaret Tighe, chair of the Australian Right to Life Committee, also wrote to Margaret: "We are all very saddened and shocked that our movement has lost a man whom we regarded as its Father." According to Liley's close colleague Herb Green (1986, 22), "his last reward was to be described at his funeral . . . by the Dean of Auckland's Holy Trinity Cathedral, in the presence of both the Roman Catholic and Anglican hierarchies, as a true agent of God."[38] Even in death, Liley's work and politics intersected in meaningful ways.

In sum, the association of Liley's medical work with abortion politics played a significant role in the making of the unborn patient in the 1960s and 1970s. Liley's clinical achievements resonated throughout a political arena in which fetuses were granted autonomous personhood and constructed as worthy of protection and advocacy. Perhaps antiabortion groups on their own would have made a conceptual connection between Liley's medical work and their own organizing efforts during this period. Yet because Liley was overtly political and had colleagues in many social worlds, he clearly facilitated the transmission of his work into other arenas. He acted as a conduit of sorts, translating and interpreting medical work on fetuses into the more accessible cultural and political language of fetal personhood. Ironically, however, his capacity to construct the fetus in this way rested on medical experimentation on human fetuses and a corresponding diminution of pregnant women's autonomy. Liley's description of some of the fetuses as "write-offs" because they would likely die anyway seems both callous and inconsistent with his public pro-life stance. There is little indication that either Liley himself, or his supporters in the pro-life movement, recognized the irony in securing fetal personhood through technical manipulation (not always successful) of fetal and maternal bodies on a dangerous new medical frontier.

"Not God's Will": Controversy and Open Fetal Surgery

Unlike Liley, neither Adamsons nor Freda were centrally involved in abortion politics. This is somewhat surprising, given that the abortion context in the United States, including Puerto Rico, was similar to the New Zealand situation historically: illegal but moving toward legalization through social and political struggle. Throughout the 1960s, abortion was a criminal act in most states. Yet a rising tide of liberalization at the state level had already begun, with New York among the most progressive states. Petchesky (1990) argues that these changes were fueled, in part, by (some) women's evolving status in the United States, by government interest in population control, and by the lack of a coherent policy on sexuality and reproduction. Because these conditions were already in place in New York, the 1973 Supreme Court decision legalizing abortion, rather than instigating widespread transformations in abortion practices, merely served to legitimate existing practices. In other states, however, *Roe v. Wade* served as a catalyst for many significant changes in abortion practices.

The situation was similar in Puerto Rico, reflecting the island's status as a U.S. colony. Abortion was a criminal offense until the law was relaxed in the mid-1960s, followed shortly thereafter by the legitimating effects of *Roe v. Wade*. Given the intense Catholicism of Puerto Rico, abortion has always been a deeply contested moral and political issue despite its eventual liberalization. In the 1930s, abortion was a "back-street procedure, shrouded in secrecy and sidestepped by both physicians and politicians as a controversial issue" (Ramirez de Arellano and Seipp 1983, 144). In the 1950s, there were approximately 5,000 abortions each year in Puerto Rico's hospitals. By the 1960s, in the context of a "deepening of conditions making it necessary for [American women] to maximize control over their lives" (Petchesky 1990, 116), women of means from the U.S. mainland began flooding the island's clinics in order to obtain abortions, increasing the annual number of abortions to around 10,000 (Ramirez de Arellano and Seipp 1983). This practice became so prevalent that these trips were known as "San Juan weekends," modeled after the "Havana weekends" that had been popular among affluent American women prior to the souring of U.S.–Cuba relations. At the same time, many Puerto Rican women were having fewer children as a result of their participation in trials of the birth control pill. By 1980, when a federal court decided that the extant Puerto Rican abortion law was actually more permissive than the federal standard, abortion was legal (although not always accessible or affordable) at any point during pregnancy.

Adamsons and Freda chose not to be involved in abortion politics during this social and legal ferment for several reasons. Because social change was already on the horizon in the late 1960s and early 1970s, they felt no inclination to enter into the often heated abortion debates. Also, in later years as abortion became liberalized in New York and then nationally, both Adamsons and Freda performed the procedure in their own obstetrical practices. Working in New York and Puerto Rico, they saw a diverse group of women with a range of reproductive needs shaped by race and class. They were perhaps more aware of women's circumstances and more tolerant of women's choices. What is clear is that neither man shared Liley's deep personal faith in fetal personhood and his corresponding antiabortion sentiment. Indeed, Adamsons told me that he has never had the same political convictions that Liley had about abortion.

Yet despite the absence of a direct connection to abortion politics, controversy pervaded Adamsons's and Freda's work in a number of ways.

Where Liley's work fascinated and was wellreceived around the world, open fetal surgery was seen from its inception as quite contested. Adamsons recounted that "many physicians felt like it was sacrilege to open the uterus." There was concern from obstetricians about maternal morbidity and mortality, as well as worry about how fetuses would be affected by such invasive treatment. The political climate surrounding any fetal research at that time, including its evocation of abortion politics, made this type of work extremely challenging. Adamsons told me that during the 1960s, the medical world collectively labeled and shunned such research as "too political, intrusive, and weird." Indeed, Adamsons's and Freda's own department chair resisted publication of the results of their initial experiments for six months, until *after* news of Liley's achievements with intrauterine transfusion technology had spread. Adamsons recalled that "once Taylor [the Chair] learned that other institutions were doing this also, some of the slack went up over the work at Columbia."

Such reproductive politics were rife at the time, with great potential to impact scientific and medical careers negatively. Adamsons told me that when he was at Columbia, he was considered "a Nazi" and "mentally incompetent" for suggesting that some fetuses resulting from superovulation be killed. He remarked, "There was a medieval notion that the uterus is a sanctuary, and it is not God's will to invade." This was "extraordinary" to him, because he wanted to consider the fetus "as a bona fide patient" that he could diagnose and treat. His efforts to do so were continually met with skepticism and resistance. For example, while at Mount Sinai Hospital from 1970 to 1975, Adamsons encountered tremendous opposition from the institutional review board for wanting to inject drugs into the amniotic fluid in investigations of fetal growth. It was not until he moved to Puerto Rico that he was able to expand his work using thyroxin for stimulating fetal maturation. Adamsons's research was poorly received by most American journals, which he felt was due to the political implications of his work on human fetuses. As a result of this unenthusiastic reception, he published many of his studies in German and Scandinavian journals. It was not until 1993 that he was again invited to write something for a U.S. journal, a bitter irony for the man who wrote a provocative introduction to open fetal surgery in an influential American medical journal in the mid-1960s (Adamsons 1966).

Controversy pervaded this work in other ways, as well. Adamsons related a story about nonhuman primate research that illustrates the contestation surrounding experimentation on both human and animal fetuses. There was very little human fetal research going on in the mainland United States in the early 1960s. Thus, there was considerable interest in Adamsons's primate research in Puerto Rico in which he was opening the uterus and removing the fetus for experimentation. In 1962, *Life* magazine heard about this work and asked if they could send a reporter and a photographer. Adamsons and his colleagues agreed, but realized that the large number of research projects at Cayo Santiago limited the availability of monkeys to use in the photo shoot. So Adamsons, his team, and the *Life* crew traveled to the Oregon Primate Center in Beaverton, which was interested in expanding its funding base by generating interest in primate research. The subject of the resulting *Life* story, according to Adamsons, was "taking a fetus out of the uterus for research; the images are of a monkey fetus lying next to the uterus." Adamsons pointed out that "they had to make sure the photograph included the monkey tail in the picture to identify it as an animal—we did not want to be accused of human experimentation." Yet at the same time, in order to placate animal rights groups, the accompanying text had to make it clear that the procedures would have an eventual therapeutic benefit in humans.

Although Adamsons and Freda were not actively involved in the abortion debates, their work was nonetheless shaped by its association with reproductive politics and indirectly with abortion debates. They pursued open fetal surgery within a context in which abortion was still illegal but gradually being liberalized. Concern about experimentation on human fetuses made physicians and other interested actors less receptive to open fetal surgery than they had been to Liley's closed technique. Although the research climate in Puerto Rico facilitated certain types of practices, it did not fully insulate Adamsons, Freda, Asensio, and their colleagues from adverse social reactions to open fetal surgery on human pregnant women. The two-decade lag between these efforts in the 1960s and later work on open fetal surgery was, at least in part, due to the profound influence of politics and discomfort with fetal research in general. Although it may have legitimated other, less invasive forms of fetal diagnosis and treatment, open fetal surgery itself has been pervaded by an aura of illegitimacy that continues to this day.

A Prophetic Debut

The renowned art historian Barbara Stafford (1991, 211) has written, "Now that the beginning and the end of life have been identified as the major biological frontiers of the twenty-first century, we need the perspective of history to help us wrestle with these unclear boundaries." Fetal interventions have indeed rearranged the boundaries of medicine, culture, and women's bodies. In this chapter, I have shown how human actors, medical work, research materials, technologies, scientific knowledge, institutions, geography, culture, and politics have been brought together vividly in the making of the unborn patient in the 1960s and 1970s. Prior to the work of the medical "pioneers" profiled here, fetuses were not considered patients in the ways they subsequently came to be perceived. The activities described—Rh research, intrauterine transfusion technology, open fetal surgery, and all of the clinical and social activities related to these innovations—shaped the development of fetal medicine on a number of fronts. Perhaps most significant, breaching the womb and "revealing" the fetal work object paved the way for the emergence of a clinical entity known as "fetal patient" and a corresponding social being named "fetal person." For some actors, notably Liley, these two identities were embodied in one and the same fetus, a unitary but universal innocent that both could be rescued by technology and should be saved from women seeking abortions.

What are we to make of Liley's place in history as the "father" of fetal surgery? Surely if he developed closed techniques and others were working on open techniques for fetal transfusion, there must be many primogenitors of what we now recognize as fetal surgery. Liley's work, supported and enabled by his numerous colleagues and patients, is deemed germinal because it was the first attempt to breach the womb. But despite his prominent position in history, his work was followed closely by those who breached the womb in even more profound ways, not only penetrating the uterus with needles but opening it and exposing its precious contents, the fetus, for medical intervention. With each iteration of fetal treatment, from the Rh vaccine to intrauterine transfusion technology to open fetal surgery, the unborn patient became increasingly more visible and accessible. What is interesting and distinctive about fetal surgery is not that one great man was responsible for its emergence, but rather that a diverse group of practitioners working in different places collectively built a new specialty and propagated a new social subject. All of the events discussed here, those seen both as "legitimate" and as "illegitimate," provided a foundation for fetal surgery upon which the making of the unborn patient could flourish.

Understanding the confluence of medicine and reproductive politics offers insight into the controversial nature of fetal practices. In the 1960s and 1970s, as now, fetal patienthood was being vigorously contested as it was also being crafted. The exile of Adamsons to Puerto Rico because people believed his work was extreme is indicative of just how difficult these struggles were. Breaching the womb both excited and troubled interested observers. On the one hand, it promised to reduce fetal deaths; on the other, it raised moral concerns about the limits of technology. Moreover, the professional and political goals of those who breached the womb varied considerably, influencing whether and how different actors manipulated the authority of science and medicine. While Adamsons and Freda recognized that there may be multiple fetuses with different meanings (i.e., those they treated in fetal surgery and those they aborted in obstetrical practice), Liley did not. By proposing a monolithic fetal subjectivity, Liley and his colleagues in SPUC located fetal medicine firmly within the context of reproductive and abortion politics, where it remains uncomfortably wedged today.

Although the making of the unborn patient was marked by controversy and illegitimacy, it is also one very important chapter in the origin story of the fetal person legitimated and naturalized by scientific medicine. That is, the fetus came to be considered "knowable" (and treatable) using the tools of science and medicine during a period in which many people were very interested in getting to know the fetus. Because of the close interweaving of medical work and cultural politics, the twin entities "unborn patient" and "fetal person" debuted almost simultaneously. And they did so at precisely the time that abortion politics were coming to the fore of public debate. The womb and its contents were beginning to be contested terrain in both medicine and cultural politics. Focusing on the many ways in which the unborn patient was imagined and animated, as I have done here, illuminates how cultural and political perceptions of the fetus permeate medical work, and how representations and consequences of medical work flow out of laboratories and hospitals into other arenas of social life.

Chapter 3

A Hybrid Practice

Traffic Between the Laboratory and the Operating Room

The previous chapter focused on ways in which medical work, culture, and politics contributed to the making of the unborn patient in the 1960s. In New Zealand, New York, and Puerto Rico, this work was clinic-based and benefited enormously from its geographic and institutional locations. As fetal patienthood was crafted and contested historically, there was considerable overlap among the animal research that went on prior to operating on human fetuses, the procedures done on human patients in the operating room, and the institutional and political contexts within which these practices occurred. Since that time, a tremendous amount of scientific, technical, and medical work has been involved in advancing fetal surgery from its attention-grabbing but somewhat limited roots to a state-of-the-art but still controversial practice today. This work, deeply social in nature, has contributed to the consequential evolution both of the specialty and of fetal personhood. In this chapter I explore the complicated character of fetal surgery by focusing on a diverse set of practices that have facilitated access to the elusive fetus, generating the unborn patient. How have surgeons and their collaborators been able to peel away the layers of flesh and convention to reveal and operate on the fetus within the woman?

Chronologically and conceptually, this chapter serves as a bridge between the historical work discussed previously and renewed interest in open fetal surgery in the late 1970s and early 1980s. I chart the proliferation of four sites and practices critical to the making of the unborn patient: fetal physiology, ultrasound, animal experimentation, and fetal wound healing. Each new site, equipped with its own tools and discourses, spawned additional cultural filaments reaching into and out of the operating room, enabling a further expansion of fetal meanings and increasing edification of fetal surgery itself. The various practices profiled in this chapter were disciplined (Foucault 1979) in the service of fetal surgery, just as each provided form and focus to the developing specialty by meeting an array of needs and functions. Examining each of these different practices as they relate to the specialty as a whole brings into focus some of the technical and cultural politics that have infiltrated and shaped the work of fetal surgery over the past thirty years.

As an experimental procedure, fetal surgery has developed within the conceptual paradigm of clinical research while also pushing at its limits. Rather than viewing experimental medicine merely as applied science, as often happens both in sociology and in popular culture, we should think of this kind of endeavor as a *hybrid practice*. Framing clinical research as such allows for an analysis of how the boundaries of medicine, science, and technology dissolve, overlap, and shift in practice and across time. None of the practices discussed in this chapter is solely responsible for the emergence of the specialty, although some are claimed to be more important than others. But taken together as a set of hybrid practices, their mobilization and intersection becomes significant in the history of fetal surgery. Indeed, it is precisely fetal surgery's hybrid character that has enabled it to advance as a medical specialty, despite persistent controversy surrounding research on human fetuses. The making of the unborn patient would likely not have been possible without the hybridity profiled here. Each practice, in its own way, has legitimated fetal surgery in its contemporary incarnation.

"Out of the Stone Age and Into the Bronze Age": Marshaling Fetal Physiology

Fetal physiology has been central both to the development of fetal surgery and to "claimsmaking" (Aronson 1984) about its legitimacy. For a variety of reasons, including its utility as a set of ideas about life, fetal physiology has become an important body of knowledge that has permeated other fetal practices in medicine and science. It provides a toolbox for understanding and defining prenatal life and a set of conceptual and practical tools that are used by practitioners in fields as diverse as fetal tissue research and fetal surgery. As we saw in the previous chapter, Liley, Adamsons, and Freda were quick to integrate physiological understandings into their work, often collaborating closely with fetal physiologists such as Liggins. In the early 1980s, fetal surgeons likewise began looking to fetal physiology for scientific answers to two tenacious problems: high fetal mortality and chronic maternal morbidity. At the same time, fetal physiologists were promoting the virtues of their science to other specialties (Gluckman et al. 1989). In actively responding to the persuasive claims of fetal physiologists, surgeons transformed their specialty by establishing what they claimed to be its scientific base. In the words of one fetal surgeon, physiology ushered fetal surgery "out of the stone age and into the bronze age." This transformation has been significant because cultural meanings—including scientific knowledge and definitions of fetal status—are located at the intersection of these different practices.

Despite their eventual appropriation of physiology, however, fetal surgeons did not immediately grasp its relevance to their clinical work. One fetal surgeon told me, "In the stone age days, we weren't making an effort to understand the physiology. It became clear to me after seeing the first couple of cases that we didn't know what we were doing from a physiologic point." A fetal physiologist echoed this assessment: "One of the problems is that surgeons were looking at this purely from the surgical point of view. They had little appreciation for what the physiological issues were." Sharp distinctions were drawn between fully understanding how fetal (and maternal) bodily processes work and merely fixing fetal anatomical problems surgically. These distinctions had much to do with the social organization of medical and scientific specialties. Most fetal surgeons are trained in pediatric surgery and thus have in-depth specialty training in surgical techniques, but they have little training in physiological principles beyond basic preclinical medical education. They see themselves as "fetus fixers" rather than as interpreters of physiological clues, more Indiana Jones than Sherlock Holmes. Understanding the basics of fetal physiology, and the physiology of pregnancy and labor, meant acquiring a brand new set of skills and concepts with which to approach their work.

In general, fetal physiologists seek to understand normal vital processes in fetuses, such as growth and development. The "father" of fetal physiology, Sir Joseph Barcroft, and his contemporaries performed the first fetal physiology experiments in the 1930s, focusing on physiological function in fetal lambs (Longo 1978). The next wave of fetal physiologists, led by Geoffrey Dawes at Oxford, continued studies of function and also expanded investigations to encompass other problems, such as fetal blood circulation. A preeminent fetal physiologist at Capital Hospital who was trained by Dawes told me, "Originally we did pretty simple procedures and then as we began to recognize that it was possible to do much more extensive procedures, we expanded our horizons and did a whole variety of studies on fetal function." Subsequent avenues of research included cardiovascular disease, hormones, the role of the placenta, and the intricacies of the birth process. The unit of analysis was always the fetus, although pregnancy and labor were often considered as adjunct or related functions.

When fetal physiologists shifted their attention to the birth process,

they began to examine fundamental processes of the fetus as an entity located inside a pregnant woman's body. The functional basis of the maternal-fetal relationship, especially the role of the placenta, became a
primary research concern (Dancis 1987). Physiologists began investigating processes such as placental transfer of molecules (Boyd and Sibley
1989), regulation of amniotic fluid (Abramovich and Page 1989), regulation of fetal growth (Fowden 1989; Johnson and Greenberg 1987), and
cardiovascular function. One reason physiologists offer for studying
such processes is that understandings of maternal-fetal function can
provide insight into fetal adaptation mechanisms that occur at birth.
Once a fetus is expelled from the womb and becomes a newborn, a host
of intricate physiological changes are believed to take place. The neonate's body must quickly assume functions that were regulated during
the fetal state by the placenta, including circulation, oxygen provision,
enzyme and hormone regulation, and temperature control.[1] By focusing
on the transformation from fetus to neonate, physiologists foster the perception that "the fetus is steadily approaching a boundary—the beginning of life beyond the womb, the termination of being unborn" (Grobstein
1988, 107). They assert, in other words, the inevitable, "normal" approach of birth and separation from the pregnant woman, and then apply that framing back to the period in the womb. This suggests a
continuity of life between fetus and neonate that obscures the significance of pregnant women.

   Yet fetal physiologists are also concerned with the pathology of fetal
function, an area of research that has had considerable impact on fetal medicine. Physiologists study problems such as abnormal labor,
preeclampsia, the etiology of congenital malformations, perinatal brain
injury, and diseases of major organs (Harrison et al. 1991; Kretchmer et
al. 1987). Historically, such research in fetal physiology was constrained
by restricted access to fetal work objects located inside pregnant
women's bodies. Inaccessibility and intense controversy over nontherapeutic research on living human fetuses (Casper 1992; Steinbock 1992)
rendered them inappropriate for much physiological research. For example, when scientists attempted to remove fetuses from the womb for
investigative purposes, the fetuses did not survive long—nor were the researchers immune from public disapproval (Maynard-Moody 1995).
Such barriers to practice have limited the types of questions scientists
can ask and the means by which they attempt to find answers.

   But the development of techniques permitting research on exteriorized (out of the uterus) living fetuses still connected to the placenta provided for a greater investigative range—and work objects that would last
longer. Researchers also developed an array of alternative practices using nonhuman animal models as well as dead human fetal material

obtained from abortions, miscarriages, ectopic pregnancies, and still-births—all highly contested practices in their own right. One technique used to conduct research on physiological problems is simulation of abnormal conditions in fetal work objects, usually nonhuman animal models constructed in the laboratory. For example, interest in congenital heart problems led one physiologist to manufacture lesions in sheep in order to study the effect of fetal defects on cardiovascular development. This technique is also used in fetal surgery and wound healing research, where sheep, nonhuman primates, and other animal fetuses are injured prenatally, repaired, and delivered for investigative purposes. These practices would, of course, be immensely controversial if performed on human models, and often are controversial even when animal models are used (Brans and Kuehl 1988).

Through their various explorations of prenatal life, fetal physiologists attempt to define—often with considerable authority—the biological parameters of human existence, parameters that also feed into cultural understandings. Physiological research produces some familiar fetal classifications, such as the division of pregnancy into stages (usually called trimesters) based on fetal development. Physiology offers us the preembryo (zero to two weeks), the embryo (three to eight weeks), the early fetus (nine to twenty weeks), the middle fetus (twenty-one to thirty weeks), and the late fetus (thirty-one weeks to birth) (Grobstein 1988). These boundaries are designed to clarify fetal status and are based on scientific accounts of organogenesis (the development of organs), behavioral function, movement, and other "natural" indicators. Such constructions are often deployed in other practices, such as legal and ethical domains, in attempts to resolve controversies over the significance of fetal life. Ironically, however, physiological research often produces ambiguity rather than clarity about definitions and periodizations of prenatal life; it contributes to, rather than resolves, the controversy surrounding human fetuses.

And controversy is increasingly the case as fetal physiology intersects with other practices focused on understanding and intervening in human development. Parameters of fetal *viability*, or the capability of a fetus to survive outside of a woman's body, shift in relation to technical "advances" in fetal and neonatal medicine. Currently, viability is considered to be between twenty-three and twenty-four weeks gestation (Grobstein 1988; Morowitz and Trefil 1992), a scientific "fact" highly relevant both to fetal research and treatment and to abortion debates. Yet as new technologies enable physicians to treat fetuses at earlier gestations, physiological understandings similarly threaten to shift. Fetal surgeons have operated on fetuses as young as eighteen weeks' gestation as well as those more than twenty-four weeks, which are hypothetically capable of

surviving outside the womb. As fetal physiology and fetal surgery continue to overlap, scientific *and* cultural understandings of fetal viability
may be altered, complicating the already hotly contested debates about
when life begins. Thus fetal physiologists are engaged not only in penetrating "the darkness of the womb to illuminate what is within"; they are
also, in significant and consequential ways, "choosing human futures"
(Grobstein 1988, ix). Fetal surgeons, themselves recharting the future of
reproduction, have been increasingly attracted to fetal physiology for
these and other reasons.

By the early 1980s, fetal surgeons building on the work of their predecessors had already executed a large number of experimental procedures in research animals, mainly sheep. Yet they had not systematically
applied, much less integrated, long-established knowledge from human
fetal physiology. They had forged ahead with clinical work in human patients with little regard for some of the key physiological consequences
of opening a gravid uterus and removing a pregnant woman's fetus. A fetal surgeon recalls:

> We were operating on this organ that nobody understands, flat out, nobody
> understands it. We thought we were doing what was right: relax the uterus,
> do the operation, close the uterus, and get out. We didn't know what we were
> doing, and we still don't know what we're doing with the placenta. There was
> no doubt that nobody understood anything at all about perioperative fetal
> physiology. And as is so often the case, you know a little bit of knowledge and
> you're very dangerous. You perturb one part of the system and the whole
> things goes haywire because you don't know what you're doing.

The primary concern, which was salient in the 1960s and remains a
problem even today, is that as soon as the primate uterus is surgically
opened a pregnant woman will almost always begin labor. Because
surgeons attempt to replace the fetus within the womb after surgery,
controlling preterm labor is fundamental to performing this procedure successfully and safely. But without physiological understanding of what causes preterm labor, fetal surgeons were helpless to
control it.

It may seem strange that fetal surgeons began operating on human
pregnant women and their fetuses despite significant physiological problems that had not yet been resolved. After all, surgeons on the final frontier have usually been very careful not to jeopardize their own research
goals. Because they had figured out how to perform fetal surgery technically and could do it with what they saw as reasonable success (i.e., at
least some fetuses survived), they were encouraged to continue even in
the absence of physiological understanding. It was only through ongoing
clinical experience—trying procedure after procedure in the operating

room—that surgeons eventually became aware of the extent of their predicament. But an overall lack of success (i.e., many fetuses were still dying) and the increasing complexity of fetal surgery compelled the surgeons to investigate other avenues. As they continued to have major problems with preterm labor, maternal complications, and fetal mortality, they turned to fetal physiology for answers. One fetal surgeon told me, "It was such an enormous undertaking early on that to have gone back to try to understand the physiology would have slowed it down by a decade or more. At the time we had success in sheep and we didn't think we needed to go back and understand the physiology. It's only now that we realize the issues exist and we have to answer the questions as well as ask them."

Fetal physiology became increasingly integrated into fetal surgery once surgeons decided to pay attention to it. Fetal surgeons began to discuss physiological issues in their publications and they developed important relationships with fetal physiologists. For example, a renowned physiologist was invited by surgeons at Capital Hospital to participate in the fetal surgery program there. As one surgeon told me, "Dr. ——— is now an intimate part of perioperative management. The really good thing about getting her involved was to get all these different groups to change their focus. Her life's work has been understanding fetal physiology, and now she has the opportunity to see it applied to human fetal surgery." One of the claimed benefits of incorporating physiological principles into this work was improved outcomes. I was told repeatedly by medical workers at Capital Hospital that applying physiology to clinical practice has made some positive improvement in terms of fetal survival, just as Rh research improved fetal outcomes in the 1960s. But fetal mortality and preterm labor remain vexing problems, suggesting that while physiology has helped, it has not been enough to secure the full safety and viability of fetal surgery.

Ironically, while fetal surgeons did not immediately jump on the physiology "bandwagon" (Fujimura 1988), another set of medical workers interested in fetal surgery had been consistently applying physiological principles in their work. Obstetricians claimed to have a solid understanding of the physiology of the maternal-fetal relationship and the birth process, an understanding that emerged historically from their clinical focus on taking care of pregnant women. Given fetal surgeons' relative lack of knowledge about these issues, one might think that they would have looked to obstetricians for advice and collaboration in attempting to solve the preterm labor problem. But they did not. Rather than recognizing that obstetricians possessed a set of skills and ideas that could be useful, fetal surgeons instead used physiology as a battleground upon which to struggle with obstetricians over which group

would define and control the new and uncertain specialty of fetal surgery. Fetal surgeons have marshaled fetal physiology in the service of
professional monopoly.

When surgeons first became interested in open fetal surgery in the
early 1980s, they assumed that obstetricians were expert in certain aspects. For example, they believed obstetricians were skilled in surgically
opening the uterus, something that many fetal surgeons had not been
trained to do. Early blueprints of the division of labor had obstetricians
opening the uterus to make the fetus available and closing it again after
the fetal surgeons completed their detailed manipulations. Over time,
however, fetal surgeons became convinced that they could learn to do
what obstetricians had traditionally done. Moreover, as one fetal surgeon
asserted, "it turns out that obstetricians don't necessarily know what
they're doing, that they don't necessarily understand what they're doing.
Because nobody understands perioperative maternal-fetal physiology. It
is clear after extensive discussions with them that they don't understand
the physiology behind it." Fetal surgeons have thus pursued a dual strategy of simultaneously denigrating obstetricians' skills and knowledge in
the realm of physiology and embracing physiological principles as their
own province.

Despite obstetricians' own claims to physiological knowledge, fetal
surgeons have used the complexity and challenges of fetal surgery as a
professional lever with which to wrest management of the pregnant
woman—or at least her uterus—away from obstetricians, whom they
cast as incompetent.[2] A fetal surgeon at Capital Hospital defined the
problem as such: "The obstetricians have painted themselves into a corner. They're frozen and unable to change, unable to adapt, unable to improve the patient's care, and unable to understand the physiology." This
quote raises the provocative question of which patient the surgeon is
talking about: the pregnant woman or her fetus. Another fetal surgeon
told me that including a fetal physiologist on the team at Capital Hospital tipped the balance of power in their direction. In this surgeon's
words, "It has been [the physiologist's] influence, as one of the most respected basic scientists in the field, that has allowed us to make changes
against the obstetricians' will. The obstetricians can't argue, they just
can't. It's like, when you're overshadowed, you're clearly outclassed. They
just can't argue." Not only is fetal physiology used to make claims about
the legitimacy of the specialty, but fetal physiologists themselves can be
used as pawns—albeit willing ones—in professional turf wars.

In sum, fetal physiology has been key to the emergence of fetal surgery because it has served as a grounds for professional claimsmaking.
Medical workers in the 1960s, as we saw in the previous chapter, worked
closely with fetal physiologists in crafting fetal treatment technologies.

Contemporary fetal surgeons, although slower to grasp the advantages of a physiological approach, nonetheless subsequently incorporated physiological principles and ideas into their work. In the face of high fetal mortality and chronic preterm labor problems, fetal surgeons turned to an established knowledge base in fetal physiology as well as to specific fetal physiologists for advice. But fetal surgeons were clearly after something beyond better outcomes in their turn to physiology: legitimacy.[3] By embracing fetal physiology, fetal surgeons were not only able to claim somewhat improved outcomes, they were also at least partially successful in defending "their" specialty against obstetricians. Now, having thoroughly integrated fetal physiology into their practices, fetal surgeons look forward to an ongoing association. As one surgeon predicted, "Once entering this bronze age, where we understand some physiology and we're able to use some techniques to monitor mom and fetus, we'll learn enough to enter the next stage where we can do better."

Pseudo-Submarines and the Dissolving Woman: Prenatal Diagnosis and the Unborn Patient

Where fetal physiology offered a mantle of scientific legitimacy for fetal surgery, prenatal diagnostic technologies have provided a different kind of boost. With the development of prenatal diagnostics, there has been an ongoing significant relationship between testing and subsequent treatment of fetuses. As Harrison (1993, 341) puts it, "As the veil of mystery is stripped away from the once-secretive fetus by powerful new imaging and sampling techniques, prenatal treatment is emerging as the logical consequence of prenatal diagnosis." Several prenatal diagnostic technologies have been integral to the emergence of fetal treatment practices, especially to fetal surgery which requires direct access to and information about the fetus prior to intervention. Yet these new diagnostic technologies often raise many more questions than they answer, even while they are transforming medical practice and offering new ways of "seeing" human bodies. As Rayna Rapp (1990, 41) has pointed out, "new reproductive technologies open a Pandora's box of powerful knowledge." Located firmly within the politics of reproduction, prenatal diagnostic technologies may certainly expand women's options as they seek healthier babies. But clinicians who use these technologies often promise more than they can deliver.

Four prenatal diagnostic techniques have been central to the development of a broad range of fetal treatment practices. One, amniocentesis, was a key element in early efforts to transform fetuses into patients, as we saw in chapter 2. By analyzing amniotic fluid, Liley and his colleagues attempted to determine which fetuses were at risk for hemolytic

disease before treating them through intrauterine transfusions. Amniocentesis is now a routine part of obstetrics for some women, specifically
those above thirty-five years of age or those at risk for genetic abnormalities, despite the fact that the technique itself may lead to miscarriage in
one out of two hundred pregnancies (Institute of Medicine 1990).[4] The
technique involves the withdrawal of fluid from a pregnant woman's amniotic sac transabdominally using a large needle, usually during the second trimester of pregnancy although it is now being performed as early
as the twelfth week of pregnancy (Gilbert 1993). The fluid, which contains fetal cells, is then cultured and analyzed, particularly for chromo-
somal anomalies and neural tube defects. Because amniocentesis is
usually performed in the second trimester of pregnancy, it raises troubling social questions about when women can make an informed and legal choice about continuing a problem pregnancy (Rothman 1986). It
also may have very different meanings among different groups of women
(Rapp 1993a; 1993b; 1994).

A second, somewhat newer, technique called chorionic villus sampling (CVS) can be used early in the first trimester and is thus often seen
as an alternative to amniocentesis. Like amniocentesis, CVS is used to
diagnose genetic abnormalities. In CVS, a catheter is inserted through a
woman's cervix and directly into the chorion, the outermost fetal membrane. Villi, or small hairlike projections on the surface of the membrane, are removed using a syringe, then separated from maternal tissue
and cultured. Although it decreases the time required to diagnosis abnormalities, CVS also has a higher miscarriage rate than amniocentesis
and may cause birth defects (Gilbert 1993). Significantly, although both
amniocentesis and CVS are *invasive* diagnostic technologies and thus invoke maternal and fetal safety issues, explicit discussion of these concerns is often muted in clinical and popular literatures.[5]

A third diagnostic technique, fetal cell sorting, is a simple test of a
pregnant woman's blood that isolates fetal cells. Still experimental, it
could potentially avoid the risks of spontaneous abortion because it is
claimed to be less dangerous to the fetus than the other techniques.[6] In
this procedure, technicians sift through a sample of maternal blood using cell sorters to find the small number of fetal cells that migrate
through tiny fissures in the placenta. The fetal cells are then examined
for genetic abnormalities using a technique called fluorescent in-situ
hybridization (FISH), which marks certain chromosomes for viewing
under a special microscopic light (Roberts 1991). Unlike amniocentesis
and CVS, which are common but not yet routine, a diagnostic blood test
could easily become an integral part of prenatal care. It would likely be
less expensive (and thus more accessible to women of lower economic
classes), could be done earlier in pregnancy, and may be used in con-

junction with other blood tests to determine the health status of a pregnant woman and her fetus. Sociologist Susan Kelly (1997) has argued that "if fetal cells could be isolated from the mother's blood, cytogenetic analysis could be performed on the developing fetus without invading the mother's body or endangering the fetus in any way. Within what might be called the collective conscience of the obstetrics community, fetal cells held the promise of a 'perfect solution' to the problem of obtaining a definitive diagnosis of fetal genetic anomalies that was beyond the scope of other noninvasive techniques."[7] But the early promise of fetal cell sorting has been hampered by technical difficulties including limited sensitivity and specificity, making its future as a screening technique uncertain.[8]

The fourth technology, ultrasound, is the most significant for fetal surgery. It differs from amniocentesis, CVS, and fetal cell sorting in that it provides a *visual* window into a pregnant woman's uterus, offering pictures of her fetus and its organs. Where the other diagnostic techniques may lead to fetal treatment of all types, only sonography has been intimately allied with open fetal surgery. Ultrasound has a rich and complex history prior to its use in medicine. It was originally developed after the sinking of the Titanic, when a British researcher filed a patent to use the technique to search for icebergs (Yoxen 1987). During World War I its use expanded to naval warfare where it was employed in the detection of submarines. Ultrasound was called sonar then, a usage that continues in seafaring today and stands for "sound navigation and ranging" (Oakley 1984). In the late 1920s, it acquired a common use in detecting fissures in metal, such as flawed seams in manufacturing. Interest in its medical capabilities was generated at about the same time, although the focus was on its curative rather than diagnostic properties (Yoxen 1987). For example, researchers believed it could be used to destroy tumors.

Use of ultrasound in mapping the human body exploded between the 1930s and 1950s as clinical researchers in several countries began experimenting with it. There was considerable impetus for this work as information about the long-term hazards of X rays became readily available and medicine began to search for safer alternatives (Cartwright 1995). Friedrich Dussik, an Austrian, began using it to diagnose neurological conditions (Yoxen 1987), and a Scotsman named Ian Donald mobilized it as an obstetrical tool (Oakley 1984). Donald had a connection in the Glasgow engineering industry and was able to obtain the necessary equipment to conduct clinical research with ultrasound. This rsearch was helpful in expanding ultrasound's diagnostic scope in the human body and working out some of the technical difficulties (Yoxen 1987). There was opposition to ultrasound by some obstetricians who believed it was too dangerous and too expensive, although most embraced it as a revolution in prenatal care. By 1970 it had become integrated into reproductive medicine, despite ongoing disagreements about what ultrasound images meant and how to interpret them. The emergence of a specialty in radiology/radiography was, in part, a response to some of these technical and professional battles.

The use of sonographic technology in fetal medicine, particularly, has expanded considerably since the 1970s. In the United States and other advanced nations, ultrasound has become a routine part of prenatal care for most women, despite its considerable cost. Charles Marwick (1993, 2025) states that "by allowing visualization of the developing fetus, ultrasound represents a major advance in perinatal care." Ultrasound images are used to detect anomalies in fetal growth, to expose birth defects, to establish how many fetuses there are, to determine gender, and to otherwise ascertain "normality" in pregnancy. Ultrasound's use in diagnosing fetal abnormalities usually centers on structural and/or organic problems rather than genetic defects. Structural defects in fetal organs are often clearly outlined in ultrasound images, paving the way for attempts at treatment. Because structural problems are most amenable to surgical treatment, ultrasound has been particularly instrumental in the emergence of fetal surgery. As Duden (1993, 76) points out, "it enabled surgeons to operate in the dark," a metaphor that nicely captures the experimental status of fetal medicine.

Oakley (1984) has used the term "pseudo-submarines" to describe fetuses revealed by ultrasound, ironically playing on Donald's (1969, 618) comment that "there is not so much difference after all between a fetus in utero and a submarine at sea." Just as ships and submarines are able to detect other vessels in the water surrounding them, ultrasound enables physicians to peer into the womb by bouncing sound waves off structures suspended in amniotic fluid. A pregnant woman, having consumed massive quantities of water, lies on her back with her abdomen exposed. A technician coats her belly with a jellylike substance and then runs a scanner back and forth across her abdomen. The scanner bounces sound waves off her "insides" and then transmits the images to an ultrasound monitor, which both displays and records the images. In fetal medicine, the ultrasound image does not "show" the mother but rather symbolically and visually excerpts and isolates the fetus from her body. In the domain of clinical decision making, these visual images of fetal bodies replace the material fetal beings still inside their mother's bodies in another part of the hospital or at home. The ultrasound representation *is* the phenomenon.[9]

While actually performing an ultrasound examination may be fairly simple, learning to interpret sonographic images is often more difficult. It is a highly technical practice and is itself the focus of a discrete med-

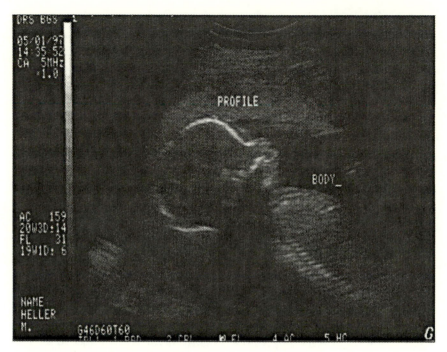

Sonographic image of a normal, healthy fetus at 20 weeks.

ical specialty. An ultrasonographer at Capital Hospital complained, "Sonography is rife with poorly trained practitioners. It is very difficult to learn. And after training people after years to do this and how difficult I've found it to be, it never ceases to amaze me how many people in the world think that they can just find the on switch to do this job. Let me assure you, that simply isn't possible." That sonographic experts are a necessary component of the fetal surgery enterprise is illustrated in the many descriptions of fetal treatment programs that stress their interdisciplinary nature, noting sonography as a key element. It is also obvious from the ways in which other practitioners, such as fetal surgeons and obstetricians, discuss sonographers. For example, an obstetrician remarked, "Dr. ——— and I developed a very good working partnership. We were doing procedures in sonography and from very early on, the concept was not always just diagnosis." These partners formed an ultrasonography group that eventually, in the early 1980s, became part of the team of fetal surgery specialists at Capital Hospital.

There is widespread consensus within fetal surgery that ultrasound has been instrumental in spurring the growth of the specialty. In discussing the origins of fetal surgery, including the lag between early efforts in the 1960s and contemporary work, most informants cited ultrasound as a key factor. In their view, fetal surgery could not have progressed from where it was in the 1960s to where it is today without ultrasound or a comparable visualization technology. It is certainly integral to much of the clinical literature on the unborn patient emphasizing diagnosis and treatment. One clinician remarked enthusiastically that it was "definitely prenatal diagnosis, primarily ultrasound" that accounted for the development of fetal surgery. A sonographer stated, "Ultrasound is extremely important to fetal treatment programs. First of all, it's crucial to identify the fetus at risk to be certain that diagnosis is correct. We wouldn't even stick a needle into a uterus today without ultrasound guidance." (Recall from chapter 2 how difficult it was for Liley, Fraser, and others to locate the fetus.) Informants at Capital Hospital point to changing conventions and standards of practice as key to the incorporation of ultrasound into fetal medicine; without adequate diagnosis of structural defects, treatment was irrelevant. It was only with the introduction of ultrasound into fetal medicine that treatment for certain conditions became viable.

Yoxen (1987, 303) points out that "explanations of the stability of technologies must take account of the social relations of work as one aspect and, in the case of ultrasound, of the reliability of the images produced." Although reliability is always contingent and subject to debate, since the specialty's inception, clinicians have focused intently on sonographic images in making treatment decisions. They eschew more "traditional" forms of fetal diagnosis involving direct physical contact with a pregnant woman's body. For example, at fetal treatment meetings at Capital Hospital where clinicians discuss problematic cases, there are no pregnant patients in the room; all eyes focus on the ultrasound image, which is given symbolic authority to represent the fetus in question. In the social organization of fetal treatment, the ultrasound image becomes something of an "obligatory passage point" (Latour 1987) around which all participants eventually coalesce. In fetal surgery, the ultrasound image has served as a symbolic prototype of the unborn patient, making visible through images what will ultimately be revealed with a scalpel.

In addition to prenatal diagnosis prior to surgery, ultrasound is also used *during* fetal surgery. A sonographer explained: "During the procedures, ultrasound is frequently used to monitor the fetus, to map the placenta, [to] make judgments about returning amniotic fluid volume, [to] guide transfusion of a fetus—all of these things are very crucial. Ultrasound will always be a major part of fetal treatment programs." Because of sonography's central role, sonographers are essential in all phases of fetal surgery from diagnosis to follow-up. Fetal treatment meetings, in which most practitioners participate to discuss cases, are in effect run by sonographers, who present sonographic images of each case for discus-

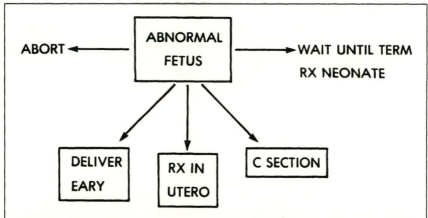

FIGURE 17–2. Prenatal diagnosis of fetal defects would have little clinical significance if the options for management were limited to terminating the pregnancy or to doing nothing until birth. Diagnosis may now alter perinatal management by allowing choices about the timing, mode, and place of delivery. In a few cases, treatment before birth may be appropriate.

Diagram showing different options when prenatal diagnosis reveals an abnormal fetus. There is a direct relationship here between diagnosis and perinatal management. Source: M. R. Harrison, M. S. Golbus, and R. A. Filly. 1991. *The Unborn Patient: Prenatal Diagnosis and Treatment.* Philadelphia: W. B. Saunders Company, p. 160.

sion and review. This is quite different from historical work in the 1960s, when ultrasound was not yet a technical reality in medicine. During the earlier era, radiologists with expertise in X rays were the key members of fetal treatment teams. The degree to which fetal medicine, especially surgery, relies on ultrasound is illustrated in Roy Filly's (1991) thorough explanation in *The Unborn Patient* of what sonographic images mean for clinical practice.

The use of ultrasound technology within fetal surgery and the development of the specialty occurred simultaneously rather than sequentially. Although ultrasound was a major tool in the formation of fetal surgery, this new specialty (and other fetal interventions) in turn bolstered the use of ultrasound in reproductive medicine. Just as amniocentesis and intrauterine transfusion were mutually reinforcing in New Zealand, ultrasound and fetal surgery have been partners in the making of the unborn patient in the United States, illustrating the shifting connections between diagnosis and treatment. Yet, despite this strong relationship, ultrasound alone is not responsible for the emergence of a new specialty; it did not technologically determine the scope and direction of fetal surgery. Without the other practices discussed in this chapter, as well as the cultural context in which fetal medicine has developed, ultrasound might not have been nearly so influential. Indeed, fetal surgery is rooted in the pre-ultrasound era; what this technology accomplished is more akin to allowing an existing practice to "upgrade" to a more intensive level. Ironically, ultrasound—like all prenatal diagnostic technologies—is capable of diagnosing far more conditions than there are available treatments, raising important questions about its routine use in prenatal care.[10]

Moreover, ultrasound and other diagnostic practices are connected to reproductive politics in terms of how these technologies affect the pregnant women who undergo surgery. Prenatal diagnosis may profoundly alter a woman's experience of pregnancy and of her fetus (Rothenberg and Thomson 1994). Following prenatal diagnosis of fetal anomalies, women are confronted with an often confusing array of "choices": abort, carry a potentially defective baby to term, opt for either nonsurgical or surgical treatment, or do nothing at all. Depending on a woman's particular circumstances, including how entrenched she may already be in the health care system, ultrasound and other technologies may shape the choices she ultimately makes about her fetus. For example, Rothman (1986) has argued that amniocentesis transforms pregnancy into a "tentative" event, contingent on the outcome of testing. Many pregnant women do not allow themselves to define their fetuses as potential babies until they have been given what I call a "diagnostic seal of approval." The allure of visual images may have implications for women's attitudes about pregnancy, including decisions to seek treatment. Routinely seeing visual images of her developing fetus may contribute to a pregnant woman's decision to select intervention rather than abortion, and ultrasound may be used by doctors as a persuasive tool in achieving women's participation in fetal surgery.

Duden (1993a) has described how ultrasound has transformed prenatal care from a potential benefit for pregnant women and their fetuses to a series of tests for certifying an absence of pathology. She writes that the pregnant woman becomes "a participant in her own skinning, in the dissolution of the historical frontier between inside and outside" (1993a, 78). But the impacts of diagnostic technologies such as ultrasound are not limited to the biomedical domains in which they are used. Often these images percolate into public consciousness through a variety of cultural channels. For example, ultrasound provides "snapshots" of a developing fetus for a pregnant woman; in this sense it becomes a high-tech method of getting baby's first picture for the family album.[11] Janelle Taylor (1993) has critically analyzed Volvo's use of an ultrasound image in an advertisement for automobiles with a reputation for safety. The accompanying tag line, "Is something inside telling you to buy a Volvo?" is obviously geared toward women consumers. Taylor (1993, 601) finds that "the equation of the image of the fetus with endangered childhood in need of parental protection is itself a highly political cultural artifact."

Fetal images may also have consequences for cultural attitudes about pregnant women. Duden (1993a, 77) argues that "the glossy photo in Joanne's hands stamps all the pregnant women before her as unenlightened, blind, unrealistic, and incompetent to relate to their own fetus in a similar way." This technology, in Duden's view, threatens to take precedence over any other means of experiencing pregnancy. Moreover, ultrasound "snapshots" are deployed by political groups intent on granting fetuses personhood in efforts to restrict abortion rights (Petchesky 1987; Rapp 1990). Antiabortion groups display these images publicly, as in the propaganda film *The Silent Scream*, using their "erasure" of pregnant women to reframe the maternal-fetal relationship as one of opposition or conflict.[12] Ultrasound works in this sense because "the maternal space has, in effect, disappeared and what has emerged in its place is an environment that the fetus alone occupies" (Stabile 1992, 180). In short, sonographic images work in the cultural and political sphere to erase women in much the same way that fetal surgery deletes women by transforming them into environments or containers for the unborn patient.

Ultrasound, then, has been a core element of fetal surgery, contributing to enhanced access to the fetus and to the development and growth of the specialty. While other prenatal diagnostic technologies have been significant in the emergence of fetal treatment generally, ultrasound holds a unique place in the diagnostic arsenal. It has been a central component of work practices organized around sighting and "siting" the fetal work object. By providing visual data about a fetus's condition, this technology offers information about anatomical defects. Fetal surgery, oriented toward repair of structural defects, was not able to proceed until adequate sonographic assessments were done. As situated within clinical practice, ultrasound is both a product and a constituent of this complex domain. While it may not be directly and causally responsible for the development of the field, it has certainly had a significant influence on the technical contours and social organization of fetal surgery in the post–Rh disease era. And it has certainly provided a critical link to reproductive politics, as different groups both in and out of medicine find meaning in fetal images and struggle over different interpretations. Ultrasound has had a crucial role in mapping the fetus and, in the process, making the unborn patient.

Tails from the Lab: Animals Model Fetal Surgery

Long before human fetuses could become "bona fide" medical patients, hundreds of animal fetuses were first made into scientific work objects. A number of scholars have examined the use of animals in research practices. Adele Clarke (1987), for example, analyzed the significance of animals as research materials in the development of the reproductive sciences. She described the collection, preservation, and use of research animals as both constraining and facilitating scientific practice. Haraway (1989), in her eloquent archaeology of primatology, narrated Western peoples' fascination with nonhuman primates. She not only described how "we" have symbolically projected cultural meanings onto primates, but she also illustrated the material uses of primates in anthropological and other scientific research. Still others have investigated different aspects of animal research, such as how animals are transformed into sacrificial scientific objects within laboratory research (Lynch 1988). All of these projects chronicle the almost mandatory use of animals as first-order experimental objects and sites in the scientific research enterprise.

Biomedical research, in particular, has been conceived and built upon animal experimentation.[13] Indeed, it is a hallmark in the history of Western medicine that clinical practice in human patients can proceed only after animal tests have rendered new techniques and treatments "safe" and "efficacious." In seeking to establish the legitimacy of experimental approaches, the number of animals tested (or "sacrificed," to use a more culturally loaded term) is an important and oft-cited benchmark. Animal research in biomedicine includes not only dissection of dead animals, but vivisection in live animals including experimental surgical operations, administration of pharmaceuticals, wounding, and a range of other tests. Animal experimentation has long been controversial and is the subject of intense ethical and political debate. Some groups are deeply concerned with the ways in which other living creatures are subjected to human practices. Here, I am interested in exploring the role of animals as technological work objects in fetal surgery, focusing in particular on how animals have been conceptualized, harnessed, and used in the pursuit of biomedical knowledge. In this section, I examine the political questions of how, why, and with what consequences animals have served as models for the human unborn patient in fetal surgery. As with other sites discussed in this chapter, animal experimentation centers around issues of access and legitimacy.

As I discussed in chapter 2, sheep and primates were essential work objects in the history of experimental fetal surgery. Sheep, widely and almost comically prolific in England and New Zealand (they wander freely in public parks and cross major roadways at whim), were used in early fetal physiology experiments as well as in subsequent research on fetal therapy. During the 1960s, both Liley and Liggins spent a great deal of time at Ruakura, an agricultural research station located near Hamilton, the major center for dairy, farming, and research on the North Island. In New York and Puerto Rico, nonhuman primates, notably Rhesus monkeys, were central to early experimental efforts. Adamsons told me that "biomedical application from sheep research was not sufficient," although he also "recognized and shared others' frustrations with primates." He described how primate models prepared at the Oregon Primate Center "deteriorated within ten days when brought to Cayo Santiago. We realized it was exposure to lights and the sounds of human activity. At Oregon, the animals were open, friendly, used to interacting with humans. The animals were treated well, like pets. At Puerto Rico, the primates had no human contact, and were kept in cages and hosed down. They really freaked out when placed in restraining chairs. So it turns out we could not do sustained observations in the Puerto Rico primates." Adamsons's recollections indicate that the social organization of animal research, such as how facilities were laid out and managed, could have great impact on the viability and indeed survival of the animals as work objects.

Other factors, including geography, could also affect animal research. In addition to his work on "standard" research animals, Liggins built a considerable body of physiological research on birth and fetal lung function through numerous expeditions to the Antarctic to study Weddell seals (Dawes 1989). I also discovered in Liley's papers that he and Liggins once attempted to acquire four armadillos from a colleague in the United States. The nine-banded armadillo was of interest to them because the animal usually has identical quadruplets, a property considered useful in experimental work on fetal nutrition, immunology, and endocrinology. Liley's correspondence with his Texas contact and the New Zealand Department of Agriculture revealed the complicated nature of animal research. In addition to arranging for the armadillos' capture in Texas, Liley would have had to coordinate their shipment to New Zealand, negotiate strict quarantine procedures, and care for them once they arrived. Because of New Zealand's relative isolation, rabies was nonexistent and its potential importation from other nations was of considerable concern to animal health officials. These arrangements ultimately proved too burdensome, both to Liley and the officials, and Liley never got his Texas armadillos.[14]

Although fetal surgeons today do not, to my knowledge, use armadillos in their work, they have experimented extensively on sheep, primates, rabbits, and other animals, building on earlier fetal research efforts and findings. One fetal surgeon told me that "there were over 1,000, maybe even 2,000, experiments done on animals before anything was ever done on humans." Sheep are widely used as research materials in the reproductive sciences for a variety of reasons. According to a laboratory researcher at Capital Hospital, "they are large animals with relatively long gestations in which to see the effects in utero. Also, their uteri are very nonreactive, unlike monkeys or humans." In other words, when an ovine uterus is opened surgically, pregnant sheep generally do not go into labor, thus allowing researchers to avoid or at least minimize one of the most significant problems in fetal surgery: preterm labor. This bodily flexibility has also made sheep useful in other areas of scientific and biomedical research. Let us not forget that Dolly, the wooly poster child of cloning, has become a contemporary icon of scientific progress, raising as many ethical and cultural dilemmas as research on the fetus.

On the other hand, because of their unique physiological qualities, investigating fetal surgery in sheep provides little *practical* assistance in solving the preterm labor problem in humans. A fetal surgeon told me, "The sheep doesn't reflect the physiology of the disease very well because it's a completely different animal. But it's chosen as the fetal model because it does not have a contractile uterus that would tend to abort." Although sheep are not so ubiquitous in most of the United States as in New Zealand, they are, according to a lab coordinator at Capital Hospital, "very easy to get." The laboratory at Capital Hospital, for example, has a contract with a farmer in the northern part of the state. Based on research needs, the lab orders sheep to be bred at specific times. Pregnant sheep are then delivered to the hospital where the animals are escorted through back corridors, out of sight of patients who might be offended, to the labs where experimental surgery takes place.

Harrison and Adzick (1991, 280) provide a graphic description of how sheep, once acquired, are used as work objects in experimental fetal surgery. They begin by asserting that in order to study the pathophysiology of a particular type of structural defect and the possibility of surgical correction, "it was first necessary to develop an animal model." This meant producing the structural defect (in this case a urethral obstruction) in fetal lambs and then attempting to correct it surgically—in other words, teratogenesis as previewed in chapter 1. Harrison and Adzick (1991, 280) write: "We produced an accurate model of severe bilateral hydronephrosis in the fetal lamb by ligating the urachus [tying off the urinary canal] and occluding the urethra with an ameroid constrictor [creating an obstruction in the urethra]. . . . Then we decompressed some of the obstructed fetuses by performing a suprapubic cystostomy [an incision in the urinary bladder] at a second fetal operation about 3 weeks later and compared obstructed, decompressed, and control lambs at birth. . . . To test whether obstruction earlier in fetal life leads to renal [kidney] dysplasia, we produced complete unilateral ureteral obstruction in fetal lambs at the beginning of the second trimester." In lay terms, these researchers tied off the urethra in an attempt to induce kidney problems that would then be experimentally treated, making the fetal lambs into a useful work object. Such techniques were worked out in sheep fetuses before they were applied to the first human fetus in 1981, and sheep research has been ongoing for more than a decade since the initial celebrated procedure.

Not only were sheep designated a necessary precursor to humans, they were also an early step in a successive hierarchy of research animals. As one researcher told me, "there is a progression of experimentation from sheep in the early stages of research to monkeys in the later stages, when techniques and procedures are almost ready for human application." Because nonhuman primates are most like us, they are the penultimate research objects and the final testing ground before human application. Brans and Kuehl's (1988) "how-to" volume, featuring prominent scientists and clinicians, illustrates the central and growing use of nonhuman primates as preferred animal models in reproductive research. Many of the volume's contributions attempt to demonstrate that nonhuman primates are "ideal" animal models because they are "closely analogous" to humans. Sheep and other animals are seen as "phylogenetically lower" and thus not useful in evaluating "the safety and feasibility of fetal intervention in humans" (Flake et al. 1988, 245). Physiologically, nonhuman primate bodies are similar enough to human bodies that experimental findings in monkeys are claimed to be especially valid and legitimate—although some researchers question how "faithfully" any animal model can replicate or model human experience.[15]

While their affinity to humans marks them as prime work objects in biomedical research, nonhuman primates are also highly placed along a moral continuum. As Haraway (1989, 3) has written, "Many people . . . have emotional, political, and professional stakes in the production and stabilization of knowledge about the order of primates." Experimenting on nonhuman primates often generates a great deal of controversy, particularly from the animal rights movement. While their "like us" quality does not protect nonhuman primates from the worst hazards of biomedical research, it may at least tweak our collective conscience and challenge our notions of moral accountability. At the very least, social discomfort with monkey experiments makes nonhuman primates difficult to access as work objects and may profoundly affect research careers of scientists and animals alike. As Blum (1994, 274) points out, "the research community and its activist critics are like two different nations . . . locked in a long, bitter, seemingly intractable political standoff,

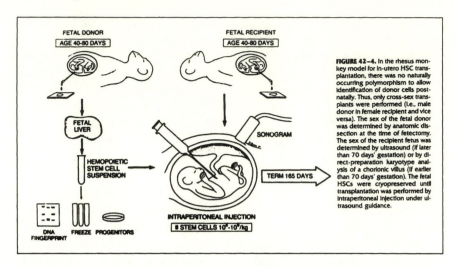

A Rhesus monkey model for in-utero hemopoietic (red blood cells) stem cell transplantation. The Rhesus monkey is a ubiquitous work object in biomedical research and has modeled many fetal interventions. Source: M. R. Harrison, M. S. Golbus, and R. A. Filly. 1991. *The Unborn Patient: Prenatal Diagnosis and Treatment.* Philadelphia: W. B. Saunders Company, p. 500.

weapons at the ready. They are fighting the monkey wars." The viability of animal models—especially our non-human primate cousins—is a key site for claimsmaking about and struggles over the terrain of experimental medicine.

In the face of these moral and political concerns, primate research in many clinical fields marches on. Of the many species of primates, the Rhesus macaque is the most popular and has certainly predominated in reproductive research. Cayo Santiago and other primate colonies were built largely around abundant Rhesus populations (Haraway 1989; Blum 1994). In describing the plight of primates in the wild and whether this has affected research practices, Blum (1994, 246) argues that "if it was simply a matter of monkey bodies, it wouldn't be a problem. The basic monkey version of a laboratory rat, the rhesus macaque, breeds easily in captivity. Some 3,000 macaques are born yearly at the country's primate centers." And Haraway (1989, 409) writes, "the rhesus monkey was a good model only partly because of its similarity to humans; its differences were also crucial, especially the differences in rates of maturation. The rhesus matured several times faster than the human child. . . . Other rate differences were also basic, like breeding times. A rhesus breeding lab can produce many more subjects per unit time than a human family" For various reasons, then, the Rhesus monkey has been constructed as an ideal tool for biomedical research and has been used throughout the history of fetal surgery.

Of major importance to any research practice involving animal models are techniques for transforming animals into appropriate work objects, as in the earlier discussion of sheep. Establishing chronic instrumentation of the primate fetus, or constructing a useful experimental work object that may be used across a specified period of time, is critical (Murata et al. 1988). One important requirement in primates is assuring that normal pregnancy can continue after a surgical procedure; this assurance is most often accomplished through sustained observation and blood sampling. Other factors that must be considered in producing good primate models are: (1) preoperative care (transportation of the animals to the research site, observation of behavior); (2) preoperative fasting (withholding food prior to anesthesia); (3) prophylactic tocolysis (administering pharmaceuticals to prevent uterine activity); (4) prechairing (placing the animal in a restraining chair before surgery so that it may adjust);[16] and (5) the use of appropriate techniques during the surgical procedure (Murata et al. 1988).

As with sheep, constructing a useful primate model for fetal surgery means first producing fetal defects in the lab. Research animals, usually Rhesus monkeys, are selected as healthy to begin with; any lesions or defects for which surgical repair is attempted must be artificially induced prior to the experimental procedure. In order to "repair" these defects, researchers prep the monkeys with anesthesia and antilabor medications. Surgery is performed over and over again, on a series of animals, to determine the feasibility of opening and resealing the uterus. The following provides some insight into how these experiments are done: "The pregnant monkey is premedicated with ketamine 10 mg/kg . . . [and] is positioned on the operating room table in a left lateral tilt. . . . Anesthesia is induced and maintained. . . . The gravid uterus is exposed through a midline incision and gently palpated to locate the two placental disks. . . . Amniotic fluid is withdrawn through a syringe, kept warm, and returned when the uterus is closed. . . . The appropriate fetal part is exteriorized and the planned operation performed. . . . The uterus is closed with a TA-90 stapling device" (Flake et al. 1988, 246–247). What is being tested here are procedures that, if efficacious, would ultimately be applied to women and their fetuses.

One fetal surgery team reported that conducting all experiments at a single site facilitated uniform care and allowed experimental groups to be compared with control groups under similar conditions. The first twenty-five cases at another center were used to develop anesthetic and tocolytic regimens that would permit fetal surgery in human primates.[17] As the surgeons at this center gained more experience through continued research, many elements in the original protocols were modified, in part because "initial results in this difficult model were discouraging.

However, results improved with modification in techniques and increasing experience over two years. We achieved the goal of being able to operate on fetal monkeys late during the second trimester and during the third trimester without significantly increasing maternal or fetal mortality compared to that of a nonoperated group" (Flake et al. 1988, 246). The results reported by this team included, but were not limited to, intrauterine fetal deaths, abortions, and "significant maternal complications" including maternal deaths, uterine rupture, and decreased fertility (Flake et al. 1988, 260). These experiments, in addition to establishing the efficacy of some fetal interventions, also indicated several problems with maternal health that the team needed to address before proceeding. Subsequent successful fertility in monkeys did not necessarily mean that *women* who underwent fetal surgery would be able to reproduce with no problems.

The credo of animals before humans is pervasive throughout fetal surgery and is illustrated in the frontis to *The Unborn Patient,* where there appears a close-up color photograph of a fetal monkey being exposed during open surgery. An especially striking aspect of this work is the way in which animal models are represented in the text. In a series of photographs, animals and pregnant women are used almost interchangeably to illustrate the accompanying narrative. One image shows a supine nonhuman primate with its uterus opened; the caption describes a technique in which "mother and fetus are closely monitored" (Harrison and Longaker 1991:191). The next page contains three graphic photographs: a "monkey fetus," "fetal hindquarters," and a "healthy neonate." Several pages later is a drawing of a human woman with her uterus opened, bearing remarkable resemblance to the previous illustration of the nonhuman primate. The article itself, while sometimes distinguishing between human and nonhuman primates, uses the terms "mother," "fetus," and "maternal" to refer to both types of patients. Textually, monkey research is presented as proof that fetal surgery can and should be attempted in women. The nonhuman primate model is the test case preceding the human model. But even visually, monkeys and women are made to stand in for and represent each other. Both types of images signify techniques, procedures, positions, and outcomes. What is elided is any critical analysis of just how representative the nonhuman primate is (or is not), and how well (or how poorly) it "models" pregnant women.

Despite discouraging results elsewhere concerning the fate of pregnant female monkeys, the fetal surgery team at Capital Hospital also has experimented on nonhuman primates in order to glean information that might prove useful when applied to humans. Throughout the past fifteen years, nonhuman and human procedures have been conducted

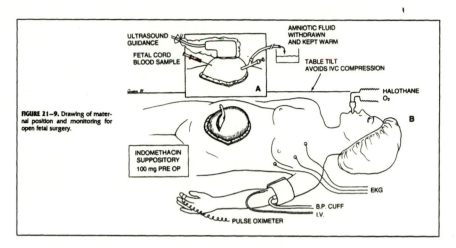

ULTRASOUND GUIDANCE

FETAL CORD BLOOD SAMPLE

AMNIOTIC FLUID WITHDRAWN AND KEPT WARM

TABLE TILT AVOIDS IVC COMPRESSION

A

HALOTHANE O_2

B

FIGURE 21–9. Drawing of maternal position and monitoring for open fetal surgery.

INDOMETHACIN SUPPOSITORY 100 mg PRE OP

EKG

B.P. CUFF
I.V.

PULSE OXIMETER

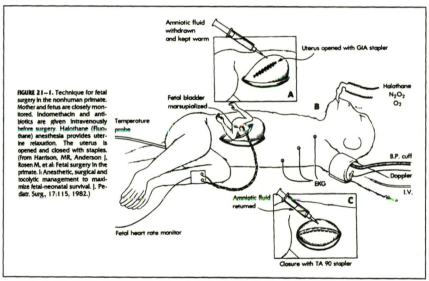

Amniotic fluid withdrawn and kept warm

Uterus opened with GIA stapler

A

Fetal bladder marsupialized

B

Halothane N_2O_2 O_2

FIGURE 21–1. Technique for fetal surgery in the nonhuman primate. Mother and fetus are closely monitored. Indomethacin and antibiotics are given intravenously before surgery. Halothane (Fluothane) anesthesia provides uterine relaxation. The uterus is opened and closed with staples. (from Harrison, MR, Anderson J, Rosen M, et al: Fetal surgery in the primate. I: Anesthetic, surgical and tocolytic management to maximize fetal-neonatal survival. J. Pediatr. Surg., 17:115, 1982.)

Temperature probe

B.P. cuff

Doppler

EKG

I.V.

Amniotic fluid returned

C

Fetal heart rate monitor

Closure with TA 90 stapler

Note the striking similarities between the image showing maternal position and the depiction of the nonhuman primate model. As represented here, women and monkeys are seen as interchangeable work objects, and animal models are made to stand in for women in terms of safety, efficacy, outcomes, and future reproductive potential. Source: M.R. Harrison, M.S. Golbus, and R.A. Filly. 1991. *The Unborn Patient: Prenatal Diagnosis and Treatment.* Philadelphia: W.B. Saunders Company, p. 199 (*top*) and 191 (*bottom*).

simultaneously there; that is, nonhuman primate experiments for some procedures occur alongside clinical trials for other procedures in humans. Although the knowledge produced by nonhuman primate research has been of mixed value in clinical practice, the very existence of the experiments—never mind their specific outcomes—is used as a legitimating strategy by fetal surgeons in making claims about the scientific basis of their work. Like fetal physiology, ongoing animal experiments are used to legitimate the human procedures with which they overlap. In the enthusiastic words of a fetal surgeon at Capital Hospital, "there is no substitute for experience and success with the nonhuman primate model."

Such uncritical faith in animal models is repeated in a video produced at Capital Hospital for viewing by potential patients; the audience, presumably pregnant women and their families, is assured that the technique of fetal surgery has been worked out in research on "hundreds of animals," including sheep and Rhesus monkeys. Positive outcomes are overstated in the video, and no mention is made of problems with maternal health in the nonhuman primate experiments, either at Capital Hospital or elsewhere. Moreover, animal research, especially in nonhuman primates, has also been used to legitimate funding for clinical trials in humans. In a proposal to the National Institutes of Health, the Capital Hospital team wrote, "In the laboratory, we have developed models that accurately reproduce the clinical features of [congenital diaphragmatic hernia], including the excessive mortality of the untreated condition. . . . With this early clinical experience based on thorough laboratory and clinical research, we stand at a crossroad for the further development of open fetal therapy. We believe that the next logical step in the development of this modality requires the assessment of its efficacy in the form of a clinical trial." Animal research may thus serve important organizational needs, including patient recruitment and acquisition of financial support.

In sum, the body of unnatural experiments done at Capital Hospital and elsewhere on nonhuman primates, in which fetal researchers produce the problems to solve—in effect, producing nonhuman "monsters"—is used to buttress and justify their claims that fetal surgery is well researched and efficacious. It is also used to support the enterprise of open fetal surgery through enhanced links to funding networks and enrollment of patients. Ironically, animal research may also insulate fetal research from the worst perils of reproductive politics by postponing experimentation on human fetuses where connections to debates about fetal life are politically salient. In many instances, animal experimentation has enhanced access to fetal work objects in humans, and it may well have resulted in at least somewhat more efficacious interventions in humans. Thus, in many ways and at several different levels, animals have served as models for the making of the unborn patient.

Fetuses without Scars: The Fetal Wound Healing Paradigm

In considering the hybrid character of fetal surgery, we must also consider the proliferation of technologies and conceptual paradigms that have emerged out of the "therapeutic" practices of fetal surgery. New sites and practices flowing from fetal surgery have in turn contributed to the legitimation of the specialty. One such practice is fetal wound healing, the scientific study of how and why many fetuses that have been operated on in the womb heal without scars. Contrary to traditional expectations of the relationship between basic research and clinical practice, in which clinical knowledge is believed to flow from experimental work, fetal wound healing is a basic research paradigm largely *derived from* clinical practice. The "discovery" of fetal wound healing processes was made possible by increased accessibility of fetuses via ultrasound and surgical technologies (Adzick and Longaker 1992a). In the 1980s, as surgeons conducted in utero fetal therapy for a range of disorders, "the observation was made . . . that the fetus appears to heal without scar formation" (Adzick and Harrison 1992, 2). Until surgeons actually opened a pregnant woman's body, removed her fetus, operated on it, and returned it to her womb for subsequent development and delivery, there was little if any recognition that fetal wound healing might differ from adult healing processes.

Unlike adult wound healing, in which tissue repair involves a series of biochemical processes that ends in scar formation, fetal wound healing is scarless. Adult wound healing is generally classified as a series of specific events, including wounding, inflammation, cell proliferation, and formation of fibrous tissue. Fetal wound healing occurs without inflammation or formation of fibrous tissue, thus making fetal wound healing more akin to *regeneration* than to the scarring process in adults. Indeed, the younger the fetal patient is at the time of surgery, the more likely it is to regenerate and to be born without scars. As one pediatric surgeon remarked about the fetal surgery experience at his institution, "the only way we could find the incisions on some of these babies was because the stitches were still in place" (quoted in Skerrett 1991, 1066). The question of how fetuses heal without scars captured the imaginations of researchers, and it has immense potential to capture the public's imagination. Of all aspects of fetal surgery, scarless healing most seems to evoke the specter of science fiction and the promise of medicine.

(Indeed, scarless healing, usually represented by passing a laser over a wound that then seems to magically seal itself, was regularly featured on *Star Trek: The Next Generation* and in other science fiction series.)

Several factors are claimed to account for the differences between fetal and adult wound healing. Most important, fetuses exist in the sterile, thermally controlled confines of the womb and are bathed continuously in nutrient-rich amniotic fluid. They also grow at a phenomenal rate: "cellular turnover and differentiation are so rapid in the normal fetus that the adult process of stimulating and recruiting normally quiescent fibroblasts may not be necessary in the fetus" (Krummel and Longaker 1991, 527). In addition, hyaluronic acid (HA), an essential component of both adult and fetal wound healing processes that promotes cell growth, is produced and sustained in fetal wound healing at much higher rates. "A prolonged presence of HA in fetal wounds may provide the matrix signal orchestrating healing by regeneration rather than by scarring" (Adzick and Longaker 1992a, 60). Although the precise physiological basis of fetal wound healing remains unestablished, there is widespread scientific agreement that it differs from adult processes in terms of cells, environment, or a combination of the two.

As with fetal physiological research, constraints on practice resulting from controversy surrounding fetal research have led scientists to investigate two major alternatives to human fetal work objects: animal models and, to a lesser extent, in vitro models. In addition to human fetuses, fetal wound healing research has been carried out on chick embryos, opossums, guinea pigs, mice, rats, rabbits, sheep, and nonhuman primates (Adzick 1992; Krummel and Longaker 1991). Despite a short gestation, the rabbit is the most widely used animal model, while nonhuman primates are considered the most rigorous in terms of applicability to human fetuses. However, "the fetal monkey model has the drawbacks of high expense and the need for postoperative monitoring and tocolysis to prevent preterm labor" (Adzick 1992, 79). As discussed in the previous section, in all animal models wounds and lesions are simulated and examined by researchers using assay systems, subcutaneously implanted wire mesh cylinders, and other "wounding" technologies, often graphically described in the literature.

In vitro models are used to study the effects of local biochemical factors on fetal wound healing. In this type of research, wounded tissue is removed and isolated from the rest of the organism and maintained in laboratory conditions using cultural media. Scientists investigate the role of circulating cells, which migrate to the wound site and are incorporated into the wound healing process. One example of the in vitro technique is the fibroblast scratch model, in which scratches are made on a layer of human neonatal skin. Fetal and postnatal calf serum are then applied to the wounded tissue and studied for significant effects and differences. The purpose of the model is "to determine if fetal serum contains unique components that stimulate the process of wound healing in a fetal-like manner" (Burd et al. 1992, 257). Another example of in vitro technology is the sheep explant model, in which pieces of fetal sheep skin are placed on gauze in culture dishes and combined with different substances. Different combinations of fetal sheep skin and growth factors are then analyzed for effects. Both models permit manipulation of fetal wound healing "in a controlled fashion," allowing scientists to "elucidate some of the individual components that participate in the phenomenal process of scarless fetal skin repair" (Burd et al. 1992, 262–263).

Fetal wound healing research is assiduously pursued by scientists precisely because it is construed as having immense therapeutic potential. Indeed, fetal wound healing is often referred to as the "blueprint" for ideal tissue repair (Adzick and Longaker 1992a). Examples of claimed potential therapeutic benefits of this knowledge include application to adult tissue repair (e.g., enhanced wound healing, control of wound contraction, development of antibodies) and to surgical correction of structural deformities such as fetal cleft lip. Scientists working in this area intend ultimately "to apply what is learned from fetal wound healing to the world outside the womb" (Skerrett 1991, 1066). Consider the following illustration of scientists' hopes for downstream application of this research: "The clinician's response to the SO WHAT question is that fetal wound healing represents a paradigm of ideal tissue repair that we would like to emulate in children and adults. As scarring and fibrosis dominate some diseases in every area of medicine, an understanding of fetal wound healing should help develop therapeutic strategies to avert the devastating consequences of excessive scar formation" (Adzick and Longaker 1992b, xi).[18]

Claims about the potential therapeutic benefits of fetal wound healing are congruent with the more traditional view that basic research leads to clinical applications. For example, when asked whether fetal surgical practices have contributed to basic physiological research, a prominent fetal physiologist replied, "I don't really think so. I think most of it has been a one-way street." Yet, as the fetal wound healing case illustrates, the relationship between research and practice may be more of a two-way street than scientists and clinicians are willing or able to acknowledge. As described, the impetus for fetal wound healing research was the emergence of the fetal work object via diagnostic and surgical practices. Constraints on the use of live human fetuses in wound healing research spawned the development of animal and in vitro models, somewhat obscuring the clinical origins of such research in human operations. Making visible the earlier, behind-the-scenes traffic between the operating room and the laboratory provides a fuller, more comprehensive view of how different practices come together in the social organization of medical work.

In sum, fetal wound healing research vividly illustrates the diversity of practices that constitute fetal surgery. Although clinical practice is often built upon physiological and other basic research in the laboratory, working on patients within the operating room may lead to scientific "discoveries." Clinical researchers must then move from the operating room back into the laboratory to seek answers to these new questions. By linking basic wound healing research to the downstream benefits of surgical experimentation, clinical researchers are able to pursue both sets of practices with some immunity from regulation and political controversy. Where fetal physiology offered a basis of legitimacy for fetal surgery, fetal wound healing legitimates by offering "proof" of fetal surgery's scientific payoffs. It also offers a compelling connection to science fiction, a cultural link that may enhance the ability of fetal surgery to side-step controversy by playing up the flashy fascination of scarless fetuses. Further, rather than being unidirectionally linked from research to treatment, the fetal wound healing paradigm embodies the hybrid nature of clinical practices. There is a continuum of research and treatment activities located within fetal surgery, with considerable overlap among the different types of work involved in the making of the unborn patient.

Hybridity in/of Fetal Surgery

A hybrid is something of mixed origin or composition. It is also the offspring of dissimilar parents, as in cross-breeding. Fetal surgery is a hybrid in both senses of the term: the specialty is a rich, complicated mixture of actors, practices, techniques, and sites of knowledge and subject production, and it was born of dissimilar parentage (despite claims of Liley's paternity discussed in chapter 2). In social and cultural studies of science and technology, the concept of hybridity is framed and used in a variety of ways. Latour (1991), for example, illustrates the common usage of hybrid as a mixture of humans and nonhumans, or rather, culture and nature. His elegant analysis traces the philosophical assumptions underlying hybridity, as well as its political consequences (such as the construction of modernity). Although fetal surgery is clearly about mixing humans and nonhumans, it is also about constructing what or who gets to count as human (Casper 1994b). It is not enough to understand that science, medicine, and even society itself are created by humans interacting with nonhumans (and vice versa), as Latour does. A more deeply political project is understanding how hybrid human activities, such as fetal surgery, produce human and nonhuman subjects, including animal models in research, the unborn patient, and fetal persons.

My use of hybridity is thus closer to that of Haraway (1997), who recognizes that hybridity is about fields of knowledge and practice, apparatuses of science and capitalism, and the production of subjects. She (1997, 128) writes,

> Objects like the fetus, chip/computer, gene, race, ecosystem, brain, database, and bomb are stem cells of the technoscientific body. Each of these curious objects is a recent construct or material-semiotic "object of knowledge," forged by heterogeneous practices in the furnaces of technoscience. . . . I am committed to showing how each of these stem cells is a knot of knowledge-making practices, industry and commerce, popular culture, social struggles, psychoanalytic formations, bodily histories, human and nonhuman actions, local and global flows, inherited narratives, new stories, syncretic technical/cultural processes, and more.

In Haraway's analysis, "sticky threads" protrude out of each stem cell and connect to the rest of the world. As she puts it, "How do technoscientific stem cells link up with each other in expected and unexpected ways and differentiate into entire worlds and ways of life?" (Haraway 1997, 130). She provides some of the conceptual tools necessary to follow the threads of hybridity, to examine and understand the links between and across sites.

In this chapter, I have profiled four generative "stem cells" of the technoscientific body of fetal surgery. Each of the practices and techniques discussed here has shaped the specialty in various ways by facilitating access to the fetus (both human and nonhuman) transforming it into a work object, legitimating the broader specialty, and enabling the debut of the unborn patient. Fetal physiology has provided scientific knowledge about developing fetuses that surgeons use both to accomplish and to legitimate their clinical work. Ultrasound technology has offered visual access to fetal work objects, making available information about structural defects amenable to surgical repair and assisting during repair itself. Extensive experimental animal research has resulted in a body of knowledge about fetal diseases and their treatments upon which fetal surgeons base clinical decisions regarding human patients. And fetal wound healing has emerged from the clinical practice of fetal surgery as a new research paradigm, providing fetal surgeons with knowledge about how fetuses heal in utero. All of these practices have been generated and used in laboratories and in operating rooms (and

elsewhere), and have themselves constituted the connective tissue joining these sites.

But how have these practices and techniques, as dissimilar they are,
ended up in the same field of knowledge and subject production? Here is
where human action comes back into the picture; after all, most technologies do not move or use themselves. Each of these practices can be
and usually are made to feed into each other by enterprising actors. Different actors are moving back and forth, to and fro, in and out of the divergent practices and sites discussed here, with the overall goal of
building fetal surgery into a successful biomedical enterprise. In order
for experimental fetal surgery to work, its human practitioners must
bring together an array of knowledges, techniques, tools, bodies, and
practices, creating a biomedical hybrid in the process. A great deal of effort is often required to marshal the different elements in fetal surgery.
Anselm Strauss (1988; 1993) has called this type of work *articulation
work* and Susan Leigh Star (1986) has labeled it *triangulation*. Regardless of what label is attached to it, this is the nitty-gritty work of hybridization in biomedicine, science, and other domains of practice.
Good examples in fetal surgery abound, including the efforts of physiologists to convey knowledge about fetal development to fetal surgeons or
the role of sonographers in performing and interpreting ultrasound images used in treatment decisions. In fetal surgery, diverse practices and
techniques are linked through the social organization and activities of
biomedical work, shaping the specialty as a whole.

I am also interested in another level of hybridity, that which *results
from* the organization of medical work and the traffic between the laboratory and the operating room, itself a multidisciplinary space. If fetal
surgery is a hybrid practice, as I have argued here, then it may also produce hybrid subjects. The unborn patient is one such subject, representing a particular type of fetus imbued with distinct meanings. I contend
that the fetus produced by fetal surgery is a *technofetus*, a hybrid creature fabricated out of diverse, highly technical practices. (Pregnant
women may be similarly configured technologically, as we shall see in
chapter 6.) As I have shown, fetuses are diagnosed via ultrasound and
other prenatal diagnostic technologies and are inscribed with particular
meanings of (ab)normality. They are exposed to the bright glare of operating room lights before they are "born," then sliced into with scalpels
and lasers. They can be "healed" (without scars!) as well as "destroyed"
by the gleaming, state-of-the-art tools of modern medicine. What I am
suggesting is that although there are many contemporary sites at which
fetal personhood is produced, the only way such subjectivity can be produced in fetal surgery is through the mobilization and activation of diverse practices such as those profiled here. In other words, hybridity

itself incites the making of the unborn patient by providing multiple nodes through which fetuses are transformed into objects of biomedical work and patients.

The power of hybrids to produce new knowledge and subjects notwithstanding, they may also create new problems. Located at the junctures between different practices, as well as within the practices themselves, are a number of cultural tensions and contradictions. Between physiology and surgery, between humans and nonhumans, between surgeons and their work objects, and between the laboratory and the operating room are spaces with considerable room for innovation and contestation. Hybridization breeds politicization. By focusing on hybrids, as I have done here, some of the politics in fetal surgery are brought into sharper view, including reproductive politics (e.g., the routinized use of prenatal diagnostic technologies), cultural politics (e.g., public struggles over the meanings of fetal images), professional politics (e.g., struggles between fetal surgeons and obstetricians over the terrain of fetal physiology), anti-vivisectionist politics (e.g., the controversial history of animal experimentation in fetal surgery), research politics (e.g., the putative value of fetal wound healing experiments), and so on. These politics are consequential for fetal surgery because they both facilitate and impinge on how work is done. Clinicians must seek ways to get their hands on the secluded fetus while also portraying their work as legitimate science. In doing so, they straddle uncomfortably some of the fault lines in fetal surgery, spaces within which some practices are constructed as legitimate while others are not. We shall see more examples of this straddling in the next chapter. Taken together, however, the practices and techniques that constitute fetal surgery have enabled its practitioners to build an enterprise crucial to the making of the unborn patient.

Chapter 4

Working on (and around) the Unborn Patient

Negotiating Social Order in a Fetal Treatment Unit

Since 1981, when surgeons in the United States successfully operated on a fetus and galvanized the field of fetal medicine, fetal treatment programs have sprouted at hospitals around the world. Most emphasize closed-uterus forms of treatment, such as the placement of shunts (mechanical devices to divert fluid that has accumulated) or selective termination. Yet a few brave centers are forging ahead with research on open surgical techniques for a range of life-threatening congenital defects. One of these institutions is Capital Hospital, a large medical center in the western United States. A rich and diverse site, it has fostered the development of a Fetal Treatment Unit (FTU) focused on the clinical needs of the fetus. Here, medical workers have created an interdisciplinary center for diagnosis and treatment, where pregnant women and their fetuses are warmly welcomed and treated by a team of specialists. Here, too, medical workers struggle with and against each other in an emergent specialty with fuzzy boundaries, jockeying for professional control and access to new patients and health care markets. This chapter explores the social organization of the Fetal Treatment Unit at Capital Hospital, specifically the complex negotiations that occur in the everyday lives of medical personnel who work on and around the unborn patient.

Where the previous chapter focused on a diversity of practices and tools mobilized to access the fetal work object, in this chapter fetal surgery is examined as an intersection of multiple practitioners with different skills and interests. Fetal surgery, despite its dazzling array of instruments and procedures, is as much about people and their work as it is about technology. I show here that fetal surgery is characterized by a diverse organizational form in which a wide variety of interactions shape what fetal surgery looks like in practice. The most significant interactions revealed in my data are but two sides of the same variegated coin:

cooperation, which makes the achievement of fetal surgery possible, and *conflict*, which threatens this achievement at every turn. Participants are well aware of their need to cooperate with each other to make the fetal surgery enterprise successful even while they may disagree loudly and consistently about how to accomplish this. They are equally aware of their many professional and political differences around which dissent erupts and which must be continually negotiated and managed. Understanding the social organization of the Fetal Treatment Unit, or how the medical personnel who inhabit it work together, sheds light on the hybrid interactional and institutional aspects of fetal surgery. Capital Hospital's ace fetal surgery team is a microcosm of the broader world of fetal surgery, which is continually disrupted and reordered through work on and around fetuses.

In addition to the concept of work objects—material entities around which people make meaning and organize their work practices—this chapter draws also on *negotiated order* (Strauss et al. 1964). Based on research in a psychiatric hospital, Strauss et al. (1964) argued that the structural life of an institution is constituted by "continual negotiative activity." Negotiations may be patterned, as for example within a web of institutional or organizational relationships, but they must be continually reconstituted through a variety of interactions as the basis for social order. Negotiations are emergent, contingent, constrained, and fluid— that is, they are ongoing, flexible, and do not exist in a vacuum—and they are essential to the coordination of medical work. The shapes of hospital wards, clinical and administrative arrangements, professional hierarchies, and institutional rules are all products of ongoing negotiations. These may achieve a relatively stable shape over time, but even stable social orders are continuously remade through commitments to certain routine interactions. Such arrangements can always be unmade if commitments flag and attention is diverted elsewhere. This chapter focuses on two types of interactions that are especially germane to fetal surgery and its unique work objects: those centered on cooperation and those involved in the negotiation of conflict.

The emerging and controversial world of fetal surgery offers a particularly fitting site through which to examine the social organization of work. Drawing on interview and ethnographic data collected at Capital Hospital from 1991 to 1994, I first describe what goes on in the Fetal Treatment Unit, painting a multihued picture of this world and its inhabitants. I then turn to the heart of the analysis: how medical workers negotiate social order in the face of tremendous diversity and outright conflict. The critical role of cooperation in creating and attempting to consolidate this new specialty is explored, focusing on how the clinical staff members of the FTU strive to negotiate good working relationships in spite of their diversity. I then focus on another dynamic aspect of this complex domain, namely, the many cleavages in fetal surgery along which participants diverge, often reflecting specialty boundaries. These cleavages include: (1) different definitions of work objects, (2) different criteria for patient selection, and (3) different views of a disease (congenital diaphragmatic hernia) and its treatment. As I show, the ongoing struggles around these differences have significant implications for work practices, for medical workers, for the health of pregnant women, for definitions of fetuses, and for the emergent enterprise of fetal surgery.

The Setting

Capital Hospital is a modern facility, outfitted with highly trained personnel and gleaming technologies. It is part of a large medical complex, where some buildings are steel and glass, and others a more antiquated yellow brick. Behind the hospital is an animal kennel where canine research animals bark loudly and frequently. Across the street is a medical bookstore where stethoscopes and skeletons hang on the walls; next door is a bustling café with striped umbrellas on the tables. Inside the hospital are long, brightly lit corridors leading to operating rooms with sterile, stainless steel equipment and to consulting rooms with subtle gray and mauve furniture designed to calm nervous patients. There is a persistent low hum in the air occasionally punctuated by announcements and calls for "Dr. Cart" (code blue) over the loudspeaker. Inside the flesh-toned walls of the hospital are people engaged in a variety of activities ranging from the mundane to the daring. The medical workers are recognizable by their crisp white lab coats and blue-green scrubs, while a worried, tired air hovers over the patients and their loved ones. Some patients, wearing revealing hospital gowns and paper slippers, slump in wheelchairs, while others shuffle along hospital corridors, dragging IVs behind them. Family members sit tensely in crowded waiting rooms, one eye on the television and the other on the door. Throughout, Capital Hospital is pervaded by an odd, familiar smell redolent of Mr. Clean, ether, and human bodies.

The Fetal Treatment Unit is located on an upper floor of the hospital, where the corridors are quieter and the view is better. It is spacious and elegantly decorated in muted shades of pink, mauve, and gray. A central reception area is dominated by a large desk and a bulletin board covered with photographs of fetal surgery's success stories—an appealing display of a dozen or more babies with rosy cheeks. There are offices behind the reception area for the fetal surgeons, nurses, and other FTU staff, and there is a medium-sized conference room with a table, chairs, projection screen, and small library. There are also several well-stocked laboratories in another area of the center. Medical workers come and go in this space, intent on the enormous, grave work of diagnosing and treating fetuses. Like cave paintings from a premodern time, fetal images abound in this space offering archaeological clues to the center's purpose. A small office is decorated with a certificate describing one of the fetal surgeons as a "Fetus Fixer," while on the wall of the conference room is an image of a fetus in a plastic bubble over the caption "Womb with a View." The FTU's logo, in black and white graphic design, depicts an outstretched hand with a tiny fetus nestled in the palm.

Unlike other parts of Capital Hospital, the main offices of the Fetal Treatment Unit are typically not chaotic. The FTU offices merely serve as headquarters for the fetal surgery team, while many activities take place elsewhere. Indeed, the quiet elegance of the FTU's reception area serves as a barrier of sorts to the noisy, bloody, controversial work that goes on behind closed doors. In addition to surgery on the fetus, the work involved in making the unborn patient occurs through meetings, consultations, telephone calls, conferences, and other sites and practices. Surgical procedures are done in the hospital's general operating rooms, and weekly fetal treatment meetings are held in a large conference room in the obstetrics department. The following are brief vignettes of the work of fetal surgery as it occurs both inside and outside the operating room. The first, a fragment from my fieldnotes recounting one of the many procedures that I watched, describes an operation on a young woman whose fetus was diagnosed with a diaphragmatic hernia:

> The surgeons sliced through [the patient's] abdomen. It was messy, and there were many layers of tissue, fat, muscle, and blood. The incisions were not neat and clean; surgeons would pull the layers apart as they ran a scalpel across [her] abdomen and the flesh and muscle would sort of rip apart slowly. As they worked their way through her body, they would pull parts of her abdomen aside and clamp them with big silver metal clips. After about eight minutes of cutting, they reached the uterus. Dr. ———— pulled the fetus partially out of the uterus and made two incisions on its left side, one about heart level and one about umbilical cord level in its abdomen. The lower incision was about two fingers wide. After making both incisions, Dr. ———— pushed the organs that had accumulated in the chest cavity downward. Immediately, a nurse placed a small device inside the fetus' chest to monitor its condition, while the organs came careening out of the lower incision and hung outside of the fetus' body.

The second vignette moves beyond the operating room to another, less visceral site where the unborn patient is crafted. The meeting described next took place in a small library located on the fifth floor of Capital Hospital; the room was crowded, noisy, and very hot, and tempers were running high following a spate of fetal deaths. Providers argued passionately about maternal management strategies and the need for better monitoring of pregnant women and fetuses both during and after fetal surgery. As we shall see, diversity is foregrounded in this vignette as multiple voices representing different specialties are heard together evaluating problems:

> A fetal physiologist remarked that the major issue in monitoring has to be umbilical blood flow reduction. An operating room nurse commented, somewhat testily, that the fetal team might "think about getting information from other operations and techniques in obstetrics and gynecology." An anesthesiologist responded that a major difference between fetal surgery and other obstetrical operations is the size of the uterine incision. Almost everyone present nodded at this, indicating wide agreement that fetal surgery is indeed different. The physiologist again took the floor and cautioned that "you should be careful about throwing things into the fetus without knowing what's going on." Speaking about a specific case, a nurse on the fetal surgery team suggested that they "need to figure out how to inhibit contractions without dangerous medications." All of a sudden, the room erupted and a number of people began talking at once. Somebody remarked, heatedly, that all procedures on the fetus are "insults." A neonatologist, with anger in his voice, asserted that "you can't compare normal labor with a woman who's had her uterus cut open and a fetus with its chest open!"

These examples provide an important backdrop for the analysis that follows. I analyze these and similar clusters of activity with an eye toward how social order is negotiated in fetal surgery through various types of patterned interactions. The remainder of this chapter explores the interactional and institutional scaffolding of fetal surgery and its role in the making of the unborn patient in the contemporary era.

"A Spirit of Cooperation": Working Together in the Fetal Treatment Unit

Like Liley, Adamsons, Freda, and their many colleagues in the 1960s— and despite persistent conflicts— contemporary medical workers *do* cooperate with each other; their cooperation indeed is a source of pride and a foundation for claims of legitimacy. From its interdisciplinary roots three decades ago, fetal surgery has continued to attract and enroll numerous different specialists through a combination of professional needs and career goals. Providers recognize that cooperation is necessary in order to bring all of their different experiences and skills to bear on complicated fetal problems. It is certainly seen as integral to the "success" of fetal surgery, such as achieving fetal survival and ensuring that pregnant women do not die during the procedure. Cooperation may also be desired as an end in itself to make working conditions more pleasant or to satisfy certain institutional requirements related to fetal surgery. For example, attempting to secure funding for research or the approval of institutional review boards is far more expedient if medical workers are able to portray the fetal surgery enterprise as cooperative rather than as riddled with conflict. But while cooperation is an important building block for "doing things together" (Becker 1986) in fetal surgery, it is by no means a naturally occurring phenomenon. Rather, cooperation, like all other human interactions, must be achieved; its existence is something to be explained rather than taken for granted. The production of fetal surgery as a cooperative enterprise is characterized by numerous institutional activities, such as regular staff meetings designed to enable and encourage people to work together. According to key actors in the field, "the institutional setting, organization, and coordination of [fetal treatment units] are elements critical to [their] success" (Howell et al. 1993, 143). What follows is a description of the cooperative components of fetal surgery that make this nascent specialty possible.

The Fetal Treatment Unit at Capital Hospital originated in the early 1980s when a pediatric surgeon, a sonographer, and an obstetrician began working together on experimental fetal surgery. Obstetricians, with input from sonographers, had already been treating fetuses nonsurgically for a variety of conditions before pediatric surgeons began to focus on the fetus, beginning with transfusions for Rh disease based on Liley's work. But for the most part, pediatric specialists and neonatologists had been unsuccessful in saving babies whose diseases were too advanced for treatment. Echoing Liley and others from the 1960s, contemporary clinicians were dismayed that they could not save afflicted newborns who routinely died at birth or shortly thereafter. This frustration, coupled with important historical precedents in fetal diagnosis and treatment, prompted the trio at Capital Hospital to consider operating on fetuses *prenatally* in order to repair defects or to prevent life-threatening conditions from developing at birth. Open fetal surgery was used in one desperate case in which a fetal catheter inserted nonsurgically to treat a blocked urinary tract refused to stay in place; replacing the catheter in order to save the fetus necessitated surgically opening the pregnant woman's abdomen. However, once a new catheter was developed it proved easier to use than the old model, rendering subsequent open surgery unnecessary for this condition.[1] By that time, however, the door to fetal surgery itself had been wedged open, and physicians had begun to consider applying this "new" technique to other diseases and conditions. Thus, a combination of concern for fetuses, technical innovation, professional goals, and institutional conditions revived interest in open fetal surgery almost twenty years after the pioneering but short-lived efforts of the 1960s.

As with the broader enterprise of fetal surgery, the Fetal Treatment Unit at Capital Hospital evolved through the interaction of professionals from many disciplines who shared an interest in the fetus. One fetal surgeon described the FTU as "a microcosm of the fetal treatment enterprise throughout the world." And like the clinical work settings of the 1960s in New Zealand and Puerto Rico, the FTU has remained multidisciplinary since its inception. From the initial triad of pediatric surgeon, sonographer, and obstetrician, the fetal surgery team at Capital has grown to include a range of practitioners with diverse skills, perspectives, and backgrounds. These include perinatologists skilled in fetal diagnosis, fetal blood sampling, and intrauterine transfusion; neonatologists, who must often intensively manage newborns after surgery and birth and during subsequent postnatal treatment; social workers who address psychosocial issues (including emotional, financial, employment, and social support issues) faced by pregnant women, their partners, and families; pediatric and obstetric anesthesiologists; nurses representing different specialties and levels of expertise; geneticists and genetic counselors; fetal physiologists knowledgeable in basic fetal biology; and medical ethicists. The feasibility of fetal surgery and the likelihood that it will become a routine rather than experimental medical practice are seen by participants as outcomes contingent upon cooperative interaction among the specialty's diverse practitioners. A successful fetal treatment center is, in the words of one fetal surgeon (Harrison 1991a, 11), a "blend of skills and expertise," and there are increasing numbers of these centers appearing in the United States and in other nations.

Practitioners of fetal surgery are acutely aware of the diversity of skills and knowledges required to diagnose and treat the fetus. Every informant I spoke with talked at length about the necessity for cooperation and working together, an issue that has also received ample attention in the clinical literature. Such cooperation and collaboration is not unusual in medicine, but the novelty and extreme risks of fetal surgery make the need to work together especially compelling. As one fetal surgeon framed the problem, "This is the most complex undertaking in surgery. We've got to enlist the aid of every person who's involved in every stage of this." An obstetrician, speaking at a professional meeting, stressed that "it's important to have a well-rounded unit for fetal surgery, including neonatologists, pediatric surgeons, and so on." One of the sonographers agreed that there is a great degree of cooperation and remarked, "Considering some of the problems we've had, generally I would say it's a reasonably orderly group of people." Another fetal surgeon remarked, "It has to be a team approach. . . . The team approach is key." And a social worker declared, "I think the days of territorialism are long gone. Because there's so much to be done for these families, everybody sort of pitches in. And I think there is a spirit of cooperation on this team that makes it reasonable to work on."

As with the Rh group in Auckland, these last comments indicate that a "team" metaphor is often used to describe working arrangements in fetal treatment units. While many medical specialties are organized around the team concept, in fetal surgery this is especially crucial as a means of achieving both efficacy and legitimacy. According to practitioners, a number of general principles have evolved since the inception of contemporary fetal surgery to guide its development. Chief among these is that "fetal surgery is a team effort requiring varying amounts of input from all team members" (Harrison 1991a, 9). As well as specifying all the requisite members of the team (e.g., obstetrician, perinatologist, geneticist, surgeon, nurse, and so forth), these principles also lay out additional rules underlying the organization of fetal surgery. For example, "although all members of the team can contribute to any particular procedure, there must be a team leader" (Harrison 1991a, 9). Who is selected as team leader may be a source of conflict and basis for negotiation, despite the rule that "the procedure is done by the team member who is most likely to produce the best outcome" (ibid.). Further, just as experimental fetal surgery is a proving ground for developing and implementing new procedures, it also provides "an invaluable opportunity to work out . . . the professional relationships that will enable the team to function smoothly. The lines of responsibility must be drawn clearly among team members before the choice of doing a procedure is offered to a patient" (ibid.). Here, team metaphors are seen as facilitating the formation of a division of labor.

At Capital Hospital, in particular, certain organizational conventions within the FTU indicate that cooperative teamwork is extremely important. At ongoing fetal treatment group meetings, all types of interested practitioners come together to discuss specific cases and strategies for treatment, evaluating past and current activities as well as planning for the future. These regular meetings, held in the same place at the same time each week, provide a forum for addressing the complexities of specific cases. Different specialists present their particular slant and, while there is much agreement, there is also much heated negotiation. In addition, regular "consensus meetings" are held among clinicians and researchers to discuss current basic scientific research as it relates to clinical practices. It is here that new fetal technologies and innovations, developed in a fetal treatment lab using animal models, are first introduced into a setting of clinicians. Fetal surgeons, obstetricians, genetics counselors, and social workers also routinely meet with potential patients, coordinating their schedules and agendas to coincide with a family's visit to the hospital. And there are ad hoc meetings on a variety of issues, such as a discussion of fetal and maternal management that took place following a rash of postoperative maternal health problems and fetal deaths. In introducing the topic of this ad hoc meeting, a fetal surgeon described those present as a "working group" convened to address the issue of maternal safety.

An illustration of the continual quest for cooperation was provided in a talk presented by one of the fetal surgeons for another group of practitioners at Capital Hospital. The presentation was given during grand rounds for obstetrics and gynecology, with most of the audience representing these two specialties. Focused on prenatal and perinatal management of anomalies, the talk was clearly designed to "enroll" (Latour 1987) obstetricians as allies, or members of the team, in the enterprise of fetal surgery. Many obstetricians are vocal critics of open fetal surgery; nonetheless, they possess the skills and expertise in maternal health issues that fetal surgeons may be lacking or seeking. For example, preterm labor is a major problem in fetal surgery, and obstetricians identify themselves as best equipped to resolve it. They are skeptical of surgeons' encroachment on this territory. The fetal surgeon strategically emphasized throughout his lecture that his team is very concerned about maternal safety. In a significant bid to establish cooperative working relationships, he invited the obstetricians to "talk about [fetal surgery] together, both its limitations and new approaches." He assured his audience that fetal surgeons are "looking to forge a new partnership." The speaker ended his talk by emphasizing that the success of the Fetal Treatment Unit at Capital Hospital "depends on people meeting in the hall, talking informally, and working together." An example of behind-the-scenes maneuvering, the presentation was a strategically delivered and polished invitation to obstetricians to participate in fetal surgery as a cooperative venture.

At Capital Hospital, then, there is an ongoing commitment to cooperation and teamwork among those who work on and around fetuses. To a large degree, any cooperation that is achieved is based in part on shared understandings of the work of fetal surgery. Regardless of what professional and political identities each medical worker brings to fetal surgery, the institutional shape of this practice situates the fetus as a primary focus of activities. Simply stated, the chief reason that people work together in fetal surgery is because a pregnant woman has been admitted to the hospital with a sick fetus requiring treatment. There are certainly many ancillary reasons for the collective nature of fetal surgery—including professional norms, organizational patterns, loyalty to colleagues, and the allure of challenging work—but these are overshadowed by the broad, public aim of "saving babies." The fetal surgery team at Capital Hospital is organized around the clinical requirements of diagnosing and treating fetuses in an experimental context. And those who work on the fragile fetus and on pregnant women made vulnerable by surgery need all the assistance, and legitimacy, they can muster.

However, given the consistent controversy surrounding human fetuses, the new and experimental status of fetal surgery, and the intersection of so many different specialties, the picture of harmony painted by medical workers in fetal surgery is too rosy. While there is certainly a great deal of cooperation, as displayed in staff meetings and in operating rooms and in the very longevity of the enterprise, it is often achieved despite profound differences between medical workers in this specialty. A prominent fetal surgeon (Harrison 1991a, 9) has written that "a special problem arises with interventional fetal procedures, especially those that require the expertise of specialists from very different fields. . . . Because no single specialty training provides the total spectrum of skills and experience, this is an area in which 'turf' battles between medical specialties and 'ego' battles among team members may sabotage the fetal treatment enterprise." This was certainly the case at Capital Hospital during the period in which I conducted my research. As any chemist (or sociologist) knows, affinity is not the only possible reaction to mixing different elements; sometimes the end result is a volatile compound.

"Folks Are Always Rubbing Shoulders": Working around Critical Differences

Although cooperation is necessary for fetal surgery to work, differences among practitioners in this domain are pervasive. There are both minor disagreements and major fights about how fetuses and pregnant women are talked about and worked on, about proper treatment plans, about postoperative procedures, about who is responsible for which work tasks, and so on. There is a seemingly infinite number of reasons why actors in the fetal surgery domain do not always "get along" with each other, some of which they themselves recognize and articulate. (They may also recognize other reasons but choose not to discuss these publicly.) Significantly, conflict is associated with failures in fetal surgery, including fetal deaths, harrowing cases with uncertain outcomes, and problems with pregnant women's health. One surgeon told me that "if everything worked right, everybody would get along fine." A sonographer stated, "If everything was red, white, and blue banners flying all the time about the successes, then believe me, there would be no conflict.

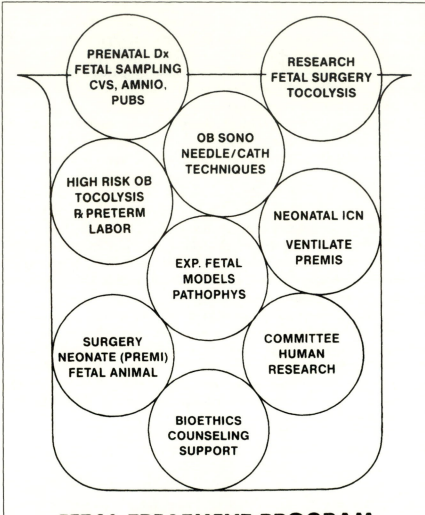

FETAL TREATMENT PROGRAM

FIGURE 2–2. The fetal treatment program is a melting pot requiring the expertise of many different specialists and specialties in an institutional setting that promotes high-level perinatal care, clinical investigation, and experimental work on fetuses.

A graphic depiction of a fetal treatment program as a "melting pot" of different specialists. Such interdisciplinarity requires extensive cooperation while also fostering conflict and dissent. It is interesting to note the placement of specialties, with prenatal diagnosis and fetal surgery at the top and bioethics counseling at the bottom, with other specialties in-between. Source: M. R. Harrison, M. S. Golbus, and R. A. Filly. 1991. *The Unborn Patient: Prenatal Diagnosis and Treatment.* Philadelphia: W. B. Saunders Company, p. 12.

Everybody would be so happy. The only conflicts would be who got to stand first in line for the laurels. We're more likely to have conflicts when we have failures." And another fetal surgeon remarked that "because things are new and things aren't worked out, folks are always rubbing shoulders. We've had terrible conflicts, arguments, and things that were strictly differences of opinion medically."

This last comment suggests that while medical failures may be seen as contributing to dissension, differences in professional training may also form the basis for conflict. For example, an obstetrician had this to say about disagreements in the program: "I think that any time you have a group of people, sort of management by committee, there are going to be problems. People just have different views, particularly when you have groups of people from different backgrounds." Yet the differences between participants in fetal surgery may be considerably more complex. One of the social workers—a somewhat unique group because they are not clinicians and are more akin to social scientists—described this rich and complicated diversity in more detail: "It was a baptism by fire. Meaning that I was surprised at how, in some ways, unprepared I was for the politics of the program. We all have a slightly different vantage, orientation, perspective, and cultural agenda. There are so many subtle ways in which we are different from one another, both because of our professional training and because of who we are as human beings." The deep-seated differences between workers in this domain, pinpointed by a number of informants, affect the shape and trajectory of this practice in often highly consequential ways both locally at Capital Hospital and in terms of the broader fetal surgery enterprise. Examining diversity at the local level of work arrangements in the Fetal Treatment Unit, I next focus on ways in which these differences are made meaningful and are acted upon in the context of actual practices.

Negotiating the "What" of Fetal Surgery: Different Definitions of Work Objects

A major site at which differences emerge and coalesce in fetal surgery is in definitions of work objects. Because operating on fetuses necessarily means surgically opening pregnant women's bodies, there would seem to be only one major human work object in fetal surgery: the pregnant woman. Yet medical workers draw a clear distinction, both in practice and discursively, between woman-as-work-object and fetus-as-work-object. Contestation centers around these often competing definitions, as well as around how much and what kind of clinical and ethical consideration to accord each entity. Moreover, although there are two recognized work objects, the fetus is positioned as the primary work object—*the patient*—within this domain, while the pregnant woman is reduced to a nonessential feature of the clinical environment. A division of labor has emerged around these different work objects, with an entire specialty now devoted to the unique clinical needs of the unborn patient.

A variety of specific practices illustrate this phenomenon. For example, every fetal operation at Capital Hospital is videotaped for research and recording purposes. Taping begins after full anesthesia of the pregnant woman has occurred and after surgeons have opened her uterus; it ends when they are finished working on the fetus but before the woman's uterus and abdomen have been sutured closed. Visually erasing women from the frame, this practice illustrates graphically what/who is considered the important work object in fetal surgery. Surgeons at Capital Hospital also hope to create a Fetal Intensive Care Unit (FICU) in the future where fetuses (and presumably pregnant women) can be monitored postoperatively. Currently after surgery the pregnant women are monitored in the standard ICU by medical workers trained in both general and obstetrical acute care. If fetuses are abruptly transformed into fragile "newborns" during surgery and not replaced in their mothers' wombs, those that survive are immediately whisked away to the neonatal intensive care unit. But, according to surgeons I spoke to, neither the standard ICU nor the neonatal ICU focuses exclusively on the needs of the unborn patient. Some medical workers, in expressing concern about inadequate fetal monitoring after surgery, have proposed intensive care of the fetus as one solution. Ironically, the FICU as conceptualized by my informants gives no indication that a fetus would still be inside its mother's body during this postoperative period. In yet another example of the intensive focus on the fetus, Capital Hospital instituted a catchy toll-free number for referring physicians and potential patients who desire information about the program: 800-FETUSRx.

Among all medical workers in this domain, fetal surgeons especially view the fetus as the primary work object. Many of them were trained in pediatric surgery and are already used to working with pint-sized bodies and doll-like body parts. They are also highly invested in building a new specialty (and a new health care market) organized around the unborn patient. A number of surgeons recounted their deep interest in learning more about the womb's tiny occupant with its own set of health problems. Echoing pro-life discourse—which defines fetal and postnatal existence as continuous—one surgeon told me that he had always understood the distinction between fetuses and infants "in geographic terms"; in his view, they are similar enough anatomically that surgeons can use similar techniques and tools to treat them. What is missing in this characterization is any sense that the fetus, unlike a newborn, is located inside a pregnant woman's body and thus much more difficult to access. Another surgeon, a resident interested in neurosurgery, explained that despite its rather obscure geographical location the fetus was a useful work object precisely because of its miniature size. Working out how to monitor and treat such a diminutive object inside an adult body is, according to this resident, excellent training for a career in heart or brain surgery, where a delicate touch is worth a great deal.

Yet as ubiquitous as constructions of the fetal patient are in this domain, not all of the actors define fetuses as their primary, or even secondary, work objects. In a number of ways, different participants attribute diverse, sometimes conflicting meanings to fetuses and pregnant women and thus organize their work activities differently. This diversity often leads to considerable strain between fetal surgeons, who define fetuses as central work objects, and other participants with different tasks and agendas. For example, most obstetricians generally consider pregnant women to be their primary work objects and are concerned with fetal health secondarily or only in relation to maternal health. Indeed, relations between fetal surgeons and obstetricians at Capital Hospital have become increasingly difficult in recent years, with the latter group, in one obstetrician's view, being "slowly pushed out" by the fetal surgeons. An obstetrician involved with the program for many years expressed her dissatisfaction with the direction of the FTU, stating, "We are having trouble with fetal surgery because we're seeing lots of complications in women. The obstetricians, of course, take care of the maternal patient." She later remarked, "Fetal surgeons don't take care of the woman after ward. We've had women who've not been able to leave the hospital, who've been in and out of labor for the rest of their pregnancies. And those are the successes!" This informant clearly foregrounds maternal health issues, which have long been paramount in obstetrics and gynecology but which are not the primary consideration in fetal surgery except as they affect and constrain fetal procedures.

One of the social workers confirmed these dynamics and described difficult relations between fetal surgeons and obstetricians: "The OBs are used to managing [maternal] patients. There is a lot of angry stuff between the OBs, such as who is going to be in attendance at these deliveries. You know, there are people who really didn't want to do it or believe in it. They think it's bad medicine to take a pregnant woman and cut her open." This is the same informant who remarked earlier that the days of territorialism in fetal surgery were now over, perhaps because much of this conflict occurs behind the scenes. Ironically, the Fetal Treatment Unit at Capital Hospital is often approached by other hospitals interested in starting fetal surgery units. One of the surgeons told me that the FTU advised a major East Coast hospital "*not* to include obstetricians from day one." As he explained, if obstetricians can be prevented from participating in new programs, then some of the problems "plaguing" the FTU at Capital Hospital might be avoided at other institutions.

Comments of fetal surgeons are especially revealing about ongoing conflict between "baby doctors" and "mom doctors." For example, the proposed Fetal Intensive Care Unit described above has proved somewhat controversial and has yet to be implemented. According to a fetal surgeon, "Anytime you have new concepts like the FICU, you're bound to encounter some resistance. That was a new concept for many people and it led to friction." When I pressed him about the source of resistance, he remarked, "Well, you know, it's just a different way of dealing with things. I'm used to doing big operations and having patients in the ICU, and some of the obstetricians and OB nurses are not used to that. They view the postoperative period as the preterm labor problem. But it was clear that patient management went far beyond just management of preterm labor, and we couldn't *not* be responsible outside of monitoring. That led to friction." Suggesting that obstetricians are not used to "big operations" is a somewhat curious criticism; they have historically, and increasingly routinely, performed cesarean sections and must have at least a passing knowledge of major surgery.

Another fetal surgeon described in far more critical terms cardinal differences between pregnant women and fetuses as work objects: "The unfortunate part is that the obstetricians have been taking care of the fetal/maternal pair for so long it's driven into them. But our patients aren't like their patients. Our patients are mid-gestation fetuses, our mom has just undergone a major operation, our fetus has just undergone a major operation, there's been prolonged anesthesia, and now there are problems with pain control, volume fluctuations, and all the normal perioperative things. Obstetricians don't understand anything about perioperative management; they don't understand anything about management of a patient in the perioperative period." Particularly striking is the distinction this informant draws between *fetal* patients/work objects as constituting the territory of fetal surgeons, and *maternal* patients/work objects as part of the proprietary but increasingly narrow terrain of obstetricians. Indeed, in his final sentence it is not even clear which patient the surgeon is talking about. But regardless of who is in charge, managing the pregnant woman means that she must remain in or nearby the hospital after surgery, often for several weeks until she delivers her baby. Throughout this period, which is characterized by cooperative efforts to ensure a successful stay for the woman and her family, there are ample opportunities for tensions to erupt among medical workers.

One fetal surgeon ascribes such heated differences to professional training and background: "Basically every group of physicians has their own personality. Surgeons tend to be a little more aggressive, we tend to push harder, get things done. It's just a personality thing. The obstetricians now have seen enough problems with fetal surgery that they're absolutely opposed to it. They don't like it. They don't want it to happen. They're against it. The only reason they're going through the moves right now is because it's protocol driven." A fetal physiologist echoes these points: "Well, I think it's again a turf issue. Obstetricians feel that they should be responsible for all prenatal care—care of the fetus *and* mother. And surgeons feel that the fetus is their patient and have therefore assumed some responsibility for the mother." Yet, although professional training may be significant, it is the implementation of such training in local work arrangements that both shapes and reinforces crucial distinctions among specialists in this domain, particularly who has access to fetuses. The availability of direct access to fetuses is an important constraint on how, by whom, and under what conditions fetuses and pregnant women are defined as meaningful work objects.

This dynamic is illustrated in a discussion in the major fetal surgery text, *The Unborn Patient*, (Harrison et al. 1991), about which specialist should perform fetal surgery, or rather, which specialist should be the team leader. Harrison (1991a) begins by stating that the most politically expedient solution would be to have each specialist do his or her part of the overall procedure. This means that obstetricians would open and close the uterus, and the pediatric surgeon would operate on the fetus. This easy solution is, according to Harrison (1991a, 10), "likely to keep team members comfortable in their accustomed roles." Yet he goes on to state that this practice is not likely to yield the best outcomes because "it assumes that traditional skills will suffice; that is, that obstetricians can close the uterus as they do in the case of an empty uterus and that the pediatric surgeon can do with a fetus what he learned in a neonate. Neither is true." He argues that "tag-team surgery is never ideal," particularly where exposure of the fetus by hysterotomy is complicated by preterm labor problems. Thus, despite the rhetoric of teamwork, it seems that a division of labor by extant specialties may not work or be construed as ideal. Harrison's answer to this dilemma is that "fetal surgery cannot develop and will not succeed unless a few *surgeons* are willing to devote considerable time and effort to developing, practicing, and perfecting all aspects of this new procedure" (1991a, 10; emphasis added). This passage is striking for the degree to which chief responsibility for this new procedure is appropriated by fetal surgeons, while the participation of obstetricians (and presumably other medical workers) is marginalized.

Another group with whom fetal surgeons struggle for territory is neonatologists, who view fetuses as potential work objects but with a very important geographical and anatomical difference. A relatively new medical specialty, neonatology provides intensive (and expensive) care for fragile newborns who are either premature or very ill. As Renée Anspach (1993) has documented, neonatologists are used to working in highly charged contexts where life-and-death decisions are made all the time. At fetal treatment meetings at Capital Hospital, neonatologists revealed themselves to be acutely interested in the fate of the unborn patient. If surgery is unsuccessful but the fetus survives—that is, if surgeons cannot replace the fetus in the pregnant woman's womb—neonatologists argue that they should then assume control over the fetus-cum-neonate. But fetal surgeons guard their work objects jealously and have demonstrated resistance to neonatologists' quest for professional control over the ambiguous fetal body. These tensions become more vivid when the fetuses in fetal surgery are the same gestational age—or older—than those being cared for in the neonatal intensive care unit (NICU). The dispute that ensued when this issue surfaced at one of the fetal treatment meetings illustrates some of the emotional and professional investments on all sides.

The fetal surgery team presented a case involving a pregnant woman carrying a 26-week-old fetus. A neonatologist suggested that resuscitation equipment be available in the operating room in the event that the fetus could not be replaced in the pregnant woman's body during or after surgery. This had only been necessary once before in the history of fetal surgery; most often, the fetuses are too young to warrant neonatal salvageability if an operation is not successful. One of the fetal surgeons responded negatively to this suggestion, declaring, "When we do our thing, it's all or nothing. We don't pull out live babies. We either put them back alive or pull them out dead." The neonatologist then demanded to know what circumstances would require removing a live fetus, and the fetal surgeon responded by citing uncontrollable labor and a contracting uterus. The surgeon then went on to say that he saw two problems in making resuscitation equipment available: "explaining it to the mother" and "having it there logistically." In a flash of anger, the neonatologist replied that "there is also a problem in that you're doing something very few people in the world are doing and we don't know what will happen!" At this point, confronted with a blatant reminder about how deadly serious fetal surgery can be, the surgeon retreated and became quite accommodating (at least on the surface), agreeing with his colleague's assessment of the situation. Several other people joined in the negotiations, and it was eventually decided that the equipment would be made available for older fetuses (those at or near the viability marker of about twenty-three weeks) and that it would be set up in the hallway outside the operating room.

To further complicate the situation regarding work objects, other participants in the FTU define their patients/clients quite differently than do fetal surgeons, obstetricians, and neonatologists. For example, many of the social workers, nurses, and genetic counselors (almost all women) were deeply troubled by fetal surgery, especially during periods of failure. In the words of one nurse, "every baby was dying. Every step of the way we've been thwarted by consequences of surgery that have high morbidity and high mortality for these babies." Because negative outcomes often create or intensify conflict, one social worker decided that she would be "an advocate for the parent." Yet differences in status within the FTU, and in medicine more widely, between social workers and physicians often made this difficult. The social worker described being frustrated in her attempts to advocate for the pregnant women by surgeons more intently focused on fetuses. For example, her judgment about a particular patient who she felt was not psychologically equipped to deal with surgery was challenged by surgeons, leading her to remark: "I was incensed about it. At that point, my confidence was shaken and I felt that if I'm going to be the psychosocial person on this team, I'm going to have to have the support of the members of the team." While her recommendation was ultimately supported by an outside psychiatrist, she described the incident as "forcing me to look again at my role and my interactions with the team."

In sum, there are a number of divergent positions on who or what are, and are not, work objects in fetal surgery. As the examples above make clear, different participants ascribe different meanings to the bodies they work on in fetal surgery. For fetal surgeons, fetuses are first and foremost patients and objects of therapeutic practices such as surgery. For obstetricians, pregnant women are (usually) the first and most important patients and objects of maternity care, while fetuses are secondary work objects. Most obstetricians do not completely reject the notion of a fetal patient; indeed, one of the striking developments in medicine in recent years is the emergence of maternal-fetal medicine as a replacement for standard obstetrics (Creasy and Resnick 1994). Nor have specialists in obstetrics and gynecology always been valiant protectors of women's health (Arney 1982; Moscucci 1990; Rothman 1982). However, conflicts between obstetricians and fetal surgeons tend to center on other aspects of treatment, such as how to keep pregnant women healthy while operating on them solely for the benefit of their fetuses. For neonatologists, fetuses may become work objects when surgery is unsuccessful and the unborn patient is transformed into a neonatal patient. For social workers, genetic counselors, and nurses, fetuses are only work objects in an ancillary sense. The pregnant woman and her family are the primary locus of care, which is defined in terms of psychosocial and ongoing postoperative care rather than surgical intervention. Yet even these practitioners may be concerned about fetal outcomes; for example, the social worker quoted above who wanted to advocate for parents was also anguished that too many fetuses were dying.

These varied constructions of pregnant women and their fetuses are consequential, as work practices are organized around the meanings that each work object has for different actors. There is a certain "logic" at work here in terms of identifying what to do next in the clinical setting (Berg 1992). That is, if the fetus is a patient, then it must be treated. If the pregnant woman is a patient, then she (and secondarily her fetus) must be cared for. If a pregnant woman and her partner need psychosocial or postoperative care, it is to be provided by the appropriate person, generally a social worker or nurse. The definition of fetuses as primary work objects is negotiated and contested in practice, and there may be significant deviations from a straight course to the making of the unborn patient. For example, obstetricians, social workers, and nurses continue to assert the importance of women's health while questioning the overall enterprise of fetal surgery. Thus, the process of negotiating social order in fetal surgery is itself shaped by several factors, including professional training, work cultures and identities, institutional hierarchies, the materiality of work objects (e.g., fetuses may die), and control over the conditions of medical work, such as access to patients. Yet despite tensions surrounding different work objects and practices, the Fetal Treatment Unit, and fetal surgery more broadly, is collectively geared toward the diagnosis, treatment, and salvation of fetuses, which continue to be institutionally and culturally defined as the most significant work objects. Pregnant women, and the medical workers who care for and about them, may thus be relegated to a secondary status in this domain; we shall explore this issue in chapter 6.

Negotiating the "Who" of Fetal Surgery: Different Criteria for Patient Selection

Not all women referred to fetal treatment units choose to have fetal surgery, which is only one, but certainly the most invasive, of several available treatment options. Other interventions include drug therapy or aborting the fetus, or even no treatment at all. Different participants in fetal surgery use a wide range of criteria for patient selection (who is considered a good candidate for treatment), based on their definitions of work objects. Clearly, if there is disagreement over who the patient is, then there is likely to be confusion and even conflict over how to select for patients. Fetal surgeons generally define selection in terms of fetuses, while obstetricians consider maternal health a priority; both groups tend to rely primarily on what we tend to think of as "clinical" criteria. In the clinical literature (Harrison 1991a), guidelines for patient selection sug-

gest that a fetus should be a singleton (i.e., not a twin) prenatally diagnosed and found to have abnormalities. The family should be fully counseled about the risks and benefits of surgery. Further, a multidisciplinary
team should be present during treatment, and high-risk obstetrical and
intensive care units should be available for women following surgery.
Bioethical and psychosocial consultation also should be made available
for both practitioners and patients. In local practices, however, these
carefully stated global guidelines are not necessarily adhered to. Depending on a variety of circumstances and conditions, some factors may
take precedence over others in the selection process. These practices reveal how "clinical" decisions, such as which fetuses are made into unborn patients, are often rooted in nonclinical priorities.

For example, one fetal surgeon outlined for me a series of selection
and treatment considerations for congenital cystic adenomatoid malformations (C-CAM). This is a condition in which a benign lung tumor
takes up too much space in the chest and can cause fetal hydrops, or excessive accumulation of fluids in the body's tissues and cavities, leading
to heart failure. The disease is particularly dangerous because fetal hydrops can cause pregnant women to become quite sick, and possibly die,
through a mechanism called placental transfer. As fluids are released
from the placenta into the woman's bloodstream, she may develop severe
preeclampsia (hypertension) or pulmonary edema (accumulation of
fluid in the lungs). The surgeon described this as "the 'maternal mirror
syndrome' because the mom's condition begins to mirror that of the fetus." After several fetuses died either during or after C-CAM surgeries,
the fetal surgery team at Capital Hospital determined that the bigger the
tumor, the less likely a fetus (and possibly the pregnant woman) is to survive surgery. As one fetal surgeon pointed out regarding the initial fetal
deaths, "Along the way, you actually learn more from things that are not
successful than from things that are successful." Laboratory research in
fetal lambs subsequently generated a technique for resecting lung tissue,
deflating the chest, and "curing" the hydrops. According to this surgeon,
patient selection for C-CAMs currently rests on a *clinical* evaluation of fetuses that includes assessment of lung tumor size, gestational age, and
the degree of advancement of fetal hydrops.

Yet clinical evaluations may also be related to the broader research
goals of experimental fetal surgery. One fetal surgeon pointed out that
there have been "a number of biologic spin-offs from this work." These
include, for example, the wound healing research discussed in chapter 3
and efforts to solve the preterm labor problem including the introduction of new drugs and technologies to prevent it. According to another
surgeon, "the preterm labor problem is to fetal therapy what rejection is
to transplantation. And we're working like crazy to come up with the

medication, like cyclosporin was for transplantation, to treat the preterm labor problem. If folks here can do it, then that would have implications beyond our little fetal therapy enterprise. That would have implications for a huge health problem." But not everybody involved with the Fetal Treatment Unit is enthusiastic about these potential scientific advances. An obstetrician complained that "the fetal surgical group constantly wants to introduce new things that have not been thoroughly tried. There's a very different approach to how experimental things should be introduced." In response to my obviously transparent probing about the ethics of experimentation, this same informant sharply queried, "Are you asking me whether I think the human pregnant woman and fetus should be used as an experimental animal? I think that is what's happening."

The contradiction between what are defined as "clinical" and "non-clinical" factors in selection is particularly evident in conflicts between fetal surgeons and their colleagues over criteria for surgery. Consider the situation, to which I alluded earlier, in which a social worker's evaluation about a potential patient was dismissed in favor of narrow clinical criteria, with particularly unsettling consequences. April, a young, white, single woman whose fetus was diagnosed with a congenital diaphragmatic hernia, was referred to the FTU for treatment. Below are excerpts from my fieldnotes taken at a meeting during which April's treatment was discussed:

> The meeting began with a description of the patient to be operated on. Ultrasound had been abnormal, indicating a possible diaphragmatic hernia. The woman smokes (mentioned by Dr. ——— as a health status indicator) and is on public aid, at which point Dr. ——— commented that the only thing that means for the Fetal Treatment Unit is they won't be paid. A social worker responded to questions about April's background and social situation. She commented that April is smart, "has religion," knows that her baby might die, and is "quite remarkable for a 19–year old," which garnered several grunts of agreement from the others present. According to the social worker, the bottom line is that April knows the risks and wants the surgery. Based in part on the social worker's assessment of April's emotional condition and the surgeons' medical assessments, the decision was made to go ahead with the surgery. They decided to schedule it for 6:00 A.M. on Tuesday. April would be admitted to the hospital on Monday evening.

It is interesting to contrast my ethnographic record of the decision-making process with an informant's recollection and interpretation of it. According to the social worker who handled her case, April "was a product of foster homes. She had a little kid, she was in a second relationship, new partner, *but she was like a perfect physical specimen. She was young,* she was strong, the baby had the right liver. And it was one of the real successes of the program. But in the end she took him home and shook him, shook her baby, and he was taken away" (emphasis added). Here the social worker alludes to some of the research motives underlying fetal surgery—young women make good clinical research materials—and points out that even when a case seems ideal from a clinical point of view, unknown and unanticipated factors may influence the outcome. In our interview, she suggested that fetal surgery may be a traumatic experience for pregnant women and consequently for their families, particularly when a pregnant woman's life circumstances and social support networks are less than optimal, as in April's case. The lesson this social worker hoped to convey is that clinical success does not necessarily translate into postoperative success; it is likely that nobody would find much to celebrate when a young woman's life is disrupted by medical intervention and she ultimately loses custody of her child. Yet, in the social worker's comment, she referred to this case as one of the "real successes" of the Fetal Treatment Unit.

While social workers and other nonsurgical providers, such as genetic counselors and nurses, do not dismiss clinical criteria or outcomes that are often quite serious, they are most interested in whether a pregnant woman will psychologically be able to withstand the rigors of fetal surgery and has adequate social support in place. These are issues that fetal surgeons and obstetricians, focused on clinical factors, consider only peripherally in practice. Emphasis on treating fetal patients draws attention away from other participants and considerations in fetal surgery, such as the physical and emotional health of pregnant women and their families. Where women are considered, it is as bodies whose proper functioning affects and constrains fetal surgery. Rarely considered beyond superficial calls for ethical analysis is how fetal surgery may profoundly affect women's health and lives. The social workers, counselors, and some nurses in the Fetal Treatment Unit, fully aware of this dynamic, strive to provide adequate psychosocial care to their constituency but are constrained in how much they can do by clinical practices aimed at "saving" fetuses and by institutionalized hierarchies of hospital care in which they typically have less power than physicians. Simultaneously, although surgeons and obstetricians do consider psychological and social factors, these issues often play second fiddle to clinical criteria and broader research goals. Thus, the prioritizing of work objects and selection of patients, essential to the social organization of fetal surgery, may have significant consequences for pregnant women, who may be conceptualized and treated as a technical means to the clinical end of fetal rescue and repair.

Negotiating the "How" of Fetal Surgery: Different Views of a Disease and Its Treatment

The third area of difference among practitioners that I focus on here concerns evaluation and treatment of fetal disease. More specifically, I discuss debates that occurred concerning what should or should not be done to correct a particular disease, namely, congenital diaphragmatic hernia (CDH). This is a condition diagnosable by ultrasound in which fetal abdominal organs migrate upward into the fetus's chest through a hole in its diaphragm. The disease is often fatal because normal, healthy lung development is impaired and fetuses die in utero of respiratory failure. Not all fetal surgical treatments are as controversial as CDH and are therefore less revealing of certain interactional dynamics. For example, repairing blocked urinary tracts is seen as a "routine" procedure in fetal surgery and it generates relatively little controversy. What makes CDH particularly contested is the very high fetal mortality rates associated with the disease, whether it is treated prenatally or after birth. At the time of my study, fetal mortality for CDH cases treated prenatally was near 75 percent and even the few fetuses who survived were not completely healthy. *All* surviving fetuses required additional postnatal surgery and follow-up.

The fetal surgery team at Capital Hospital began pursuing prenatal surgery for CDH with the hope and expectation that early treatment would prevent the condition from worsening. That is, they anticipated that prenatal surgery to repair the hernia would enable an adequate growth period in utero for fetal lungs and would prevent a cascade of related structural problems from developing. Following a series of animal experiments, surgeons decided that they were ready to attempt CDH repair in human fetuses in 1983. They performed a handful of operations with no success; of the first five cases, all fetuses died either during surgery or shortly thereafter. As one surgeon observed subsequently, "The learning curve in fetal surgery is steep." Through the ensuing years, surgeons attempted additional CDH operations, often modifying their techniques in practice. In 1993 they developed a procedure called PLUG (discussed more fully in chapter 5), which proved equally problematic. Mortality statistics did not improve significantly, and prenatal CDH repair eventually receded as a major focus of the Fetal Treatment Unit. This does not mean that all CDH repair has ceased; sometimes an infant born with CDH can be operated on successfully and many CDH cases are treated after birth. Yet despite low success rates and opposition from some of their colleagues, surgeons have not given up hope for the resuscitation of prenatal CDH repair. It is useful to examine the debates around CDH not only for what they reveal about the internal politics of fetal surgery, but also for how they have contributed to the demise of one type of surgical procedure in a constantly evolving specialty.

Because it was so unsuccessful, CDH became a sort of rallying cry around which critics of fetal surgery organized their resistance while fetal surgeons struggled to meet the challenges posed by this easy-to-diagnose but difficult-to-treat disease. Fetal surgeons were very enthusiastic about the promise of prenatal treatment for CDH, even while recognizing that their lack of success marked the procedure as controversial. They were thrilled when the Fetal Treatment Unit received a grant from the National Institutes of Health in 1991 to conduct a controlled trial of CDH cases. They believed there was a great deal at stake in the study. As one surgeon told me, "We've just begun this NIH trial, and we've been in starts and stops, moratoriums, you name the process, we've been through it. It's been extremely frustrating, and it's hard to know if formal diaphragmatic hernia repairs will be possible before birth. We're hoping that this trial will have the answer, so we can tell the rest of the world that yes, this is worth doing, or no, stop doing it, and you have to just take your chances after birth." Initial outcomes of the study were discouraging to surgeons because many fetuses died. Yet the fetal surgeons, and the women enrolled in their study, kept trying and hoping. As one surgeon pointed out, "Most of the mistakes, or most of the things we've learned, have been the result of frustrations doing the first few clinical diaphragmatic hernia repairs. And things that you couldn't have predicted no matter how many fetal animals you've done. So that's a very controversial area of treatment." When I mentioned that I had heard some negative criticism about the CDH cases from other practitioners, a fetal surgeon remarked: "But that's fine, that's good, at least now we can sort of put it to the test and see once and for all, after incredible painstaking review by the NIH. That's the way it gets sorted out."

While fetal surgeons continued to investigate and advocate surgery for CDH, other participants became increasingly outspoken in their criticisms of the practice. An obstetrician declared, "I think now you'll get divergent opinions. They are still enthusiastic about CDH, we are definitely not and I'm willing to go on the record saying that. I would not recommend that any of my patients have open CDH surgery. The chance of survival is much greater to not have surgery and deliver in a tertiary center [general hospital] than the surgical survival is right now. There are just problems that have never been solved." When I asked him if he thought the conflict had to do with different professional training, he replied angrily, "It's not a disciplinary split! Get the actual numbers of how many CDH cases have been done and what the success rate is, and how many of those kids are living. Then compare that to the fact that if you come in here and have a CDH that we diagnose prenatally, and you deliver in a tertiary center, there's very good evidence that you will have a 40 percent survival rate. And you will draw your own conclusion as to whether you would ever have such surgery or whether you would ever suggest to a patient that they have it." With respect to *postnatal* surgery for CDH, he went on to assert that "the pediatric surgeon still gets to operate on them, but it's a less sexy thing and it's something everybody's doing."

Social workers, nurses, and genetic counselors, who disagreed with physicians about selection criteria for treatment, often found themselves on the same side of the CDH debate as obstetricians. Many were deeply disturbed by these cases. In the words of one informant, a nurse, "I found myself feeling like maybe this wasn't the best thing we were doing. It would be a relief to me if they weren't doing fetal surgery for the diaphragmatic hernia." Her reasons were similar to the obstetricians' and had to do with the mortality rates. She points out, "I can't recall very many healthy survivors of the fetal surgery program [for CDH]." Also like the obstetricians, other nonsurgical practitioners expressed a certain amount of distrust of the fetal surgeons. One social worker remarked, "I was wondering about the presentation and whether we hadn't been manipulating statistics in a way to make it sound like this was an alternative to these kids going to term. I really felt although they were trying to be honest, it was very hard to really paint an accurate picture and expect that anybody would actually do a thing like this, put themselves through this." As we spoke about the CDH cases, she grew visibly upset and finally remarked, "I don't know how many more moms and babies we can bring up to the altar of fetal surgery with the outcomes that we're having. It's not as though you go through this and you're gonna have a healthy kid at the end!"

Several obstetricians, nurses, genetic counselors, and social workers I interviewed suggested that the CDH cases were in part motivated by professional interests of fetal surgeons. Fetal surgery has often been referred to as the "final frontier" in reproductive medicine, and it has certainly been a career-making enterprise for fetal surgeons (Kolata 1990), if not for other medical workers. Those with whom surgeons work are acutely aware of these professional issues. In response to my question about why fetal surgeons continue to do CDH surgeries in the face of high mortality rates, one obstetrician replied bitingly, "Well, they believe in themselves. They believe they're going to stamp out disease and save babies. And I think what they're doing at this point is unfair and it borders on being immoral. Therefore our group is no longer part of it." This is yet another example of the split between obstetricians and fetal surgeons discussed earlier, although here professional differences transcend definitions of work objects and cut to the core of whether fetal surgery should even be pursued.

One of the critical care nurses also put her finger on the pulse of professional interests, remarking that "there are kids who have hernias the size of the Grand Canyon. And Dr. ——— is the kind of guy who really likes to take on something like diaphragmatic hernia. It's one of the most vexing problems. Sometimes I look at [the fetal surgeons], I step back, and I think, Can't they see that this isn't really going very well? When are we going to say, gee, this isn't really working? Maybe we need to move on to something else. But the further along they get, the more dogged they get in their determination to meet every problem with a solution." This last statement was said with a tone closer to admiration than criticism; regardless of how else their colleagues feel about the fetal surgeons, they seem to recognize them as deeply committed to the work of salvaging fetuses. But given the professional ethos of surgery, which differs from that of other specialties, the most difficult problems are often seen as the most challenging and rewarding. And it is the difficult problems and cases that generate the most conflict among practitioners.

How treatment of fetal diseases such as CDH is defined and negotiated relates to definitions of work objects. Because surgeons define the fetus as the primary work object, attempting to correct a lethal disease surgically is seen as the most logical course of action. But neither obstetricians nor other medical workers necessarily consider fetuses to be primary work objects. For them, work practices center not on saving the fetus surgically, but rather on rescuing fetuses from fetal surgeons through activities that promote maternal health (physical and emotional) and fetal well-being. These activities may well include criticizing fetal surgeons for pushing certain treatments, such as prenatal CDH repair, that seem inconsistent with overall goals of healthier women and babies. During the period when CDH was most intently debated, the potential benefits of prenatal CDH repair were perceived as far too few to outweigh the considerable costs. Thus CDH, which has proved remarkably resistant to prenatal treatment, also proved to be a charged issue among certain medical workers in fetal surgery who were more cautious than others about forging ahead. Despite many practitioners' concerns about maternal health and dismal fetal outcomes, surgeons diligently pursued prenatal surgical repair of diaphragmatic hernias until the NIH grant ended. This indicates that some medical workers—in this case, the more powerful surgeons—were able to dominate the trajectory of fetal surgery as a practice focused on rescuing the unborn patient, even where the "treatments" themselves were highly controversial and contested by their colleagues.

The Politics of Difference in Fetal Surgery

Fetal surgery is a negotiated yet fluid order, given institutional and practical shape through the interactions and work practices of its participants. As a dynamic and diverse enterprise, fetal surgery is characterized by cooperation, conflict, and a range of other ongoing interactions. Participants coalesce around fetuses and pregnant women in different ways, and there is both agreement and dissent surrounding who or what is the work object in fetal surgery. These interactional patterns shape such aspects of fetal surgery as patient selection and definitions of diseases and their treatment. Differences between practitioners are thus mobilized in certain ways to produce a negotiated order, an outcome that supports the overall institutional goals of the Fetal Treatment Unit—saving babies—while differences may continue to rage internally. This *politics of difference*, a key component of negotiating order, refers to how diversity is mobilized and articulated by social actors in different ways and for various purposes. Such politics are an extension of the hybridity I discussed in the previous chapter; in this case, however, hybrid refers to the multidisciplinary practitioners in fetal surgery and their complex interactions. Cooperation and conflict, endemic to fetal surgery, are two possible types of interactions through which the politics of difference are played out.

The politics of difference also means that while there are many participants in this domain, some are heard and seen more clearly than others in the making of the unborn patient. Focusing on how different actors define work objects and organize their work practices highlights the many alliances and cleavages formed in this world. Fetal surgery may well be a negotiated order, but it is continually evolving in response to other factors shaping negotiation. A context in which fetuses are defined as primary work objects leaves little room for the practical differences among actors to filter up to the institutional level. Most significant, surgeons have been successful in framing fetal surgery in line with their own commitments and interests, while resistance by other medical workers has been muted. As one surgeon remarked, "None of [the other practitioners] would be needed, it would be down to a single group of physicians, if we could just make them realize the goal is to get the fetus to survive the operation. We need a czar. We need to be the czar." The point here is not to demonize fetal surgeons or to impugn their commitments to healthier babies, but rather to show how negotiations are patterned within and by institutional hierarchies, access to work objects, and professional investments in human fetuses.

It is likely impossible for fetal surgeons to ever gain complete control over fetal surgery when the cooperation of other providers—especially obstetricians, neonatologists, nurses, and social workers—is essential to the enterprise. Indeed, there is some indication that a few of the most egregious differences described here have been worked out since I conducted this research. In follow-up interviews with some of my informants, I was told that while my characterization of the conflict between different participants involved in fetal surgery is accurate, it reflects a specific period of time in the evolution of the fetal surgery program. There appears to have been a normalization of some conflict over time, a common occurrence in medicine as new techniques are introduced and subsequently routinized (Koenig 1988; Reiser 1982; Reiser and Anbar 1986). Yet, according to many informants, the salient differences related to definitions of work objects continue to occupy participants in this field, even while they strive cooperatively to meet the Fetal Treatment Unit's institutional aims of rescuing fetuses from certain death. How, and if, these differences will be resolved is contingent upon an array of factors. There is little reason to believe that contestation will simply cease should fetal surgeons, or any other group, become "czars" over the terrain of fetal surgery. Is is far more likely that fetal surgery, as both a set of practices at Capital Hospital and as a new specialty, will continue to be shaped by negotiations involving an array of different interactions and struggles.

Focusing on the politics of difference also means carefully considering the broader implications of fetal surgery and how local work practices might seep out of the operating room and into other spheres of social life. For example, surgeons' emphasis on fetal work objects constructs pregnant women as barriers that must be passed through in order to reach the primary patient. Although there are workers in this domain who advocate for pregnant women, such as social workers and nurses, the interactional fabric of fetal surgery is woven in such a way that being an advocate for anybody other than a fetus is very hard work. The social workers, self-proclaimed "handmaidens" to the clinicians, are often unable to address psychosocial concerns of pregnant women because clinical criteria applied to fetuses take precedence and because social work is positioned well below surgery within the medical hierarchy. While obstetricians also attempt to advocate for pregnant women, their more circumscribed clinical orientation often precludes attention to important psychosocial and emotional issues. These dynamics have a number of implications, including possible compromised maternal health and well-being and even fetal survival.

This is not to suggest that if social workers or nurses or any other group interested in the broader implications of fetal surgery had more power and were able to advocate for pregnant women, fetal surgery would be without problems (although it would be marvelous if the decision to treat a pregnant woman with a sick fetus included *all* of the many social, cultural, psychological, economic, and clinical factors affecting her life). The issues here are much more complex than simply replacing "clinical" concerns with "social-psychological" ones. Rather, an important task in fetal surgery, as in any medical practice, is to determine where the "social" and the "clinical" overlap, and how the politics of difference impact on both the ongoing emergence of medical specialties and the health and well-being of the patients they serve. As I have shown, it is in these intersections, rich with the intricacies of work, cultural practices, and politics, that the unborn patient has been made and contested. The next chapter explores these organizational dynamics further, focusing specifically on the human subjects approval process at Capital Hospital as an important site of contention.

Chapter 5

Clinical Trials in Fetal Surgery

Making, Protecting, and Contesting Human Subjects

During the same period that different specialists at Capital Hospital were negotiating and contesting the shape of fetal surgery, another set of actors was drawing important connections between the work itself and its controversial objects, as well as its broader social implications. As bioethicists John Fletcher and Albert Jonsen (1991, 14) have asserted, "Experimental fetal therapy is the occasion for several significant ethical problems." Fetal surgery is indeed troubling, but who gets to determine what is "ethical"—and for whom—on this biomedical frontier is itself a source of contention. I address this issue through an examination of the lively but tense working relationship between members of the Fetal Treatment Unit (FTU) and the Institutional Review Board (IRB), a committee charged with protecting human subjects used in biomedical research at Capital Hospital. Here, I introduce an oft-hidden set of work practices and actors as a key site in the formation of an experimental medical specialty and its patients. As an object of sociological inquiry, the complicated process of seeking and obtaining IRB approval embodies the hybrid shape of medical work including local and extralocal politics, cultural meanings, and organizational dynamics.[1]

In general, IRBs serve as organizational mediators between the federal agencies responsible for protecting human subjects and the scientists and clinicians researching them. All biomedical institutions covered by federal regulations or supported by federal funding, such as Capital Hospital, are required to establish an IRB to evaluate research on humans in accordance with federal guidelines and ethical principles (discussed more fully below). There is broad recognition that the relationship between a medical researcher and her subject is very different from the traditional doctor-patient relationship. As Rothman (1990, 193) observed with respect to the origins of IRBs in the 1960s, "conflict of

interest marked the interaction of investigator and subject [and] what
was in the best interests of one was not in the best interests of the other.
The bedrock principle of medical ethics, that the physician acted only to
promote the well-being of the patient, did not hold in the laboratory"—or
in clinical settings. Thus, biomedical *research*, unlike routine or innovative practices, cannot proceed without IRB oversight and approval. To
secure approval while minimizing conflict of interest, clinical researchers must adhere to broad federal guidelines, but they do so by negotiating their compliance with local IRBs (sometimes called ethics
committees). IRBs are authoritative, if not always effective, institutional
actors uniquely positioned for potential clashes with the medical researchers they oversee. Guided by a larger regulatory framework but
working within concrete settings such as hospitals, IRBs and medical researchers wrangle over what constitutes "ethical" (or, rather, acceptable)
research procedures. Assuring accountability of researchers—a key task
of IRBs—is consequently shaped by ambiguity, tension, and conflict, all
of which must be continually negotiated and managed.

The IRB at Capital Hospital is composed of about fifteen members
representing a variety of specialties, including pediatrics, internal medicine, radiology, cardiology, immunology, oncology, surgery, psychology,
medical anthropology, and many others, illustrating another aspect of
the hybridity discussed in chapters 3 and 4. There is always at least one
community member on the committee, and all members serve two-year
terms. IRB negotiations have been particularly intense at Capital Hospital, where efforts to secure human subjects protection for women and
their fetuses have, at times, dominated the work of the IRB. This emphasis is rather extraordinary given that Capital Hospital is a major research
and teaching facility with hundreds of scientific protocols ongoing at
any one time.[2] But as a new specialty plagued by high failure rates and
linked to broader social and political issues, fetal surgery has been
fraught with controversy. Conflicts over the work of fetal surgery are prolific and, as we have seen, occur both inside and outside the Fetal Treatment Unit. Disagreements involving the IRB represent special challenges
to the development of fetal surgery and to the making of the unborn patient. While approval of fetal surgery protocols facilitates the growth of
the specialty, the IRB's insistence on accountability both slows the process and shapes what kinds of practices may proceed.

IRB members, like the providers discussed in chapter 4, are deeply
concerned about the fate of human work objects in fetal surgery. They
too collectively engage in a type of work central to the making of the unborn patient. But for the IRB, as we shall see, fetal surgery itself is the
work object in question; while IRB members care about fetuses and
pregnant women, their focus is on the actual research practices. They

look not only at what surgeons can do, but also at what they should (or should not) do and at potential consequences of their actitivies. No matter their training or specialty prior to serving on the IRB, once on board they become ad hoc ethicists. The IRB considers such problematic issues as definitions of the patient, the viability of operating on fetuses, the social implications of operating on pregnant women, informed consent, risks and benefits, costs, and, perhaps most significant, the blurred boundaries among experiments, innovations, and standard treatments in medicine. Because their perspective often differs substantially from that of the fetal surgery team, the process of obtaining a green light from the IRB to conduct research has involved many iterations of protocol submissions, denials, revisions, approvals, and renewals.

The IRB at Capital Hospital has been a crucial constraint on the making of fetal surgery there. For example, by 1993 the IRB had grown increasingly concerned about the implications of fetal surgery for human subjects and believed that the fetal surgery team was minimizing these concerns and failing to respond in the most appropriate manner. Several committee members remained unconvinced that fetal surgery offered *any* positive benefits to society, stating in one document that "what remains unclear are the potential benefits of the studies for the babies, the mothers, and society. Simple 'survival' of the child and mother until the expected time of delivery is not an adequate measure." As an entity charged with regulating biomedical research, the IRB did the only thing it could do when faced with perceived threats to human subjects: it suspended all fetal surgery protocols. (Anticipating the IRB's punitive action, fetal researchers had already voluntarily suspended activity on their protocols.)

Before it would consider reinstating the protocols, the IRB demanded better explanations of criteria for inclusion and exclusion, more accurate reporting of results, and more comprehensive informed consent procedures. Importantly, it also mandated the formation of an Oversight Committee (OC) for fetal surgery, the first time ever that such an organizational innovation had been proposed at Capital Hospital in relation to an experimental procedure. The OC is testament to the complicated issues surrounding fetal surgery. It is equal parts interpreter, liaison, and watchdog, and is charged with providing intensive peer review of fetal surgery protocols. After the OC's inception, the IRB only reviewed protocols that were first approved by the committee, although it retained the power of approval or rejection over these. By agreeing to meet the IRB's requirements and to work closely with the OC, the fetal surgery team was rewarded with restoration of its protocols later that year. But the circumstances surrounding the suspension and reinstatement assured that relations between the IRB and the fetal surgery team would be marked by ongoing contention. As the suspension illustrates, the IRB approval process is an ideal site for examining important factors and perspectives that are built into—and left out of—experimental treatment of fetuses.

The analysis in this chapter reflects a deep concern with issues traditionally identified as the domain of bioethics, but the analysis is sociological and situated within a broader critique leveled against bioethics by many social scientists (e.g., Weisz 1990). All too often, these critics argue, bioethical pronouncements seem to float down from the sky—usually requiring scriptural interpretation by bioethicists—and are devoid of any connection to what is really going on in a particular social situation. Traditional bioethics approaches have been "top down," moving from theory to practice with a core focus on abstract, universalizing principles. In contrast, the newer approaches move from the study of actual practices to an empirical interpretation—from practice to theory. In focusing on how ethical decisions in medicine are *actually made*, critics have attempted to counter persistent bioethical abstractions. Following these approaches, I reframe "ethics" as a set of concrete social practices that can be captured ethnographically, examining the social processes and judgments underlying what comes to count as an acceptable practice. This approach is different from most standard ethical analyses of fetal surgery, which tend to render sweeping judgments based on moral or religious principles and typically focus on fetal status (Chervenak and McCullough 1985; Mastroianni 1986; Sgreccia 1989; Twomey 1989; Walters 1986).[3] I argue instead that ethical formulations about what can be done to pregnant women and their fetuses are social rather than reflective of some inherent natural status or order unveiled by medicine. The "ethics" of fetal surgery, including human subjects protection, has as much to do with routine work practices as it does with morality.

Guidelines for Protecting Human Subjects: An Overview

From the polio vaccine to penicillin, biomedical research has resulted in amazing and significant contributions to human life. But medicine and science, for all their promise, also raise pressing moral and political questions. With each exciting discovery or achievement, such as fetal surgery or cloning, come new quandaries. These concerns have to do not only with our capacity to alter and redefine human destiny, but also with the implications of doing so. Bioethical dilemmas often have as much to do with how research is done as with its dazzling and beneficial products. Such dilemmas are intensified in experimental medicine, where research subjects are human beings—often at their most vulnerable due to sickness. Research on humans, no matter how beneficial the outcome, continues to be haunted by the legacy of Nazi medicine and its flagrant human rights abuses, including grisly experiments on and euthanasia of concentration camp prisoners (Alexander 1949; Proctor 1988). After World War II, collective horror and a resolute desire to prevent such violations in the future prompted the development of standards for research involving human subjects. The Nuremberg Code of 1947, emerging from the Nuremberg War Crime Trials, established an international code of practice for judging physicians and scientists who had engaged in medical research violating human rights. This code served as a prototype for subsequent standards, including policies formulated in the United States in the post-World War II era.

In the 1960s, a number of disturbing reports about human experimentation in the United States became public knowledge, reinforcing cultural anxieties about the power of medicine and science in people's lives. These included the notorious Tuskegee study (Jones 1993)[4] and a series of research abuses on servicemen, prisoners, and vulnerable populations such as the institutionalized elderly and mentally disabled (Beecher 1966; Rothman 1990).[5] Rothman (1990, 190) argues that these graphic and shocking reports did for Americans what the Nuremburg Trials did not; namely, they brought "the ethics of medical experimentation into the public domain and [made] apparent the consequences of leaving decisions about clinical research exclusively to the individual investigator." One of the outcomes was the formulation of the U.S. National Research Act of 1974 and its offshoot, the National Commission for the Protection of Human Subjects of Biomedical and Behavioral Research. The latter body was charged with identifying bioethical principles and developing guidelines to assure compliance with those principles for federally funded research in the United States. The commission was given the task of considering such issues as the boundaries between biomedical research and the routine practice of medicine ("standard of care"), assessment of risks and benefits, appropriate guidelines for selecting human subjects, and the meanings of and standards for informed consent to be a research subject. The resulting federal guidelines contain a set of broad bioethical principles and have served for two decades as a basis for evaluating biomedical research in terms of its treatment of human subjects—a core task of IRBs.[6]

The first principle has to do with the distinction between standard practice and research, a distinction that is often unclear because these activities can and do occur together, as in experimental therapies like fetal surgery. Here, *practice* refers to medical interventions designed to enhance patient well-being that are likely to be successful and that already enjoy routine or regular use. By contrast, *research* is defined as any activity designed to test something and is usually described in a formal protocol as distinct from practice and innovation: "when a clinician departs in a significant way from standard or accepted practice, the innovation does not, in and of itself, constitute research. The fact that a procedure is 'experimental,' in the sense of new, untested or different, does not automatically place it in the category of research" (*Belmont Report* 1979, 3). But, the federal guidelines go on to say, innovations should be made objects of research at an early stage to determine whether they are safe and effective, and it is up to IRBs to insist on this early testing. When research and practice are carried out together, such activities "should undergo review for the protection of human subjects" because they contain an element of research.

The second principle concerns respect for persons, beneficence, and justice. *Respect for persons* means that individuals should be treated as autonomous agents and that persons with diminished autonomy are entitled to special protections. As we shall see below, this principle is complicated by protocols where fetuses are research subjects. In most research, respecting persons requires that subjects voluntarily participate in the research and are given adequate information upon which to base their decision to participate. According to the federal guidelines (*Belmont Report* 1979:4), "respecting persons, in most hard cases, is often a matter of balancing competing claims urged by the principle of respect itself." *Beneficence* refers to a researcher's obligation to make every effort to protect and secure the well-being of her subjects. This is expressed in the injunctions to do no harm and to maximize benefits while minimizing risks. Yet, as the guidelines point out (1979, 4), "even avoiding harm requires learning what is harmful; and, in the process of obtaining this information, persons may be exposed to risk of harm." In other words, the task is to determine when it is justifiable to seek larger clinical and social benefits through research despite the risks involved. *Justice* refers to inequities in who participates in research and who ultimately benefits. The burdens of research historically have often fallen upon the poor and illiterate, such as in the Tuskegee study, while others with more resources benefit downstream. The federal guidelines require that "the selection of research subjects needs to be scrutinized in order to determine whether some classes [of patients] . . . are being systematically selected simply because of their easy availability, their compromised position, or their manipulability" (*Belmont Report* 1979, 5).

The third general principle concerns the *application* of the other principles in relation to informed consent and risk/benefit assessment.[7] *Informed consent* means that human subjects must be given the opportunity to choose what will and will not happen to them; that is, subjects must be provided with enough information to make an informed decision, including the purpose of the research, risks and benefits, costs, and alternative procedures. Informed consent is both controversial and extremely important because "research takes place precisely when a common understanding does not exist. . . . The research subject, being in essence a volunteer, may wish to know considerably more about risks gratuitously undertaken than do patients who deliver themselves into the hands of a clinician for needed care" (*Belmont Report* 1979, 5). Guidelines are designed to ensure that information about risks should never be withheld to gain a subject's cooperation, and the requirement of voluntariness is supposed to be respected at all times. Moreover, information should be presented in a manner that subjects will be able to comprehend. For subjects defined as "incompetent" (e.g., the mentally disabled, young children, infants, fetuses), informed consent should be sought from third parties who are most likely to act in the subject's best interests. The more serious the risks and the more vulnerable the subjects, the greater the obligation on researchers to adhere to the federal guidelines—or to not do the research at all.

Assessment of risks and benefits refers to the balance of possible harms and anticipated benefits. In other words, is it worth it—on any number of levels—to pursue a particular research protocol? This has been especially germane to fetal surgery and other consequential "state-of-the-art" practices, where concern centers on who benefits from certain procedures. Risk/benefit assessments occur through a thorough analysis of existent data, close examination of protocols and research designs by researchers and IRBs, and thoughtful analysis of whether risks are justified in light of probable benefits. Risks are defined as potential harms, while benefits are conceived as something of positive value related to health and welfare. The human subjects process itself, through the ongoing accumulation and assessment of information, is designed to provide systematic analysis of risks and benefits.

Two additional ethical codes apply to risk/benefit assessment: brutal or inhumane treatment is never morally justified, and risks should be reduced to those necessary to achieve the research aims. These codes are especially relevant in situations where human subjects are deemed "incompetent" and somebody must represent their interests. But as with all of these ethical principles—and bioethics more generally—determination of "risks" and "benefits," as well as what is considered "inhumane," is relative, situated, and contingent. For example, most of modern medicine has been criticized as dehumanizing in its reductionist focus on body parts and diseases rather than whole persons. How, then, are certain procedures singled out as inhumane or excessively risky? And for whom are they considered as such? As we shall see, in fetal surgery these issues have been hotly contested.

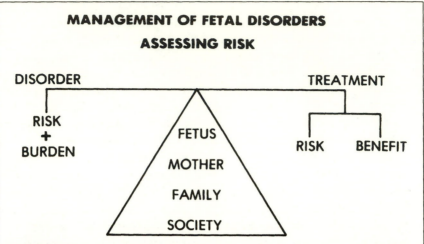

FIGURE 17–4. In counseling and management, the risk and burden of the untreated disorder on the individual and his or her family is compared with the possible benefit of treatment. The risk of the treatment itself may not be known when a procedure is new. It includes not only the possibility of injury to the fetus and mother, but also the possibility that a fatal lesion will be "corrected" to a nonfatal, but disabling one.

Participants in fetal surgery attempt to strike a balance between the risks and benefits, for both women and their fetuses, of fetal disease and its treatment. Achieving such a balance is extremely difficult, as some critics of fetal surgery point out. Risks often exceed benefits to the fetus, the pregnant woman, and society in general. Source: M. R. Harrison, M. S. Golbus, and R. A. Filly. 1991. *The Unborn Patient: Prenatal Diagnosis and Treatment.* Philadelphia: W. B. Saunders Company, p. 163.

The federal guidelines reviewed here are important because they constitute, in part, the criteria for gaining IRB approval. In ongoing interactions between IRBs and the clinical researchers they monitor, the guidelines are a crucial procedural compass. Yet extant standards for protecting human subjects may be inadequate to deal with complex situations, such as fetal surgery, because they are often too broad and thus difficult to interpret or apply. In addition, although the guidelines distinguish between research and therapy, these are *never* clearly drawn in clinical research practices (as we saw in chapter 3) and debates often center on *"how* experimental or *how* therapeutic" a new procedure is (Kaufman 1997, 28; emphasis in original). Renée Fox (1959, 47) described some of these difficulties in her pioneering study of metabolic research, noting that "the physicians of the Metabolic Group often found it difficult to judge whether or not a particular experiment in which they were engaged 'kept within the bounds' delineated by these principles." At the time of Fox's research in the 1950s, the metabolic researchers did not have an IRB to consult—or to be accountable to.[8] Feminist ethicist Susan Sherwin (1992, 168) has suggested that "the fine line separating therapeutic research from 'established' therapies" may be especially permeable in women's health care.

Ironically, today's IRBs—which depend on the federal guidelines to do their job—are also charged with filling in the often wide gaps between standard rules and actual medical research situations involving clinical researchers operating at the edges of what is technically possible and morally acceptable. Indeed, such formulations occur at the very complicated juncture of what constitutes "clinical" and "research" practices. This confusion of boundaries creates a process of ethical oversight that is definitionally ambiguous, leaving ample room for negotiations shaped by local settings and institutional dynamics. Thus, although IRBs and researchers ostensibly structure their practices around established formal guidelines, the actual working out of what is considered ethical and acceptable in biomedical research is contingent, contested, and not at all determined prior to negotiations. Such has certainly been the case at Capital Hospital. Investigating how IRB approval has been sought, contested, achieved, maintained, suspended, and terminated offers up particular incarnations of the fetal surgery enterprise and those who care about it.

A Complex Case: Who are the Human Subjects in Fetal Surgery?

Fetal surgery is particularly complex in terms of IRB approval practices because the most relevant terms—"human" and "subject"—are rendered problematic. First, there is no cultural consensus on the humanity or personhood of the fetus. The contemporary abortion conflict, as well as controversy over the use of human fetal tissue, hinges precisely on this contestation over fetal status. While the fetus may be defined as a human organism by virtue of its DNA, as many have suggested, it is not a thinking, speaking agent. The observation that fetuses respond to stimuli, as argued by Liley and others in the antiabortion movement, does not imply that fetuses are people. Fetuses are incapable of social action, and somebody must always speak for them in a culture in which speech, autonomy, and action are requisite for civic participation. Moreover, fetal subjectivity is not a natural, preexisting ontological status but is rather relational and acquired within specific contexts (Casper 1994a, 1994b; Morgan 1996; Sherwin 1992). If fetuses are seen as human subjects in research, this is a social category into which they have been placed by pregnant women, surgeons, ethicists, lawyers, and others. The fetus is not merely an "incompetent" research subject; it is a deeply relational subject whose varied social status is conferred by other actors. This raises some important questions: When, exactly, does a fetus become a "person" in the sense referred to in the federal guidelines? When does it require special protection? And from whom or what is it being protected?

A second complicating factor in the IRB process is that there are two (interrelated) work objects in fetal surgery: the pregnant woman and her fetus. But only one of these objects is also a "subject" capable of choosing to participate in biomedical research. In most research, human subjects speak for themselves when they either accept or deny treatment—at least theoretically. Both the risks and the benefits are theirs alone, as Fox (1959), Fox and Swazey (1974), and many others have so eloquently demonstrated. In fetal surgery, however, pregnant women consent to surgery on behalf of both themselves *and* their fetuses. As we shall see in chapter 6, women assume a great deal of risk in fetal surgery but gain no personal clinical benefit. Fetal surgery focuses solely on the assumed clinical needs of the unborn patient. Or, as one fetal surgeon told me, "We tend to view the fetus as independent. We're not looking at the mother; we see her as a carrier for the fetus." Thus, pregnant women are recognized as human subjects in terms of informed consent and risks, but research *benefits* are directed solely toward their fetuses. This creates a complicated situation for IRBs, which must attempt to sort out the distinctions and connections among fetal risks and benefits, maternal risks and benefits, and informed consent of pregnant women.

Although pregnant women are the most obvious spokespersons for their embryonic progeny, the politics of reproduction ensure that women's authority is highly contested. Third parties—as contrasted to pregnant women themselves—increasingly claim to speak on behalf of fetal rights and interests (Macklin 1990; Nelson and Milliken 1990; Ryan 1990; Steinbock 1992). Fletcher and Jonsen (1991, 15) suggest that consent for fetal treatments may be obtained from the pregnant woman *or* (not *and*) from "an impartial physician, involved in the fetal medicine team, to 'speak for' the fetus."[9] In research where the benefits are not clearly defined, a woman's refusal of fetal therapy may be considered ethically and legally sound." Yet Fletcher and Jonsen (1991, 16) go on to suggest that "the prospect of efficacious therapy suggest[s] a serious reflection on the issue of conflict between fetal well-being and maternal autonomy." This is remarkable given the substance of the federal guidelines reviewed above. How can somebody other than the human subject herself, who will experience the surgery and mother a surviving child (disabled or not), "consent" to fetal surgery? Does pregnancy—particularly one involving a vulnerable fetus—diminish a woman's capacity as a human subject? Why, in this instance, is the personhood of women contingent? And, according to what bioethical logic can we describe as "impartial" a partisan physician involved in fetal medicine and advocating for the fetus?

Because of the challenges it poses, any research on pregnant women and/or their fetuses is treated as a special case in the federal guidelines for protecting human subjects. It is useful to consider the terms used to define who is affected by these principles and when. *Pregnancy* is defined as the period from confirmation of implantation until expulsion or extraction of the fetus. A *fetus* is defined as the product of conception from the time of implantation until a determination is made, following expulsion or extraction of the fetus, that it is viable. (Fetus is not distinguished from embryo in these guidelines.) *Viability* is defined as the ability of the fetus, after either spontaneous or induced delivery, to survive given the benefits of available medical therapies. All of these definitions are salient in fetal surgery, but they are challenged there, as well, as they shift with new technical practices. Pregnancy is *not* continuous in fetal surgery; the procedure actually ruptures pregnancy when a woman's uterus is opened. The fetus is extracted during fetal surgery and then replaced within a pregnant woman's uterus, confusing notions of fetal status and viability. Once a fetus has been removed from a woman's uterus, is it still, technically, a fetus? At what points during fetal surgery is a fetus viable, and how might the technology itself refigure this determination? The guidelines are no assistance on these complex matters, and it is left to IRBs to negotiate definitions in concert with clinicians.

There are two distinct categories of research highlighted in the federal guidelines that are germane to fetal surgery: activities directed toward pregnant women as subjects and activities directed toward fetuses in utero as subjects. Pregnant women can be subjects only if "the purpose of the activity is to meet the health needs of the mother and the fetus will be placed at risk only to the minimum extent necessary . . . *or the risk to the fetus is minimal*" (DHHS 1991, 13; emphasis added). Fetuses in utero can be subjects only if "the purpose of the activity is to meet the health needs of the particular fetus and the fetus will be placed at risk only to the minimum extent necessary . . . *or the risk to the fetus imposed by the research is minimal*" (DHHS 1991:13; emphasis added). In addition, fetuses can be subjects "only if the mother and father are legally competent and have given their informed consent." (Consent of the father is usually explicitly sought, but it is not needed if his identity cannot be ascertained, he is not available, or the pregnancy resulted from rape.) By distinguishing between these categories—research on pregnant women and research on fetuses—the guidelines reinforce the notion that pregnant women and their fetuses are distinct entities. Moreover, the guidelines imply that research on fetuses does not even involve pregnant women, framing the problem as if fetuses were in fact autonomous entities who simply need their parents' permission to undergo surgery.

In terms of human subjects *protection*, what is even more astonishing is the absence of *any* reference to maternal risk in these guidelines; in both cases, risk is considered only in relation to fetuses. Apparently, pregnant women and fetuses both can be research subjects as long as *fetuses* are not unduly harmed. While there is an obvious logical fallacy here, this disregard is consistent with a bioethical (and clinical) framework in which research on fetuses in utero appears to take place outside of women's bodies, which are conceptually erased (e.g., Bowes and Selgestad 1981; Purdy 1990). Nowhere does the section on fetal research cite maternal safety as a consideration, nor does providing informed consent for research on their own bodies guarantee that pregnant women will remain free of harm. Could the guidelines' authors simply not imagine—in the years prior to fetal surgery—any type of fetal research that might also harm pregnant women? It is unsurprising that as we shall see, concern for maternal safety has not been paramount in fetal surgery; after all, even the federal guidelines on fetal research do not recognize maternal risk. In fetal research, then, the category of "human subject" and its attendant implications is quite murky. This has ramifications for how local IRB permission to do fetal surgery is sought and obtained. It also sheds light on how a local IRB can address maternal safety in the absence of explicit federal language of concern.

Experiment, Innovation, or Standard of Care?

One of the most significant issues concerning interpretation of principles by the IRB is whether or not fetal surgery is indeed *research*. This determination is consequential because of the meanings attached to each salient category—experiment, innovation, or standard of care—in terms of the making of fetal surgery. For example, medicine is full of innovations, some more radical than others. Indeed, in the age of the technological imperative (Fuchs 1968), the *absence* of medical innovation would be remarkable. While innovation embodies certain cultural meanings related to progress, it does not always trigger moral hand-wringing; indeed, there may even be a strong "moral imperative" (Koenig 1988) to use medical technologies. That is, if the technologies exist it may be seen as unethical for clinicians *not* to do everything they can. The categories of experiment and standard of care are weightier both ethically (in terms of protecting human subjects) and economically (in terms of insurance reimbursement). Generally speaking, if an innovation is deemed experimental and included in a research protocol, particularly at a public institution, the study is subject to the federal guidelines regarding human subjects protections. But for a clinician to classify his work as research means sacrificing some degree of professional autonomy and submitting to routine evaluations by an IRB. While the rewards may be great in experimental medicine, restrictions on clinical practice may also increase considerably. Thus, there are pressing reasons why a clinician may be reluctant to abandon the comfortable (and even lucrative) ambiguity of innovation, including limited accountability to human subjects, for the potentially constraining domain of research. But when procedures are especially innovative and consequential, as with fetal surgery, clinicians may have little choice but to classify their work as experimental, at least in the initial stages.

When an innovation or experiment becomes standard of care, the issues are equally complex. If an innovation has never been studied in a formal protocol, questions may surround its appropriateness in routine medicine. Even if it has been researched, this does not guarantee that all of the ethical wrinkles were ironed out. Once a practice or procedure is considered standard of care, there are usually two institutional mechanisms for determining how ethically acceptable it is: informal peer review and ethics committees mandated by hospital accreditation. An IRB does *not* have jurisdiction over routine medicine, although it may mandate the creation of a committee to oversee an innovation's transition from experiment to standard of care. Also, in standard practice patients are *not* considered human subjects and thus are not protected by federal guidelines. It is almost always up to researchers themselves to classify their work, and their motivations for selecting a particular category may vary. There may be important economic reasons for classifying medical practices as standard of care. Most health plans and insurance companies will refuse reimbursement of experimental treatments and will only cover routine medical procedures. This financial imperative raises additional questions, especially regarding clinicians' or institutions' motivations for moving a practice or procedure to standard of care. The obvious risk here is that concern for the patient can get lost in the negotiations between providers and insurers.

The above rules apply to all biomedical research, but in surgery distinctions among these categories are especially ambiguous. Unlike the introduction of new medical devices or drugs requiring FDA approval, where formally establishing efficacy is rigorous and legally must be done before routine use,[10] in surgery the boundaries among experiment, innovation, and standard of care are blurred. Throughout the history of medicine, clinicians have attempted new, sometimes radical therapies in the hope of eradicating disease and curing patients. Consider the classic surgical aphorism: "A chance to cut is a chance to cure." Since they often in-

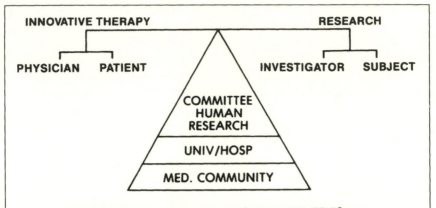

FIGURE 2–3. The institutional setting is important for a fetal treatment program. At this stage, fetal treatment involves elements of both innovative treatment (a physician-patient relationship) and research (an investigator-subject relationship). Deicisons pertaining to treatment must have the support of the Committee on Human Research, the hospital, the university, and, in the long-term, society. Although a decision to attempt treatment may be a matter of medical judgment, it implies an inflexible obligation to report all results, whether good or bad, so that the benefits and liabilities of the treatment can be established as soon as possible.

Here, the balance between innovative therapy and research is seen as hinging on the participation of the institutional review board (IRB), the hospital itself, and the broader medical community. Note the clear distinctions drawn between "physician and patient" in innovative therapy and "investigator and subject" in research. Such distinctions are never as clear-cut in actual practice, where clinical researchers shift among their various, sometimes competing, identities and obligations. Source: M. R. Harrison, M. S. Golbus, and R. A. Filly. 1991. *The Unborn Patient: Prenatal Diagnosis and Treatment*. Philadelphia: W. B. Saunders Company, p. 12.

volve unique situations or single cases, not all surgical innovations have been subject to peer review or IRB approval, nor have they occurred within the context of formal research protocols. Many such innovations occur in the often urgent day-to-day context of attempting to heal sick or dying patients. For these reasons, experimental surgery has had much more latitude than drug therapy. Often in these cases, oversight is determined by informal peer review within each institution. Certain activities may never come within the purview of an IRB simply because clinicians may choose not to classify their work as research. Researchers must seek

IRB approval if their innovation is federally funded, but if it is not, there is a fairly broad scope of permissible treatments. According to an IRB administrator at Capital Hospital, "until an activity is classified as 'research' or 'experimental,' the human subjects issues are less contested."

These issues are significant in terms of fetal surgery's movement among the three categories. Recall from chapter 2 that the history of fetal surgery included a range of innovative treatments that were never part of formal protocols. Indeed, some of the impetus for experimental work carried out in Puerto Rico was precisely to avoid the restrictive ethical regulations being implemented in the mainland United States. In New Zealand, fetal therapy occurred within a context of local, not national, peer review with both the Rh Committee and the Fetal Medicine Advisory Panel offering ongoing evaluations. At Capital Hospital in the late 1970s and early 1980s, many innovations in fetal surgery were tried before they ever became part of formal research protocols. Even then, for many years several different procedures were grouped under one study protocol. We know from chapter 4 that diaphragmatic hernia cases were studied under a clinical trial funded by the NIH, but this procedure was the exception rather than the rule in fetal surgery. In short, fetal surgery at Capital Hospital has not developed in any straightforward progression. Rather, different protocols have been defined as innovation, experiment, *and* standard of care, often at the same time. This has been consequential for the specialty itself and for the making of its human subjects.

A Case Example: The PLUG Odyssey

The trajectory of PLUG ("plug the lung until it grows") offers a good example both of fetal surgery's rather convoluted course at Capital Hospital and of the ways in which a new procedure passes from one category to another. The PLUG procedure, used for the treatment of congenital diaphragmatic hernia (CDH), involves creating a temporary obstruction of the fetal trachea using a floppy sponge. The sponge is removed after birth in a procedure known as EXIT (ex utero intrapartum tracheoplasty). Researchers claim that tracheal obstruction accelerates fetal lung growth and could ameliorate the often fatal pulmonary hypoplasia (underdevelopment of the lungs) associated with severe CDH. In the early 1990s, fetal researchers developed a formal protocol for PLUG after conducting a series of experiments in lamb models. Prior to submission, informal peer evaluation by colleagues at Capital Hospital produced two critical reviews, both of which pointed to the potential for tracheal damage. One concerned reviewer noted in his response, "This matter is treated very briefly if not casually by the investigators." In response to the peer review, fetal researchers modified the protocol to include an expanded consent form, information about follow-up and delivery, and an indication that surviving babies would require ventilation support after delivery. They then submitted the modified protocol to the IRB.

But in the ensuing weeks, *before* the IRB formally responded to the protocol, the fetal researchers performed the PLUG procedure in clinical practice. Recall from the previous chapter that surgeons were eager to solve the vexing diaphragmatic hernia problem and had already tried numerous techniques. When faced with a complicated case, they responded with what Koenig (1988) calls a "desperation reaction": the need to do something immediately to solve the problem. In reporting their results to the Oversight Committee, the surgeons stated: "if one of these alternatives proves to be safer experimentally, we will come back to your committee for permission to pursue it clinically. We are trying our hardest not to get into that uncomfortable situation where we are surprised at the time of surgery." In this instance, surgeons seemed to be implying that formal experiments only make sense if a procedure performs well during an informal, unregulated examination period. In the language of IRB approval, this translates into an assumption that human subjects matter only if a procedure has been formally defined as research. That the team performed surgery at all was rather remarkable given that a research protocol had been submitted to the IRB but approval had not yet been granted. By pursuing the PLUG as an innovation rather than as research in this case, the fetal researchers may well have jeopardized not only the well-being of the pregnant woman they operated on (and the safety of her fetus), but also the viability and legitimacy of their own study.

The IRB was not happy about this breach and sharply reprimanded the fetal surgery team, chastising the researchers for how the decision to proceed had been made and requesting all data on the surgery. The fetal surgeons responded by attempting to work around or bypass the jurisdiction of the IRB: "First, a response to the general problem of trying to evolve a surgical procedure that is not yet technically mature under IRB guidelines. It is essentially impossible which is why surgical innovation which occurs in multiple small steps *simply cannot function under these guidelines*. In this case, we know what we want to accomplish. . . . Exactly how to accomplish it is evolving" (emphasis added).

By using the language of evolution rather than development, the surgeons seem to be subtly attempting to convince the IRB that fetal surgery simply moves ahead—or evolves—with no active agent.[11] This would have obvious implications for who is responsible in and for fetal surgery. The surgeons are clearly rejecting the application of federal guidelines (and thus IRB intervention) in their work, which they define as incremental. In addressing the IRB's charge of noncompliance regarding the unauthorized surgery, the fetal surgery team wrote, "Since we are in the process of evolving the surgical technique that will prove safest, I hope we can exercise some judgment about what to do in any individual case." In other words, fetal surgeons reiterated their appeal for professional autonomy to determine whether a particular case is innovative or experimental. They met with some success. After careful review of the modified protocol, the IRB approved the PLUG procedure and the study proceeded as originally intended by researchers.

Yet two years later, many of these same concerns again came to the fore when fetal researchers attempted to renew their protocol. The results of the experiments were not sufficiently good to warrant continuation of the study; in fact, they were quite discouraging. The chair of the IRB wrote to the fetal surgery team (emphasis in original):

> In reviewing the results of this study to date (that is, with this procedure there have been eight deaths and one severely impaired child, but with routine care there have been seven survivors), the members believe that the likely outcome with surgery is so poor that there is no suggestion you can expect a significant reversal in the pattern in the future. So far, you have not quite proven that the use of the PLUG procedure is *worse* than routine care, but even if it were *equal* to routine care, given the risks to the mother, there is not sufficient justification to continue this study. The risks to both the mother and the fetus appear to outweigh the benefits and the importance of any increased statistical significance you may obtain by continuing this study at this time in its present form.

In other words, the study proved that fetal surgery using the PLUG technique was a much worse option than routine care. The study was not reapproved and fetal researchers were ordered to follow up with the lone survivor, a premature baby delivered at twenty-seven weeks with chronic lung disease requiring prolonged support with supplemental oxygen. The baby, clearly not one of the successes of fetal surgery, also suffered from hypercapnia (carbon dioxide in the blood), scoliosis (curvature of the spine), gastroesophageal reflux, perforation of the esophagus, bilateral severe retinopathy (degeneration of the retina), a hearing deficit, central nervous system problems, and spinal cord damage.

One week later, fetal researchers submitted a modification of the now defunct PLUG protocol for use in fetuses *after* twenty-eight weeks' gestation, framing the proposed surgery as if it were a different procedure altogether. Specifically, they wanted to operate on a woman who was already scheduled to travel to Capital Hospital for a PLUG procedure. Yet the only difference between this woman and the prior cases was the age of the fetus, suggesting that the surgery team was looking for a loophole through the original ruling. The IRB refused to grant an exception to its prior decision, and its response drew clear distinctions among research and innovation:

> The members suggested that you use your best professional judgment as a physician and treat this particular patient according to what you consider to be in the best interests of the fetus and the mother. If that treatment includes the use of the PLUG procedure, then you would be treating this patient using innovative therapy, but not under an approved research protocol. In this case, the IRB would have no jurisdiction over the treatment procedures. However since you would not be treating under an approved protocol, the data could not be used for research purposes. If you decide to treat this patient using the PLUG procedure, then it is imperative that the family be fully informed about the procedures and the previous results. The patient must be told that the IRB could no longer approve continuing the use of the procedure as a research protocol because of concerns that the documented risks outweigh any hoped-for benefits.

While recognizing the autonomy of surgeons to categorize the procedure as they saw fit, the IRB also delineated the conditions under which the operation could proceed. Human subjects protection would be salient for research, but not for innovation that would have no application in the research community. In other words, surgeons had to choose one set of practices and consequences or the other; the procedure could not be both innovative and experimental in terms of IRB guidelines, no matter how much these categories overlapped in practice. This exchange captures nicely the dual role of surgeons as clinical researchers, as well as the obligation of the IRB to protect potential human subjects in research.

While "the PLUG odyssey," as fetal researchers have termed it, is a rather extreme version of the zigzag course of fetal surgery protocols, it offers insight into the process by which innovative procedures pass in and out of different phases of research and treatment. Other procedures have had different trajectories. For example, fetal surgery for congenital cystic adenomatoid malformation (C-CAM) passed relatively smoothly from innovation to experiment to standard of care. After extensive investigation, the fetal surgery team was convinced that the C-CAM procedure was sufficiently safe and effective to become a routine offering. Fetal researchers justified this move in a letter to the IRB, noting the role of insurance companies:

> Open fetal surgery for C-CAM associated with hydrops should no longer be considered experimental at Capital Hospital and should not be an IRB-reviewed therapy. . . . All comparison cases have died. . . . Maternal health in all

nine [fetal surgery] cases has been excellent. . . . In the majority of cases, insurance carriers have recognized open fetal surgery as a therapeutic option for treatment of an otherwise fatal birth defect.

Persuaded by the researchers' impressive findings, the IRB had no objections to redefining C-CAM as no longer experimental—despite other extant fetal surgery protocols still at other stages. But the committee made it quite clear that while it accepted the surgeons' findings, it could not endorse a transition to routine care—regardless of the views of the insurance industry. The chair of the IRB wrote: "We almost never question a researcher's decision to consider a research project finished, and the members saw no obstacles to ending this study. The goal of showing the advantages of open fetal surgery for congenital cystic adenomatoid malformation appears to have been achieved. The members commented, however, that the IRB cannot establish or endorse a particular treatment as standard of care." Standard of care, then, seems to be negotiated, here at least, between providers and insurers.

In sum, fetal surgery at Capital Hospital has followed a rather serpentine course, moving among innovation, experiment, and standard of care. In part, this course has been determined by the sheer novelty of the procedures involved in fetal surgery and the research goals of the surgery team. But the trajectory of fetal surgery has been shaped also by the interventions of the IRB and its efforts to protect human subjects, key elements of the social context in which these procedures take place. While at least one procedure has proven its mettle, other protocols have consistently troubled IRB members. Despite the relatively smooth transition of the C-CAM procedure, almost all fetal surgery protocols encountered difficulties with the IRB approval process, such as those related to the PLUG procedure. Yet in spite of the IRB's chronic objections, all protocols for fetal surgery research had expired by 1995 and were not subsequently renewed by researchers. This means that surgeons have abandoned some unsuccessful procedures while shifting all others to standard of care. At Capital Hospital, fetal surgery is increasingly considered "innovative care" rather than experimental therapy. But its technical difficulty, limited application, and social consequences—as well as the attention it receives in popular cultural forums—suggest that fetal surgery is anything but routine.

By pushing fetal surgery toward standard of care before all, or even most, of the ethical conundrums were resolved, fetal researchers circumvented the very process designed to ensure their accountability to human subjects. Is fetal surgery today so very different from fetal surgery five or even ten years ago? Some critics argue that it is not, that fetal mortality from most procedures is still quite high. A procedure, then, may rely on exactly the same techniques regardless of how it is defined; that is, techniques may become standardized while attention to social consequences may vary. The difference lies in the meanings of the work: whether or not the patients/subjects—pregnant women and their fetuses—are defined as human subjects and protected by federal guidelines. Five years ago, many protocols were defined as experimental; today, they are not. As we have seen, procedures that are considered standard of care are no longer under the purview of the IRB. For such procedures at Capital Hospital—no matter how innovative, risky, or untested—there is no protection for patients outside of local peer review as determined by hospital policy and professional norms. This presents a rather disturbing scenario: whether fetal surgery is considered innovation, experiment, or standard of care, a number of urgent issues remain regarding its use. How are "ethics" for standard practices formulated? Who protects patients in routine but still quite risky medicine? And, more broadly, who controls medicine itself?

Manufacturing Informed Consent in Fetal Surgery

Informed consent is a significant component of efforts to protect human subjects in research, and thus crucial to the making of fetal surgery. Along with the research protocol itself, informed consent documents—or, what information potential research subjects will be given toward eliciting their participation—are a cardinal focus of evaluation by the IRB at Capital Hospital. Informed consent documents convey, in textual form, what both the fetal surgery team and the IRB deem important for pregnant women and their families to know. What gets included in the documents by clinical researchers may be guided as much by the principle of nonmalfeasance (to do no harm) as by fears of malpractice should fetal surgery go awry. After the fetal surgeons submit an informed consent document for approval, the IRB responds with its assessment of what has not been adequately addressed, what is missing, and what needs clarification. Depending on a number of factors, such as the level of risk in a procedure, documents will be either approved or, more commonly, sent back for revisions. It is in researchers' best interests to "get it right" as soon as possible so that they can begin conducting experiments on human subjects. But in almost all fetal surgery cases for the period I studied, informed consent documents went through many iterations before approval was granted, suggesting that getting it right is by no means obvious. Examining the paper trail between the fetal surgery team and the IRB reveals hidden meanings and institutional politics related to human subjects protection, as well as some of the conditions that must be in place for the creation of a new specialty and its patients/subjects.[12]

Contested Definitions, Multiple Iterations, and Chronic Omissions

I begin by examining the first version of a consent form for congenital diaphragmatic hernia (CDH) submitted to the IRB by fetal surgeons. On the surface, the document seems to provide enough information for pregnant women and their partners to make an informed choice. The form clearly conveys the potentially grave outcomes of carrying a fetus with CDH and it lays out some of the risks involved in surgery. Consider the following:

> Because this treatment is new, its effectiveness is not known. . . . The role of open fetal surgery in treating CDH is unclear. For a fetus like mine where the hole in the diaphragm is large and the diagnosis is made early, the fetus is likely to die and fetal surgery may offer the only hope for survival. My doctors do not know, however, if open fetal surgery is worth the risks involved, or if the results will be any better than with the standard care that is now used after the baby is born. . . . Open fetal surgery is major surgery and has risks associated with it. . . . There is even a slight possibility that I could become infertile or that I might die during this procedure. Even if the surgery is successful the fetus might die.

While the uncertainty of the treatment and potential risks are highlighted, so too is the threat of fetal death if no action is taken. Moreover, fetal surgery is portrayed as the "only hope for survival." Clearly, what is included here is designed both to allay potential subjects' concerns and to encourage their participation.

The consent form also outlines the procedures to be performed, both during and after surgery. For example:

> The surgery is like a cesarean section, with an incision made in my lower abdomen and womb. . . . I will be kept at Capital Hospital until I am well enough to leave the hospital. . . . After I am discharged, I will stay in a nearby residence to make sure that I am well enough to be out of the hospital. . . . I will remain on medication to prevent premature labor . . . When I am ready to deliver my baby, I will return to Capital Hospital.

The document offers an alternative treatment trajectory should a pregnant woman not choose fetal surgery, and it also explains procedures for ensuring confidentiality. The "costs" section emphasizes that expenses not covered by the patient's insurance company will be paid by a grant from the National Institutes of Health. The form further promises that treatment will be available if the patient or her fetus is injured as a result of participating in fetal surgery, although it does not specify who will pay for such treatment.

Now let us consider the IRB's response to this form, in which a number of omissions in the surgeons' first version are pointed out and clarifications are requested. IRB concerns include costs ("please discuss whether families might seriously or completely deplete their lifetime cap for insurance benefits as a result of participating in this study"); statistics ("the statement that 'six out of ten babies die even with the best treatment currently available after birth' is misleading and misstates your own experience");[13] and description of procedures ("the IRB members were disturbed to realize that the protocol being reviewed does not actually describe the fetal surgery procedure for correction of diaphragmatic hernia"). In its response to the next, almost unchanged, version about a week later, the IRB again expressed concerns about costs ("please clarify what costs have to be covered by subjects themselves"); benefits ("because it is not clear that open fetal surgery offers a better chance of survival than carrying the fetus to term, the members ask that you delete the sentence which implies that fetal surgery offers more hope"); maternal risk ("among the risks to the mother please discuss the possible need for medications to forestall premature labor"); and alternatives to surgery ("the alternatives section should be revised to make it clear that prospective subjects can refuse *all* participation in the study"). After several more iterations, a much more thorough version was submitted and approved.

At around the same time, fetal surgeons submitted a separate protocol for sacrococcygeal teratoma (SCT) that closely resembled their initial consent forms for other procedures—that is, containing minimal information. What was particularly striking about the ensuing communication between the fetal surgery team and the IRB was how reluctant the investigators appeared to incorporate the IRB's suggestions about costs, risks (especially maternal risks), outcomes, quality of life issues, and reporting procedures. For example, in the margins of the documents I examined, "not done" was written in black ink beside almost every point raised in the IRB's prior response. (This could have resulted from unclear instructions on the IRB's part, but in almost every letter I read the IRB's instructions seemed clear, concise, and very detailed.) Although the fetal surgery team eventually (after three more rounds) modfied the informed consent documents in line with the IRB's suggestions, they also challenged the IRB on several important points. In one letter to the IRB, the surgeons wrote: "We have found that the most effective way to transmit information about the details of the procedure and the associated risks is via a thorough patient education videotape. Many of the Committee's concerns about delineating the risks and/or discomforts in the consent form are thoroughly covered in the patient education videotape." This correspondence raises the question, effective for *whom*—the patients or the surgeons? The IRB, which had no prior knowledge of the videotape, demanded that it be submitted for review immediately. Fetal surgeons did so, and ultimately the tape was *not* approved for use as an informed consent tool.

What can these examples tell us about patterns in the informed consent process in fetal surgery? For every experimental procedure, several iterations were necessary before the IRB approved the final document. The fetal surgery team consistently left out important information, and the IRB invariably demanded that this information be included in subsequent versions. Often it was the same kinds of information left out of subsequent applications. After reading hundreds of pages of documents, certain chronic omissions become particularly striking. Maternal risks, fetal risks, and poor outcomes were either understated or completely ignored; costs were minimized and related issues, such as insurance, were evaded; and fetal surgeons often represented their specialty as "new" rather than "experimental." They also consistently portrayed fetal surgery as far more hopeful or beneficial than it is, often defining it as a positive alternative for women who have difficulties becoming pregnant or who are opposed to abortion.

From these data, it is clear that the fetal surgery team and the IRB have very different standards regarding what is ethical or acceptable in fetal surgery. The documents reveal an ongoing struggle between two very different kinds of work: medical experimentation on human subjects and efforts to protect human subjects. As Rothman (1990, 199) has written, "ethics in medicine has become everyone's business. . . . To an unprecedented degree, physicians must now share authority in medical decision-making." But they certainly do not have to like it, and they have considerable leeway in how (and how quickly) they adhere to federal guidelines, even when those guidelines are adjudicated by an IRB comprised of fellow physicians. Surgeons' ongoing resistance to incorporating the IRB's suggestions can be read as efforts on their part to maintain a degree of autonomy in this process, outside the purview of the IRB. The multiple iterations of informed consent documents illustrate that fetal surgery is a site at which professional, cultural, *and* ethical perspectives and meanings both intersect and conflict.

"It's a Reality Dump": Practicing Informed Consent

Despite chronic omissions and a seemingly endless stream of iterations, informed consent documents are eventually produced and deemed suitable by the IRB. When these forms enter the clinic-based world of experimental fetal medicine, their hard-won clarity may still be insufficient to protect research subjects fully. The actual practices of informed consent and the maintenance of records can remain ambiguous and uneven, partly because physicians themselves shoulder responsibility for conveying information once IRB approval has been gained. Why assume, as the IRB procedures ultimately do, that surgeons would be any more forthcoming with their research subjects than they were with the IRB? Conflicts of interest between clinicians as healers and clinicians as researchers exist whether a practice is part of a formal protocol or not, but the stakes for patients/subjects may be much higher in research where the benefits of medicine are questionable. In addition, "medical speak,"—what actually gets said rather than what is written on a form—tends to distance patients from their doctors, and even thorough discussions (or videos) often do not clearly provide the necessary information. The *practice* of informed consent thus raises a number of important concerns about the power of medicine in the immediate lives and well-being of patients/subjects—particularly where there is ambiguity concerning who is the human subject.

There is a vast literature on physician-patient relationships as often problematic, and these problems may be compounded in clinical research situations. For example, patients may become overwhelmed or intimidated by the terminology or by physicians' attitudes, making them afraid to ask questions (Fisher 1988; Todd 1989; West 1984). Differences of class and culture also may serve to impede successful communication, including the informed consent process (Kaufert and O'Neil 1990; Thong and Harth 1991). Further, medical practitioners may simply withhold or minimize information as we have seen here in order to enroll or maintain human subjects in their protocols. As Fletcher and Jonsen (1991:15) have written, "Due to the possibility that some pregnant women may be likely to disregard their own well-being for the sake of the fetus and also to the possibility that clinical investigators will convey enthusiasm about new but unproven approaches to fetal therapy, special precautions for the consent process [are] recommended." In short, as many in the bioethics community recognize, the concrete practices of informed consent often do not conform to the ethical guidelines administered by IRBs, which emphasize abstract ideals rather than actual situations. Perhaps this is why anthropologist Sharon Kaufman (1997, 26) calls informed consent an "elusive project."

Elusive though it may be, the fetal surgeons I studied seemed well aware of the need to provide informed consent whether or not they managed to do so in practice, and it is likely that the IRB approval process was what made them aware. For example, one surgeon told me: "I think we can give the parents and referring doctors a great deal of information about the natural history of diseases, what the mode of surgery should be, what the timing of surgery should be, whether the timing of the surgery should change depending on clinical circumstances. Giving parents a better idea about the outcomes, that's a tremendous service to be able to do that, to counsel a family."

Another surgeon was somewhat more nonchalant about the need for informed consent: "At least at present, women choose to come to us for our help. We feel that the parents have control over what to do." But simply recognizing that women and their partners voluntarily seek fetal surgery does not guarantee that pregnant women, as human subjects, will be protected. Ironically, it is the rigorous IRB review process and not surgeons' own activities that seem most likely to ensure adequate protection of human subjects in fetal surgery.

Such was the situation at Capital Hospital, where a number of my informants indicated that pregnant women who consent to fetal surgery are, in fact, neither fully nor adequately informed. For example, a team of obstetricians and bioethicists at Capital Hospital not directly affiliated with the Fetal Treatment Unit began a project in 1995 explicitly examining informed consent in fetal surgery. They planned to interview former fetal surgery patients retrospectively, using a survey instrument. Their guiding assumption, according to one participant, was that "it is easy for the informed consent process to become corrupted. Can patients really know what it's all about?" This informant also pointed out that when fetal defects are potentially fatal (as in *all* cases where fetal surgery is an option), women become more vulnerable to arguments that a decision in favor of treatment will "save" their babies. Women for whom abortion is not an option may be especially vulnerable to persuasion (although they may also be among the most enthusiastic participants in fetal surgery, as we shall see in chapter 6).

This concern was echoed by several informants, including one social worker who told me that "there are a lot of people who have waited a long time to have a baby. To discover that they have a lesion like this, they're desperate to do something about it. And they just want to believe so much that it's going to be all right." Because the women and their partners are so desperate, there is no guarantee that they even read the entire informed consent document or that they are able to process the information given to them in meetings. Another informant went on to tell me, in an anguished voice:

> Although [fetal surgeons] were trying to be honest, it was very hard to really
> paint an accurate picture and expect that anybody would do a thing like this,
> put themselves through this. We have become increasingly honest and forth-
> right with people because of the consequences of not being that way. But we
> cannot give informed consent, and no matter how much we tell them, they
> are still surprised by the discomforts, risks, lack of privacy, and enormous
> time commitment involved.

Here, this informant points to several aspects of fetal surgery left out of
informed consent documents even *after* IRB approval, such as the lack of
privacy and the lengthy time commitment that patients will face. She
seems to be suggesting that no matter what the intentions of the fetal
surgery team, it may be impossible to convey just how disruptive the
procedures are for the pregnant women who undergo them. Another informant, a nurse, remarked:

> The surgeons' worry is always that we nearly pummel people to death with
> the truth. It's a reality dump, these consent forms. And some people are
> daunted by that. We had a doctor who came here, a doctor couple, who re-
> ally knew what we were talking about. I mean talk about informed consent.
> These were physicians. She was willing to do it and go for it. So we didn't re-
> ally tell them everything.

This seems ethically dubious and raises the question of what information is withheld from patients when they do *not* have any medical training. It also suggests that members of the fetal surgery team may cut a
few procedural corners in an attempt both to access the unborn patient
and to expand their specialty. If pregnant women *really* knew what to expect, would they consent to fetal surgery?

One informant offered a sociological interpretation of why fetal surgeons may not be as forthright as possible:

> I think one of the problems is not that [the surgeons] are dishonest by any
> stretch, but that they are surgeons. And I think that surgeons have to be up-
> beat or they couldn't get out of bed in the morning. You know, they come
> here and they cut people open. If they didn't believe in what they did and be-
> lieve there was a positive outcome at the other end, I think they would be-
> come immobilized.

In other words, the demands of salvaging fetuses and the professional
culture of surgery shape how fetal surgeons approach their work, including implementation of informed consent guidelines.

As with the iterative process of producing informed consent documents, their use in the actual clinical practice of fetal surgery is shaped as
much by professional autonomy and the social organization of work as by
broad ethical conceptions. Implementation of informed consent may also

be shaped by gender and a certain lack of respect for women's capacity to make important and consequential decisions in medicine. As we saw with respect to formulation of the federal guidelines, the social status of pregnant women is often framed as contingent, an issue we shall return to in chapter 6. Yet pregnant women are not simply "fetal containers" (Purdy 1990). As a class, they are certainly capable of making informed choices about their own bodies and fetuses. Fully informed consent—that which may discourage women from participation in fetal surgery protocols—may be seen by clinical researchers as an unacceptable constraint on the viability of study protocols. Surely surgeons' activities in relation to the IRB seem to straddle a fine line between partially and fully informed consent provision. In sum, certain aspects of fetal surgery, especially those related to informed consent such as full disclosure of risks, may be neglected in favor of others that contribute more centrally to the making of the unborn patient by securing women's participation.

Assuring Accountability

Informed consent was not the only area of strife between the fetal surgery team and the IRB at Capital Hospital represented in the documents that I studied. There was also considerable disagreement and confusion about statistics, suggesting that a rather different kind of accountability is also at stake in fetal surgery. Contention existed along several different lines, including the actual numbers themselves (how many operations have been performed, how many fetuses have died, and statistical comparisons between fetal surgery and standard treatment), how study results are reported to the IRB and presented to research subjects, and what other kinds of information is obscured by quantitative rather than more fully descriptive data. The IRB was able to pose these challenges to fetal researchers because it had access to information about outcomes that did not appear in published articles. For example, one of the fetal surgeons told me that "we only discuss the published results," begging the question of who has access to nonpublished results and under what conditions. (Indeed, because the fetal surgery team was reluctant to share this data I could only obtain access to this information by going directly to the IRB files.) By reviewing the documents related to the human subjects approval process, we (like the IRB) are privy not only to statistics that may not be available to a wider audience, but also to the behind-the-scenes process by which quantification comes to matter in terms of ethical accountability. As with almost all other aspects of fetal surgery, this process embodies some of the complicated meanings and politics related to the making of the unborn patient.

One of the first disagreements centered around how best to organize the fetal surgery studies. In the earliest stages of the Fetal Treatment Unit, all "innovative" procedures were covered under one protocol, "Experimental Fetal Surgery." As the program grew and distinctive procedures became available for different fetal defects, investigators wanted to include new procedures under the same existing protocol. From their perspective, this would simplify almost all aspects of the research, including informed consent and reporting of results. It would also limit their accountability to the IRB by reducing the number and scope of procedures and issues. The IRB, however, had a different idea, demanding that each procedure be studied under its own, distinct protocol. From the IRB's perspective, delineating the various protocols separately would provide more complete information about each one. For example, rather than simply assuming that one informed consent document would apply to several different protocols, the IRB wanted to ensure that each procedure to be utilized was fully and adequately explained to potential research subjects.

Organizing each protocol as a distinct study also made sense in terms of the reporting of study results. In a letter to the principal investigator on the original protocol, the IRB asked that he formally withdraw the open fetal surgery sections of the protocol: "The members became concerned that your protocol is very general and does not clearly delineate the conditions to be treated and medications and procedures to be used. Given the recent experiences of the open fetal surgery program, the IRB will not be inclined to approve such general protocols in the future." In other words, inconsistencies in the data could easily remain hidden in one complicated protocol encompassing several procedures. But if each procedure were treated separately, it would be more difficult for medical researchers to mask poor outcomes. The importance of numbers to the review process was thus intimately tied to the reorganization of the studies themselves. Fetal surgeons had not necessarily been doing anything wrong prior to this request. But they needed to change some aspects of their work so that the IRB could better determine the risks and benefits of each protocol. In this case, accounting and accountability went hand in hand.

Contention also surfaced over how and when study results were to be reported, both to potential research subjects and to the IRB. The committee members were concerned about inconsistencies in the statistics included in the applications, and asked that researchers clarify the actual number of surgeries to date and the survival rates. The committee also asked that patients be told what the differences in fetal mortality rates were between fetal surgery and alternative treatments. Several informants echoed the IRB's concerns about how study results were reported and discussed their connection to informed consent. One physician told me that "pregnant women and their fetuses are being used as experimental animals. We don't have to be up in the forties now [number of surgeries performed] with as few survivors as there are. We know that there would have been, out of that forty, at least sixteen survivors if we did nothing. We don't have sixteen survivors after [fetal] surgery, so how can you ethically tell the next woman that she should have surgery?" When I asked about informed consent specifically, the informant went on to imply that fetal researchers are less than fully forthcoming with patients: "Patients don't know about the forty cases that have been done because the number of survivors has not been published. I don't think anywhere but in [a nurse's] desk can you get survival rates. All that information should be published and available." What this informant might not have known is that at least some of this information *was* made available to the IRB if not to the patients themselves.

In another letter to researchers offering a broad indictment of certain aspects of fetal surgery, the IRB wrote:

> It is almost impossible to determine the precise number of subjects enrolled on each protocol, let alone the outcomes for all the patients operated on and outcomes for appropriate cases. The numbers provided in individual summary reports are often inconsistent. Numbers developed by IRB members attempting to quantify the results often differ from the fetal surgery summary reports. Trying to understand these inconsistencies places an undue burden on the IRB, which must evaluate the risk and benefit ratio of each separate protocol.

In an effort to improve reporting procedures and thus secure greater accountability, the IRB requested that fetal researchers create a streamlined accounting process that clearly indicated enrollment and outcomes for each protocol. In his response to the IRB, the chief surgeon wrote: "I agree that our system has become immensely convoluted and difficult as a consequence of repeated requests for information which we have complied with sequentially. We need to cut the Gordian knot and get down to the information that will be useful to the IRB." Here, the surgeon is clearly blaming the IRB itself—with its "repeated requests for information"—for the confusion.

But in an unusually responsive move, the fetal surgery team changed their reporting procedures and developed a clearer and more informative table format, which included fetal disease/defect, type of surgery, delivery date, outcome, and insurance information. The team also began actively recruiting a biostatistician. The new format was indeed easier to understand, and it had an added benefit of providing qualitative data that previously had been either buried in the protocols or missing altogether. For example, quantitative data had always been useful for certain information, such as outcomes: 84 percent fetal mortality for CDH; 100

percent fetal mortality for SCT; 44 percent fetal mortality for CCAM; and 55 percent fetal mortality for miscellaneous procedures. But the new reporting format revealed richer data about these cases. Reviewing CDH cases, for example, we learn that "intraoperative demise" occurred in 25 percent of the cases; in another case, "preterm labor was poorly controlled"; one fetus "died 2 wks postop due to pulmonary hypoplasia" while another "died @ 2 hrs of life"; physicians "withdrew support on day of life #3" from yet another fetus; and one former patient "now attends preschool. Eats everything by mouth." This type of qualitative data, which reveals some of the consequences of the making of the unborn patient, had previously been much harder to locate in the flood of numbers accompanying each protocol.

The new reporting format also, at least partially, fulfilled another consistent suggestion from the IRB: better long-term follow-up. Addressing fetal researchers, the IRB wrote, "We need more informative longer term followup data for both the fetal surgery cases and the appropriate comparison patients. Ultimately, the benefits of fetal surgery and alternative therapies must be evaluated based not only on fetal survival but also on the quality of life of survivors and families." The IRB recognized that providing this data would increase researchers' work load, but underscored the importance of monitoring fetal surgery's patients long after the operations are done. It also suggested that surgeons prepare a separate protocol for this follow-up data that would be collected from participants in all of the fetal surgery protocols. The new reporting format offered narrative data about the long-term consequences of each case: one former patient "now attends kindergarten. Has high-freq. hearing loss"; another is "a healthy 8–year old. Continues intermittent urinary catheterization 2x day"; another had "abdominoplasty, orchiopexy, urinary tract revision @ 7 months."[14] This is precisely the kind of data beyond stark numbers that the IRB—as well as other concerned participants such as funders, bioethicists, and sociologists—need in order to evaluate the consequences of fetal surgery adequately.

Yet, despite all these changes and surgeons' general willingness to alter their accounting practices, the IRB's discomfort with fetal surgery intensified, eventually culminating in the suspension of all protocols discussed earlier. Assuring accountability, it seems, ultimately proved too difficult for both the IRB and clinicians alike.

The Fate of Human Subjects on Biomedical Frontiers

This chapter has focused on the human subjects approval process at Capital Hospital as an essential site of negotiation, interaction, and conflict in fetal surgery where "ethics" are worked out in everyday practices. Within and through these various practices, human subjects—the lifeblood of research—are made, protected, contested, and even unmade by different sets of actors with consequences for fetal surgery itself. Among fetal surgeons and their colleagues in the Fetal Treatment Unit (FTU), the important work of fetal surgery could not proceed without human subjects —pregnant women patients and their fetuses—on which to operate. But in their struggle to build fetal surgery, fetal researchers seemed to view the IRB and its demands as a hindrance, or a kind of "clinical trial," to their real work of surgically rescuing dying fetuses and advancing biomedical knowledge. Their correspondence to the IRB is a hallmark of professional autonomy, revealing a chronic reluctance (or inability) to incorporate the IRB's suggestions into their protocols. In pursuit of the unborn patient, other considerations such as maternal risks, costs, informed consent, and follow-up fell by the wayside. This approach is exemplified in the shifting of all fetal surgery procedures from experimental to standard of care or routine medicine, outside the authoritative scope of the IRB.

For the IRB, on the other hand, the work of fetal surgery (if defined by investigators as experimental) could not be allowed to proceed without protecting the human subjects who would be part of it. This is a rescue operation of a different sort: saving women and their fetuses from risky, unacceptable practices. During the years of my study, the IRB attempted to secure the protection of human subjects in fetal surgery by requesting revisions in documents, demanding additional data, creating an oversight committee, maintaining its authority as ethical arbiter, and policing fetal surgeons when they overstepped the bounds of acceptable practice. And it performed these activities within a rather complicated framework in which various definitions—of human subjects, of maternal-fetal relationships, of fetal surgery itself—were ambiguous and in flux. The working relationship between the IRB and the fetal researchers at Capital Hospital thus resembled a kind of tango, with both sides pursuing their own aims while locked together in a rather awkward institutional embrace. Each was simply doing its job, but in many instances, these jobs were incompatible. One set of actors was made to be accountable to another set of actors, which was able to impede, and even shut down, the making of the unborn patient—but only temporarily. In the end, fetal surgery has emerged from these struggles as standard care. It is still limited in scope with respect to fetal medicine more broadly, but it is no longer considered to be research at Capital Hospital.

What can we make of this tangled and complicated process? First, fetal surgery may tell us something about surgeons as an occupational group and their apparent unwillingness to subject themselves to ethical (or any other kind of) regulation. Although many physicians may be resistant to ethical oversight, surgeons inhabit a notoriously arrogant specialty; they are technically rigorous, highly paid, and endowed with the godlike power to save people's lives. Charles Bosk (1979, 28) has argued that the features of surgery that make surgeons into heroes also make them into symbols of what scares people about medicine. Surgery, once done, usually cannot be undone. Surgeons are often singled out as "prime abusers of the public trust," and surgeries gone wrong make for compelling media coverage. (And, given the awed media coverage that fetal surgery has received in the past few years, we can be certain that a major failure, such as the death of a pregnant woman, would make headlines.) In part, this is because what surgeons do is "precise and definitive. . . . So clearly are the surgeon's actions connected to the patient's condition that the only warrant for surgery—the only acceptable reason to subject a patient to the risk and trauma of surgery—is the expectation that the operation will cure or palliate the patient's condition" (Bosk 1979, 29). These issues are considerably more complex and potent when surgery is experimental and when it takes place on (or, rather, inside) one of the final frontiers in medicine: the womb. It is this immediate connection between operations and outcomes (both inside and outside the operating room) that makes human subjects protection in fetal surgery so important, and fetal surgeons' ongoing dismissal of ethical guidelines so problematic.

Fetal surgeons are certainly not unique in advocating for their professional autonomy; after all, the medical profession itself was built out of the struggle for such autonomy (Starr 1982). Nor is it unusual for clinicians to conflict with IRBs over the shape of medical research. But fetal surgery is unique in a number of ways, not least of which are the specific kinds of concerns that are evaded or ignored. No other intervention involves the complicated, contested issues of operating on fetuses still in the womb. In fetal surgery, the human subjects process and all of its components have the added task of accounting for pregnant women's needs and interests, as well as those of the "primary" patient, the fetus. To ignore the issues of risk, costs, consent, and follow-up is, as the IRB consistently argued, to put women and their fetuses in certain kinds of danger. Why, then, is it left up to the IRB to advocate for women's health? Where is the accountability of fetal researchers to raise these as serious concerns in the first place? What important ethical issues will be sidelined as fetal surgery becomes a routine operation rather than an experiment? Can we assume that fetal surgeons will be any more accountable outside of the research setting than they were inside of it? Given the thrust of the material presented here, there is some cause for concern that many issues raised by the IRB may be discounted by clinicians' relentless focus on the making of the unborn patient.

This story also tells us something about the human subjects approval process for biomedicine in general. The example of fetal surgery suggests that the *process* of IRB approval may be far more important than its eventual outcomes. As I have shown, the "ethics" of fetal surgery has much to do with everyday work routines: researchers endeavored to get their protocols passed, while the IRB labored to secure adherence to federal guidelines. Despite its numerous objections, concerns, and requests for revision, the IRB never simply said no to fetal surgery protocols. Even when it suspended all protocols, it reinstated them after surgeons agreed to comply with the federal guidelines and the IRB's own institutional demands. (Subsequent data revealed that the surgeons' compliance *never* ceased being an issue for the IRB, which routinely had to remind the fetal surgery team to work more closely with the Oversight Committee.) However resistant or critical of fetal surgery in the years leading up to the "routinization" of fetal surgery, the IRB at Capital Hospital was central to its emergence. The example of fetal surgery suggests that the human subjects approval process has "no real teeth," to borrow Barbara Koenig's wonderful phrasing.[15] As such, the fate of human subjects in fetal surgery as well as on other, equally complicated biomedical frontiers may be precarious.

I am reminded of Bosk's invocation of Everett C. Hughes's (1971) phrase "the rough edge of professional practice." As Bosk (1992, xxi) frames it, "ultimately, that edge is the space where the patient's unique tragedy meets with the professional's everyday routines." As we have seen, navigation of this space is propelled by institutional and professional politics, as well as cultural meanings about women, fetuses, and medicine. I close with some unanswered questions about the "ethics" of fetal medicine, or what is considered acceptable—and by whom—on this frontier. Does fetal surgery represent the kind of medicine we want? Is clinical research the best way to ensure healthy babies? How can we assure accountability that goes beyond statistical reports to protect human subjects and patients at the "rough edges" of medical practice better? And, invoking reproductive politics, what do we learn about medicine and culture when a practice moves to standard of care without ever fully convincing those who are designated by the nation to oversee it that its human subjects will be protected? We shall address this last question in the next chapter, which focuses on those who have the most to lose and to gain in fetal surgery: the pregnant women.

Chapter 6

Heroic Moms and Maternal Environments

Pregnant Women on the Final Frontier

Prologue

Susan and Jim Davis were desperate. They already had two children, a four-year-old girl and an eighteen-month-old boy, when Susan became pregnant in 1992. Initially thrilled about the pregnancy, Susan was devastated to learn in the fourth month that her fetus had a tumor growing in its chest, crushing its heart and lungs. This condition, called congenital cystic adenomatoid malformation (C-CAM), is fatal if left untreated because it prevents vital organs from developing properly. But local doctors in their large midwestern city said there was nothing they could do. Susan, ardently pro-life, did not want to have an abortion. She and Jim researched other options and eventually learned about experimental open fetal surgery. They contacted Capital Hospital and forwarded their medical records for review. A short time later, they were invited for an evaluation and possible treatment.

Susan and her fetus met the program's selection criteria (both clinical and psychosocial) and underwent surgery soon after their arrival, at about twenty-three weeks' gestation. Susan admits that surgery was "a very hard thing to do physically" and that she was "tapped out" often. As in all fetal surgery cases, preterm labor was a major concern both during and after the operation. Twelve days after surgery, Susan prematurely went into labor and her fetus was delivered by cesarean section. The newborn weighed less than two pounds and was immediately whisked off to the Neonatal Intensive Care Unit. After several rocky months of additional treatment and monitoring, including care for a collapsed lung and open heart surgery, the fragile baby was well enough to leave Capital Hospital. Elizabeth weighed just under four pounds when Susan and Jim brought her home.[1]

I interviewed Susan and Jim at their home on a brisk fall day in 1994. At the time, Susan was in her late twenties, a big-boned, pretty woman with short brown hair and a lot of energy. Mark, in his early thirties, had a receding hairline and a passionate oratorical style. They worked together in a family business and seemed to enjoy a comfortable, middle-class lifestyle. The Davises identified themselves as religiously conservative, including adherence to a pro-life platform, and they discussed fetal surgery primarily in the context of abortion. For example, Susan told me that "if women stopped making decisions based on their own convenience, then abortion might end." Having made just such a sacrifice on behalf of her own daughter seemed to bolster Susan's belief that women who choose abortion are selfish. Jim described abortion as murder, the killing of an unborn child, and became quite heated in his defense of an antiabortion position. At one point, he began pacing the living room floor, speaking faster and louder in his excitement and fervor about the absolute wrongness of abortion. I was moved by their obvious political and emotional commitments. The Davises see their daughter Elizabeth as a "miracle baby," living proof that a surgical intervention is preferable to abortion as a means of dealing with an ailing or defective fetus.

When I asked Susan and Jim how they felt about fetal interventions in general, fully expecting a homily about letting nature take its course despite the choice they had made, they surprised me. They argued that "it is a form of human arrogance *not* to take advantage of the technology that God has given us. Medicine and science are gifts of God, designed to make our lives better and to create miracles." The Davises expressed enthusiasm about any scientific or medical practice that fosters the notion of the unborn patient. In fact, they started a private philanthropy to support endeavors such as fetal surgery and hoped to raise money through their vast network of antiabortion connections, as well as through family ties. Susan and Jim's insight into how their foundation might serve the antiabortion movement was smart and sophisticated. They believe that traditional pro-life politics are "virtually bankrupt," in Jim's words. He pointed out that the specter of RU-486, the newish abortion drug that can provide nonsurgical abortions earlier and at medical sites other than abortion clinics, threatens to render images of so-called aborted fetuses less effective in the political realm. He and Susan feel that emphasizing "fetal patienthood" is a better way to assert "fetal personhood," and they are enthusiastic about any practice that will facilitate constructions of fetuses as full-fledged human beings. In this regard, their positive experience with fetal surgery and the successful birth of their daughter sustains and invigorates their political views and activities. They believe, in Susan's words, that a "legitimate, scientific foundation, not directly linked to the antiabortion movement except through funding, advice, and support," will be critical to the future of antiabortion politics. But their intent to portray the foundation as a "nonpartisan" organization is belied by its numerous informal connections to antiabortion politics and by the Davises' own politics.

In talking to fetal surgeons and their colleagues about the connections between their work and reproductive politics, I learned that overtly linking fetal surgery with abortion makes the fetal surgery team at Capital Hospital quite uncomfortable. Fetal surgeons there are nervous about clients like Susan and Jim, even while they welcome the support the couple offers to the program. When they learned that I would be interviewing the Davises, the fetal surgeons carefully pointed out that Susan and Jim are not representative of all fetal surgery patients. One surgeon told me that although most patients tend to be opposed to abortion, not all share the "extreme views" of the Davises. But, as we have seen throughout this book, most physicians (with the exception of Liley) tend to downplay the political nature of fetal surgery, recognizing that controversy poses a threat to the longevity of their work. As one surgeon astutely pointed out, "The only issue now, the biggest fly in the ointment, is political. If we are squelched at Capital Hospital, it will be for purely political reasons." It is one of the great ironies of fetal surgery that some of the most enthusiastic patients (e.g., women like Susan Davis who want to help build the specialty) are those whose support also prods reluctant medical workers into the political arena.

Rethinking Maternal-Fetal Relationships

The story of Susan and Jim Davis embodies many of the complicated reproductive politics associated with fetal surgery, some of which I have touched upon in previous chapters. Here, I focus in greater detail on pregnant women's participation in and experiences of fetal surgery. As we have seen, the fetus is not the only work object in fetal surgery; pregnant women too are work objects and they also act on behalf of their fetuses. In treating the unborn patient, clinicians work *on* pregnant women's bodies, but they also work closely *with* the women without whose cooperation the specialty would not exist. As the physicians, nurses, social workers, and other specialists are at work in the fetal surgery setting, so too are the pregnant women. A number of tensions are engendered by these women's multiple identities as both subjects and objects in fetal surgery. I show in this chapter that women like Susan Davis are engaged actors, fully participating in the making of the unborn patient, and not just passive technologies of fetal access. But they are also configured in many different ways within and by fetal surgery, as a distinctive kind of colonization of women's bodies occurs on this reproductive frontier.[2] Pregnant women are represented both as "heroic moms" and as "maternal environments," and there is ongoing confusion among all participants about the relationship between women and their fetuses.

In order to grasp some of the contradictions surrounding pregnant women's varied positions in fetal surgery and how these are represented, it is helpful to understand the *maternal-fetal conflict* paradigm as a ubiquitous institutional and disciplinary form. Within ethical frameworks, for example, fetuses are accorded interests on the basis of their moral value as potential persons (Chervenak and McCullough 1985; Steinbock 1992). But because fetuses are located in women's bodies, assignment of fetal interests is often construed *in opposition to* pregnant women's interests. Among many ethicists, the difference between a fetus and a newborn is often construed as "merely geographic." But as Sherwin (1992, 106) argues, the only way in which this framing makes sense is if pregnant women are conceptually erased from the experience of pregnancy or, in the case of fetal surgery, reduced to a penetrable flesh and muscle barrier separating fetal surgeons from their true patients. A similar perspective exists in the American legal system, which has witnessed an expansion of the fetal rights framework in recent years and a corresponding diminution of women's reproductive autonomy (Daniels 1993; Johnsen 1986). Fetal rights are increasingly conceptualized as being in direct adversial conflict with pregnant women's rights and interests (Chavkin 1992). A hallmark of both ethical and legal approaches is the construction of distinct, binary, and opposing subjectivities for the woman and her fetus.

Within medicine, as in ethics and law, the interests of the unborn patient are increasingly seen as quite different from those of the pregnant woman who is increasingly disregarded or erased. As Mattingly (1992, 13) argues, before the appearance of fetal diagnostic and treatment technologies, clinicians could only address fetal anomalies through "the maternal environment. Unable to interact with the fetus in clear distinction from its host, physicians conceptualized the maternal-fetal dyad as one complex patient, the gravid female, of which the fetus was an integral part." Although the biological relationship itself has not changed, its metaphorical representation has shifted to one of difference and opposition. Mattingly (1992, 13) points out that "clinicians no longer look to the maternal host for diagnostic data and a therapeutic medium; they look through her to the fetal organism and regard it as a distinct patient in its own right."

This framework pervades fetal surgery, where the interests of the fetal patient are seen as paramount and pregnant women are conceptualized either as inert tools for enhancing fetal access or, conversely, as barriers restricting fetal access. When women's own clinical needs are recognized, these may be seen as competing with the needs of the unborn patient. Pregnant women's autonomy in such a framing may be severely diminished. According to some observers, "Autonomy must remain a key factor in any arguments about intervention on behalf of the fetus. The 'slippery slope' only gets further greased, and issues become progressively more complicated and cloudy when one focuses on the potential benefits to a fetus" (Evans et al. 1990). In other words, as the needs and interests of the fetus grow, those of pregnant women seem to shrink correspondingly.

But what happens to formulations of the maternal-fetal conflict paradigm when we put women back in the picture, recognizing their agency as well as their erasure in fetal practices? One way of addressing this question is by emphasizing the work that women do in fetal surgery. I draw on synbolic interactionist perspectives to situate the pregnant women as *engaged* actors in the sense of being actively involved in or committed to the enterprise of fetal surgery.[3] An ongoing theoretical focus in interactionism is how people take account of or orient themselves toward other people and things in meaningful ways. People have a variety of commitments, interests, and desires toward what (or whom) they find meaningful. They act on these commitments to the extent that they are able and within contexts that may be constraining and imperfect in various ways. Pregnant women assume an engaged stance toward their fetuses and act on the basis of their fierce commitments, not because of essential maternal instincts but, at least in part, because their fetuses are extremely socially meaningful to them (Rothman 1989; Sherwin 1992). Just as the fetus has been a work object for medical workers, so too do women engage in work on behalf of their fetuses, ranging from eating better to undergoing surgery. In short, women care a great deal about their fetuses.

In this chapter I address women's engaged participation in fetal surgery and raise important questions about the implications of *their* work and *their* commitments to the unborn patient. By focusing both on women's engagement with fetal surgery and on the ways in which women are shaped by clinical practices, the maternal-fetal conflict paradigm is challenged by the recognition that women are multiply configured in fetal surgery. Pregnant women are simultaneously subjects and objects, engaged and implicated. They act with conviction and in many ways on behalf of their fetuses, while simultaneously being treated as merely maternal environments for the unborn patient. I do not attempt to resolve these tensions, for they are very much a part of the fabric of fetal surgery and many other reproductive practices. But I do suggest that a simple conflict model is insufficient for making sense of these practices. Unlike ethical and legal perspectives, which emphasize an abstract, decontextualized version of maternal-fetal conflict, what actually happens in practice is far more complex as women alternate among a variety of shifting positions. Indeed, fetal surgery is as much about the making and unmaking of maternal bodies as it is about the making of fetal bodies. Paraphrasing Nelly Oudshoorn (1994, 12), I show how pregnant women's bodies have been manipulated—by themselves *and* by others— in the pursuit of the unborn patient. In doing so, I reframe fetal surgery as a women's health issue with significant implications for women's reproductive experiences and lives.[4]

"Anything We Had to Do to Give the Baby a Chance": Women Engage Fetal Surgery[5]

In the 1960s in Auckland, New Zealand, obstetrician Florence Fraser encouraged pregnant women to talk to their fetuses. She suggested that women "think of their babies as personalities" before birth, as this would enhance the bonding process in the neonatal period. Fraser believed fetuses to be "people from a very early stage," and she saw no conflict in helping pregnant women do the same. She found very little resistance to this idea from her patients, who were eager to do anything to facilitate a healthier pregnancy and better bonding after birth. Fraser told me, "The mothers were very involved with their babies and what was happening. I believed that was terribly important. [Bonding] is not scientific, I know, but it did make a difference."[6] She felt that women's involvement with their fetuses was especially useful in fetal surgery cases, where procedures were sometimes complicated, fetuses routinely died, and Rh-negative women often needed to return to National Women's Hospital for subsequent fetal transfusions. Fraser found the fetal transfusion patients to be engaged and enthusiastic about interventions that might help rescue their fetuses from hemolytic disease.[7]

As in New Zealand in the 1960s, fetal surgery patients in the United States in the 1990s are a committed group of women. They are in the operating room because they have made a very complicated decision to seek treatment for an ill or defective fetus that they want to carry to term. As one of the fetal surgeons at Capital Hospital told me, "Why is the fetus a patient? It's not a patient unless mom says it's a patient." Although simplifying the historical, technical, political, and cultural processes through which the fetal patient has emerged, this surgeon's comment nonetheless highlights the crucial role of pregnant women in birthing this new social entity. Throughout their experiences with fetal surgery, from initial prenatal diagnosis through postoperative recovery

and delivery, these women do an extraordinary amount of work on behalf of their fetus. Although to date only a small number of women have
encountered fetal surgery, its increasing routinization suggests that the
pool of women affected may expand.

Most pregnant women who come to Capital Hospital on behalf of a
sick fetus are also presented with other, perhaps equally agonizing, decisions: abortion, a range of nonsurgical treatments, postnatal treatment,
or no treatment at all. Prenatal diagnosis plays a significant role in shaping these pregnant women's desires and choices. Fetal diagnosis and
treatment occurs within a context of women's (un)willingness or (in)abil-
ity to bear and raise an impaired baby in a society where this is a most
difficult task. In Rothman's (1986) poignant study of amniocentesis,
many women who chose prenatal diagnosis did so out of fear of fetal disability. Is fetal surgery, like prenatal diagnosis, seen by pregnant women
as a way to increase their odds of having a healthy baby? If so, there is a
cruel irony in that fetal morbidity statistics for fetal surgery suggest that
even *with* treatment, if there is any baby at all, an impaired baby is
highly likely. Women who choose fetal surgery are indeed "moral pioneers" (Rapp 1987) on a rather precarious frontier, assuming great risk
on behalf of their vulnerable fetuses.

Given the uncertain nature of fetal surgery and the significant risks
associated with the procedure, it is easy to be curious about the range
of women's motivations to seek intervention. Of all the motivating factors described by informants that may lead a woman to choose fetal surgery, the most significant seems to be the desire to save her baby from
almost certain death. All of the conditions currently being treated by fetal surgery are considered terminal if left untreated, and medical workers remind women of this continually through the use of diagnostic
technologies and clinical discourse. This is a powerful incentive for
women who forgo other options in order to reconceptualize their fetuses
as patients. It is reflected (and reinforced) in the introduction to the
now-defunct patient education video discussed in previous chapters:
"This videotape follows a number of courageous mothers, struggling
with the decision of *how to save the life of their unborn child*" (emphasis
added). It is also articulated in women's own voices as they explain their
intensive focus on their fetuses. One patient, Debbie, recalled, "I was so
focused on the fetal surgery and her [the fetus's] operation and what it
entailed, that I don't think it dawned on me that *I* was going to go
through major surgery." Marla, a patient whose fetus died one month after surgery, stated, "You can look at statistics any way you want. When it
came down to it, it was more an intuitive feeling, that this was the way to
go. Because you can look at facts and analyze the risks, and in the long
run you just have to go with your gut reaction."

A fetal surgeon echoed these sentiments: "We're not dealing with a standard mom. In fetal surgery, mom has taken this penultimate sacrifice. I ask them all [why they want to do this] and they all want to do it because they want their baby. It's not really complex for them. It's typical of most women." In addition to invoking cultural assumptions about the gendered nature of maternal sacrifice, this clinician's comments underscore how important fetuses are to the women who choose fetal surgery. Yet this version of reproductive politics, resting on the presumed inevitability of women's sacrifice, may ignore that fetuses are important to men as well. Marla's husband, Dan, succinctly and emotionally described their reasons for selecting fetal surgery: "We *really* wanted this baby." Marla agreed: "Don't second-guess yourself. Just go with whatever decision you make because it's the best one with the information you have at that particular time." In short, the "best" decisions for these women and their partners involved selecting an intervention that transformed their fetuses into patients rather than certain casualties. But the context in which these decisions occurred is shaped by notions of maternal (not paternal) sacrifice, medical uncertainty, cultural anxieties about disability, and the value attached to fetuses.

Medical workers in fetal surgery offered additional interpretations of why women opt for fetal surgery. Some informants acknowledged that women engage fetal surgery within the broader context of their lives. One informant illustrated this well with a detailed dramatization of pregnant women's decision making:

> What's the story? "I'm Catholic, I wouldn't have an abortion, I want this baby no matter what, I love this man in spite of what my mother says, I want this baby, I know it seems crazy but I really want this baby to have every chance. I've thought about this, I am committed to this, I know the baby may not live, but I don't want to take the chance of going to term, I don't want to carry a baby with a potentially lethal lesion. If I'm going to do something about it, I want to do it now." That's a very common story from women at eighteen and at thirty. "I don't want to spend the rest of this pregnancy agonizing over this, I want to do something about it now. This is something to do, and if it works it's going to change the course of this baby's outcome. And even if there's only a small chance that it'll work, I want to do it." There are many women who do it because it's there, because it exists, because there's someone like Dr. ——— who says, "This is a shot. Stick with me."

This informant went on to suggest that in addition to women's desire to save their babies, they may also be motivated by the perceived benefits of involvement in an experimental protocol (see chapter 5). She told me, "There are people who are just transfixed at the prospect of coming out here." She situated the women's desire within the context of major efforts by the fetal surgery team to invite patients to participate: "We do a number, I tell you. We take care of them, we feed them, we worry about them. There are people who go through this process who get more attention in the course of time they're here than they have in their lives or ever will again. We are an incredibly nurturing bunch. We're very nice to people. And we are intentionally nice."

A nurse told me that some patients were so impressed by the surgeons that they based their decisions on admiration and loyalty. She said, "The ones who come here are very committed. They are adoring of Drs. ——— and ———, and there are a lot of babies named after these guys. Because they are extraordinary surgeons, and they have integrity, they're kind, they're devoted, they're committed to their work, they're really extraordinary people to work for." She felt that patients were excited about becoming part of a clinical research team with these charismatic fetal surgeons at the helm. She remarked, "Everybody takes something away from this. Patients are part of the team. It gives them a sense of meaning. They become part of medical science and it jacks them up." In this sense, reproductive politics are present in the ways in which pregnant women are actively enrolled in fetal surgery as research subjects on behalf of fetuses. They must provide detailed informed consent for the treatment, as we saw in the previous chapter. Even more than that, however, reproductive politics refers to women's perceived pleasure, assumed by medical workers, at being "captured" and perhaps captivated by the research process itself.

Reproductive politics mold women's engagement with fetal surgery in other ways. Almost every informant discussed the relationship between women's beliefs about abortion and their decision to seek fetal surgery. Like Susan Davis, many of the women who choose fetal surgery hold antiabortion political views and likely would not choose abortion as a treatment option. But this is not necessarily the case for all women undergoing fetal surgery. When a pregnant woman carrying a potential fetal surgical candidate arrives at Capital Hospital, she undergoes a battery of prenatal diagnostic tests and is presented with an array of options. A pro-choice woman whose fetus has a serious, potentially lethal defect may be more likely to select abortion as an option than a woman who is opposed to abortion (Rothman 1986). Yet a pro-life woman may decide to eschew technology and do nothing at all, while a pro-choice woman experiencing what may be her last pregnancy may be quite reluctant to abort her fetus. For example, Marla and Dan were both in their forties and did not already have children, making their ailing fetus—possibly their last chance at parenthood—that much more valuable to them. Its death a month after surgery devastated them. These issues are extremely complex (Rapp 1994; Sandelowski and Jones 1996), and it is not easy to map a woman's choices—particularly when she is faced with a severely ill fetus.

A fetal surgeon framed these complicated connections to reproductive politics in this way:

> You know, it's an incredible commitment that the parents, particularly the mother, makes with this intervention. Because she has a big operation, because the medicines we give her to prevent labor make her absolutely miserable. And it's an incredible sacrifice. We try to let them know that preoperatively, and so I think that an easier option would be to opt for abortion. And I think by the nature of that, the women tend to be less pro-choice. But at the same time, our philosophy is that if we really cannot fix the problem, then we do a fetectomy, we take the fetus out [during surgery]. I suppose there are a lot of real ardent antiabortion camps out there who would probably feel that we shouldn't do any intervention on the fetus. I think [fetal surgery] could potentially become a real hot spot in the abortion debate.

This informant went on to say that abortion is problematic both inside and outside the clinical setting. That is, not only do "pro-life" women tend to select fetal surgery rather than abortion, but women who select fetal surgery, in this surgeon's view, may be considered more "pro-life" than women who do not. In this sense, fetal surgery is a type of work—both clinical and cultural—that may resonate with abortion politics in multiple ways, including women's motivations for selecting intervention and medical workers' evaluations of the women. Here, fetal surgery is defined as a life-affirming act, a definition that imputes a certain moral countenance to the pregnant women who choose it.

Unfortunately, I was not able to collect enough data from the pregnant women and their families to develop a more detailed understanding of the relationship between abortion politics and women's decisions.[8] The medical workers I interviewed shared a consensus that most women who choose fetal interventions are "pro-life." But even this framing is contested: a pro-choice woman who aborts her severely defected fetus may very well consider her decision to be life-affirming. And as fetal surgery becomes a standard procedure for certain fetal anomalies, a wider range of women (and not just "pro-life" women) may see intervention as a more viable option. The experience of dealing with a doomed fetus may itself confound women's political identities. Perhaps further research will shed light on the multiple trajectories of the hundreds of women who are counseled at Capital Hospital and elsewhere each year, including how only a few women wind up at fetal treatment centers while others never get beyond their local physicians. Once there, how do factors like timeliness of diagnosis, gestational age of the fetus, the woman's own age, the severity of the fetus's condition, and cost affect women's decisions to abort, let nature take its course, opt for postnatal treatment, or venture into the domain of fetal interventions? It would also be useful to track how the maternal-fetal conflict paradigm plays out along these different trajectories, with a range of interventions from diagnosis to abortion to treatment evoking issues of maternal sacrifice and women's "opposition" to fetal interests.[9]

Because reproductive beliefs are so deeply held by people, women's politics and medical workers' politics can sometimes clash in fetal surgery. A fetal surgeon outlined some of the ethical and legal challenges posed by fetal surgery: "Biologically we're treating the fetus as a patient, as part of mom, and it's a patient because mom says it's a patient. If she says it's not a patient, it's not a patient. The legal framework is that it could still be aborted. I think more than anything else it shows how artificial the framework is. But it never happens. And the reason it never happens is that mom has never decided to make it an abortion. Mom still has a say." I asked the surgeon what would happen if one of the women did choose to have an abortion following fetal surgery. He replied, "Who decides to abort? It's her decision." I then asked him how he would *feel* about it. He admitted, "I would be upset, mostly because we'd have invested time, energy, and effort in the fetus's well-being. And I would feel that mom's shortsightedness had really ripped off that fetus, as well as our investment of time. It would be a terrible thing. The truth is it will probably never happen because these moms are just fantastic." It is not difficult to appreciate this surgeon's frustration in such a hypothetical situation, although it seems ironic that the surgeon would portray a woman who aborts after fetal surgery as "shortsighted," given her investment in fetal surgery in the first place. Again, women are paradoxically positioned along a continuum of choice, and some of their decisions about the same fetus may be seen as valid while others are not.

Regardless of their motivations for engaging fetal surgery as a treatment option, pregnant women usually must reorganize their lives profoundly once they select it. Because the procedure is offered at only a handful of facilities in the United States and globally, this type of intervention involves travel, large time commitments, living in a different city for several weeks, financial expenditures, and often leaving other family members behind. Amber, a young woman whose twenty-eight-week fetus was diagnosed with polyhydramnios (excessive water in the amniotic fluid), was referred for treatment after having amniocentesis at her local hospital—more than four hundred miles away in a different state. After having this diagnosis confirmed at Capital, she was asked to return one week later for follow-up. Beatrice, a seventeen-year-old from a town two hundred miles away, was referred with fetal encephaly, or bowel loops in the amniotic cavity. She underwent prenatal diagnosis at Capital Hospital, which revealed normal chromosomes and hydronephrosis (swelling of the kidneys resulting from obstructed urine flow) in her fetus. One month later she had to return for follow-up diagnosis, which determined that the fetus's condition had worsened.

Once they have been operated on, women are expected to remain near Capital Hospital for the duration of their pregnancies, sometimes up to two or three months. They are told to make financial arrangements prior to traveling to determine their eligibility and coverage. Pregnant women must also cope with being bedridden immediately after surgery. To prevent premature labor, they are discouraged from moving around. Boredom and frustration may become real problems. All of these factors take a considerable toll both on the pregnant women and on their partners and families. One patient, Marie, made the following remark to her caretakers after surgery: "I had *no idea* it would be like this." A nurse told me, "It takes a certain kind of person to do it. I still find it fascinating to see people make these kinds of sacrifices, even in the face of statistics that are not at all reassuring." As did the fetal surgeons, this nurse invokes cultural meanings related to maternal sacrifice, although here it is the risky nature of fetal surgery that frames women's actions as sacrifice. Whereas the surgeon's assumption seemed to be that all women would "naturally" make such a sacrifice on behalf of their fetuses, the nurse sees these pregnant women as special because they chose a dangerous procedure.

But while they may sacrifice a great deal for their fetuses, these women are also average women attempting to cope with a serious medical problem. One nineteen-year-old patient's story, told by a social worker, illustrates both the complexity and the ordinariness of the women's lives. Shortly after her operation and needing a break from the intensity of fetal surgery, April went on an outing with her sister, prompting considerable outrage by her doctors. A social worker told me, "She went ahead and went to Great America. Her sister took her. You know, she's wearing a terbutaline pump; it was madness."[10] April's story illustrates that, although these women work hard to save their babies, they do so within the broader framework of who they are and what they are willing and able to do on behalf of their fetuses. It also shows that these women struggle to maintain many aspects of their identities across sites and may not be willing to limit their lives for months on end to the role of patient on behalf of their fetuses. Why wouldn't a young woman undergoing a difficult and prolonged series of medical procedures want to take a day off and visit Great America?

The pregnant women who undergo fetal surgery may also be forced to leave their families behind and to take extended leaves of absence from their jobs. In this vein, one of the fetal surgeons described just how disruptive fetal surgery might be for some families: "It's an incredible commitment the mother makes with this intervention. There are an incredible number of medical bills. Usually what has to happen is the mother has to stay out of work. It disrupts everything in the family." Susan Davis is a good example of this. She told me how hard it was for her to spend several weeks at and near Capital Hospital, far away from home and her family business. Although her husband, Jim, joined her for most of the postoperative period, she had to leave her other two children at home in a relative's care. Her son was very young at the time, and she found leaving him to be very difficult. Often such hard choices are made bearable only by the support of the patient's partner or family. Another patient, Marla, talked about how important it was to her to have her husband, Dan, at her side the whole time. She stated emphatically that "it would have been impossible without him." In addition to providing psychosocial support, a partner may also provide family income so that a woman can take time off from work to travel to a distant hospital for treatment. But what about women who do not have partners or who cannot afford to miss work? Would they be more likely to abort a sick fetus than to travel hundreds of miles and undergo surgery requiring a lengthy recovery period? This raises the issue of access and what kinds or classes of women will be able to "choose" fetal surgery.

In Praise of Heroic Moms

One of the striking aspects of fetal surgery is that women are routinely praised by medical workers for their commitments. A fetal surgeon told me, "The moms who decide to do this are in every way heroic. I mean, they are truly heroes." But what does it mean to describe these pregnant women as "heroic moms?" Unraveling the reproductive politics embedded in this terminology tells us much about some of the cultural meanings attached to fetal surgery. I first consider the term "mom," a standardized, almost clinical label that many medical workers—especially fetal surgeons—use to refer to the pregnant women. This term performs a certain kind of cultural work in defining these women as mothers *before* they have given birth. Many women do consider themselves "moms" while still pregnant, but motherhood is usually contingent on the presence of children. Mothering a fetus is a bit more complicated. Describing the pregnant women in fetal surgery as "moms" taps into a range of cultural assumptions about motherhood and maternal sacrifice, while also linking fetal surgery to warm, apple-pie images of hearth and home rather than the high-tech, sterile operating room.

Moreover, when medical workers use "mom" terminology to describe the women, they also discursively identify with fetuses. This is obvious, almost comically so, in one surgeon's electronic mail address: "fetus@ —— —." Perhaps, in man's eternal quest to return to the comfort of the womb, operating on fetuses is the next best thing to being one.

Describing pregnant women in fetal surgery as "heroic" adds another dimension of meaning to these practices. In exalting women who choose fetal surgery, acceptance of surgical intervention is seen as something to be rewarded. The women in fetal surgery are indisputably brave, and their engagement with fetal surgery has been integral to the making of the unborn patient. Yet the many more women who opt to fore go fetal surgery in favor of a different treatment or who choose to abort their fetuses are faced with decisions every bit as daunting and complex. All reproductive decisions, regardless of their outcome, are fraught with ambiguity—particularly within the current zeitgeist of abortion struggles, gender role confusion, and restricted access to health care. But medical workers' use of the term "heroic" to describe *only* the pregnant women who choose fetal surgery reinforces the cultural significance of maternal sacrifice on behalf of a living fetus. At the same time that many women in the United States are vilified for choosing to abort their fetuses, a small group of fetal surgery "moms" are promoted as reproductive heroes. Thus, fetal surgery celebrates and embodies the Western myth of "the ever-bountiful, ever-giving, self-sacrificing mother" (Bassin et al. 1994, 2), a myth that can all too easily transform maternal engagement and sacrifice into duty.

Use of the term "heroic" also suggests that fetal surgery may be more dangerous than surgeons are willing to acknowledge publicly. Heroes are usually legendary, noble figures who risk their own lives to save others. They walk through burning buildings to rescue small children; they emerge from war zones bloody and exhausted, carrying their fallen comrades on their shoulders. Heroism in fetal surgery, as medical workers define it, seems to embody these mythic qualities. The pregnant women who choose surgical intervention are esteemed for selfless acts on behalf of their fetuses, and their courage is duly noted by everyone involved. As pioneers on a new, hazardous frontier, the women risk their own lives on behalf of their fetuses and often emerge, like soldiers, bloody and exhausted from their ordeal. Like the bold heroes of action films, they enter into an unknown territory where their fate is uncertain and they could die. Is fetal surgery—increasingly considered a "standard" treatment as we saw in the previous chapter—so risky, dangerous, and scary that women undergoing it on behalf of their fetuses could be considered heroes in traditional framings of that term? Certainly medical workers seem to be implying as much in their veneration of "heroic moms," despite their assertions in other contexts that the procedures are safe and efficacious.

"We Haven't Lost a Mom Yet": The Risky Business of Operating on Fetuses

Women's engagement with fetal surgery involves danger, risk, and unfavorable odds. Indeed, many informants in fetal surgery *claim* that maternal risk and safety issues are paramount in spite of evidence presented in chapter 5 that maternal risk is downplayed. Several fetal surgeons proudly told me, "We haven't lost a mom yet!" Risk is important for several reasons, the most significant being the ever-present possibility of maternal death. Although fetal death affects everyone involved, especially the women, it is not unexpected in fetal surgery; after all, more fetuses have died during during fetal surgery than have been rescued by it. Moreover, most fetuses would likely die anyway even without treatment, making fetal loss a regular feature of this practice and helping to prepare the women for such a possible outcome. But if a pregnant woman were to die during fetal surgery, it is likely that fetal surgery could not continue, at least without serious reappraisal. It is ironic that in a specialty in which pregnant women are routinely erased, one maternal death could have major consequences. This points to the fragile balance medical workers attempt to strike between safeguarding maternal health while doing everything they can to salvage fetuses.

The longevity of fetal surgery as a new specialty rests on establishing satisfactory levels of maternal risk. But satisfaction in this case is relative. In a risk-benefit analysis applied to fetal surgery, some maternal morbidity may be considered acceptable and inevitable by some practitioners. Maternal mortality is clearly *not* acceptable, at least for oversight committees, funders, and most medical workers. Moreover, given that there is *no* clinical benefit of this surgery for pregnant women *at all*, even some maternal morbidity is seen as too great a risk by many participants. Yet somewhere between death and safety is an ambiguous gray zone, in which medical workers define risk through their innovative practices of operating on pregnant women and fetuses, and where some pregnant women "heroically" accept risk as part of their commitments to saving their babies. In other words, as Lisa Jean Moore (1996) has argued, there is no standard meaning of acceptable risk and assessments must be negotiated in practice.

The following account describes how pregnant women are prepared for fetal surgery, illustrating some of the potential vectors of risk:

Maternal preparation begins with a 100-mg suppository of indomethacin before operation and placement of an epidural catheter for postoperative anal-
gesis. . . . Maternal intraoperative monitoring includes a blood pressure cuff,
large-bore intravenous catheters, a bladder catheter, electrocardiographic
leads, and a transcutaneous pulse oximeter. . . . The mother is positioned
supine with towels placed under the right side to lift her uterus off of the in-
ferior cava to avoid compromise of venous return. The uterus is exposed
through a low transverse abdominal incision and delivered into the operative
field. A large abdominal ring retractor is used to maintain exposure . . . The
position and orientation of the hysterotomy is planned to stay as far away
from the placenta as possible and still allow exposure of the appropriate part
of the fetus. (Harrison and Adzick 1991, 287–288)

Pregnant women are positioned here as physical barriers to be traversed,
a flesh and blood organism that must be surgically opened and clinically
monitored for the sake of the unborn patient nestled inside. Extraordinary technical maneuvers are required to access the fetus surgically. The
very graphic nature of this description belies notions of maternal-fetal
conflict, illustrating instead the visceral overlap between women and
their fetuses. In operating on fetuses, women are *always* at risk at numerous points throughout the procedure.

Harrison and Longaker (1991, 189) suggest that "the main deterrent
to direct fetal intervention by hysterotomy is not the risk to the fetus
(who will benefit if the intervention is successful) but the risk to the
mother." Maternal morbidity in fetal surgery is roughly equated to that
posed by cesarean sections, "except for the ongoing problem of a contin
uing gestation (e.g., preterm labor) after surgery" (Harrison and Longaker 1991, 199). That is, fetal surgery is seen by some medical workers
as not that different from a routine cesarean section. Yet among the complications that occurred in one sample of thirteen women who underwent fetal surgery between 1981 and 1989 were amniotic fluid leaks,
premature rupture of membranes, chorioamnionitis (infection in the
amniotic sac) requiring a cesarean section, enterocolitis (inflammation
of the intestinal membranes), hyperplacentation syndrome (overattachment of the placenta), pulmonary edema (excessive fluid in the lungs),
persistent oligohydramnios (insufficient amniotic fluid), and premature
labor (Harrison and Longaker 1991). Amazingly, the authors of this article suggest that "Fortunately, there has been no maternal mortality, and
significant morbidity has occurred in only one case" (Harrison and Longaker 1991, 199). Here, risk is seriously minimized: low risk is defined as
no maternal deaths and overall morbidity assessments exclude serious
complications experienced by many of the pregnant women. It is striking
that ruptured membranes, emergency cesarean sections, edema, and

TABLE 21–8. Maternal Outcome with Open Fetal Surgery

		Preoperative		Operation				Postoperative					Pregnancy Outcome	
		Gestational age		Hosp. Stay Postop. (days)	Procedure	Operative Time (min) Fetal/Total	Blood Loss (mL)	Tocolysis	Hospital Stay	Gestational Age (wks)		Type of Delivery	Complications	Subsequent Pregnancy
Pt	Age	Dx/Op (wks)	Dx							Labor	Delivery			
1.	18 yo G1P0	22/23	Bladder	9	Bilateral ureterostomies	28/165	900 2 units Tx	Indomethacin Ritodrine	9	35	35	C/S	None	2 normal pregnancies Cesarean deliveries; normal male and female
2.	19 yo G1P0	22/25	Bladder	9	Bladder vesicostomy	22/90	800	Indomethacin Ritodrine	9	30	32	C/S	Amniotic fluid leak at 26 weeks Fx with 1 suture Premature rupture of membranes at 30 weeks	1 normal pregnancy; cesarean delivery; normal male
3.	30 yo G1P0	24/27	Diaphragm	5	Diaphragmatic hernia repair	60/110	1,000	—	5	—	—	—	None	1 (currently pregnant)
4.	17 yo G3P2	22/26	Diaphragm	5	Diaphragmatic hernia repair	55/180	600	—	5	—	—	—	None	None
5.	31 yo G1P0	22/24	Bladder	8	Bladder vesicostomy	15/90	600	Indomethacin Ritodrine	8	33	33	C/S	None	None
6.	26 yo G2P1	22/24	Diaphragm	9	Diaphragmatic hernia repair	60/120	350	Indomethacin Ritodrine IV Terbutaline PO	9	30	33	C/S	Amniotic fluid leak Chorioamnionitis requiring a cesarean section	1 pregnancy complicated by uterine rupture at 37.5 weeks; cesarean delivery, normal female
7.	38 yo G3P2	18/20	Diaphragm	6	Diaphragmatic hernia repair	60/180	500	—	6	—	—	—	None	1 normal pregnancy; cesarean delivery; normal male
8.	30 yo G2P1	25/27	Diaphragm	13	Diaphragmatic hernia repair	35/120	200	Indomethacin Ritodrine IV Terbutaline PO	13	30	30	C/S	None	1 normal pregnancy; cesarean delivery; normal female
9.	35 yo G1P0	17/18	Bladder	7	Bladder vesicostomy	10/75	350	Indomethacin Ritodrine IV	7	28	31	C/S	None	None
10.	27 yo G4P3	17/20	Bladder	14	Bladder vesicostomy	12/90	300	Indomethacin Magnesium IV Terbutaline PO	14	30	31	C/S	Clostridium difficile enterocolitis treated by vancomycin PO	None
11.	30 yo G3P2	20/23	Teratoma	15	Sacrococcygeal teratoma excision	25/80	200	Indomethacin Magnesium IV Nifedipine IV	15	25	25	C/S	Hyperplacentation syndrome and pulmonary edema Premature rupture of membranes 12 days postoperatively	None
12.	25 yo G1P0	22/23	Bladder	16	Bladder vesicostomy	17/80	1,000 2 units Tx	Indomethacin Magnesium IV Terbutaline PO	16	25	25	C/S	Persistent oligohydramnios requiring 500 mL NS amnioinfusion on postoperative Day 5 POD no. 11 reoperated and fetectomy	None
13.	34 yo G1P3	22/23	Bladder	8	Bladder vesicostomy	10/90	700	Indomethacin Magnesium IV Terbutaline PO	8	25	25	Vaginal	Poor compliance with discontinued PO maintenance tocolytic leading to premature labor and delivery	None

premature labor are not seen as "significant" problems. What, then, are the major risks?

As we have seen in previous chapters, "premature labor remains the largest obstacle to a successful outcome in the postoperative course" (Harrison and Adzick 1991, 288). Tocolysis, the pharmaceutical management of preterm labor, is required for all patients undergoing fetal surgery. But, ultimately designed to benefit fetuses which would otherwise be expelled by a contracting uterus, tocolysis presents major risks to pregnant women. Among the different tocolytic agents are β-mimetic drugs (ritodrine, terbutaline), magnesium sulfate, calcium channel blockers (nifedipine), progesterone, prostaglandin inhibitors (indomethacin), ethanol, and oxytocin or vasopressin analogs.[11] These agents act on women's bodies by affecting the response of the uterus to stimulation or intervention (Scheerer and Katz 1991). Maternal complications from these drugs may include pulmonary edema, cardiac arrhythmia, myocardial ischemia (constricted blood flow in the heart), hypotension (reduced blood pressure), altered metabolism, decreased muscle tone, respiratory problems, nausea, vomiting, dyspepsia (gastric indigestion), and cardiac arrest (Scheerer and Katz 1991).[12] Tocolysis may also pose risks to fetuses and newborns: terbutaline may lead to higher rates of tachycardia (rapid heartbeat), magnesium sulfate may lead to neuromuscular depression, and indomethacin may lead to cardiovascular and renal problems (Scheerer and Katz 1991).

Tocolysis is extremely important in the postoperative period, thus increasing a woman's risk far beyond the operating room. The following describes a typical strategy for postoperative management using tocolytic agents:

> Once the initial period of uterine contractions has subsided (usually within 5 days), oral tocolytics gradually are substituted for intravenous drugs and then continued throughout the remainder of the pregnancy. Perioperative antibiotics, generally a cephalosporin, are continued for 3 days after the operation. The patient is kept at bedrest for at least 3 days following surgery and then begins a progressive ambulation program. . . . Generally the patient is discharged on only oral tocolytic therapy within 10 days of the procedure. (Harrison and Adzick 1991, 288)

(Opposite) Maternal outcomes in thirteen open fetal surgery cases. Of particular interest are the columns of complications and subsequent pregnancies, most of which were delivered by cesarean section. Complications were present in more than half of these cases, and in one case (#13), the patient was identified as noncompliant, most likely because she delivered vaginally. Source: M. R. Harrison, M. S. Golbus, and R. A. Filly, 1991. The Unborn Patient: Prenatal Diagnosis and Treatment. Philadelphia: W. B. Saunders Company, p. 200.

The need for daily, ongoing tocolysis, even after patients are discharged, is a crucial but contested component of fetal surgery. An obstetrician complained that *all* of the patients require tocolysis postoperatively: "They go into labor the minute they come off of tocolytics! The patients must stay on pumps giving them tocolytics for the rest of their pregnancies." In this informant's view, tocolysis is yet another example of the dangers of fetal surgery. Another obstetrician described the first few days after surgery as the hardest for pregnant women: "They've been bombarded with medications, bombarded with general anesthesia, they've had an incision in the uterus, and they're *still* pregnant." And they must remain pregnant if the fetus is to have any chance at all of growing enough to survive, hence the need for tocolytic agents.

While women are recovering from surgery and preparing for what will most likely be an early birth, they must monitor their contractions and administer their own tocolytic drugs daily using an infusion pump, and they usually must commit to continuous and complete bed rest. One fetal surgeon told me, "Keeping the kid inside until he's big enough and ripe enough to come out and be a good kid—that's a struggle. A guaranteed struggle for the mom." According to many informants, tocolysis may contribute to women's discomfort after surgery. A patient, Wendy, recounted her rather painful postoperative experience: "I was using the morphine button because they give you a button to control it. I guess I pushed it like fifteen times in an hour." Women's self-surveillance may have additional consequences, such as medical workers blaming the women for poor outcomes. A social worker discussed one problem case: "She finally did go into labor at about thirty weeks, which seemed unnecessary at the time, although in retrospect it seems as if everybody goes into early labor. So maybe it was about April and maybe it was about just what this is." It does seem likely that the pregnant women, like the social worker quoted here, would experience similar dilemmas of attribution of causality with respect to preterm labor. Who is at fault when preterm labor occurs after surgery despite everyone's best efforts: the doctors who performed the surgery, the nurses responsible for postoperative care, or the women who administer their own drugs?

Because of the risks to pregnant women, contention surrounds the use of some tocolytics. For example, in the early 1990s the fetal surgery team at Capital Hospital began to use nitric oxide to control preterm labor. A fetal surgeon enthusiastically told me, "Nitric oxide makes your smooth muscles relax, and the uterus is a smooth muscle. We have very compelling experimental evidence that the use of nitric oxide—nitric, not nitrous—medications can relax the uterus. Extremely promising."[13] Yet despite fetal surgeons' excitement about nitric oxide, other medical workers view with suspicion its use in fetal surgery. An obstetrician complained that "the surgical group constantly wants to introduce new things that have not been thoroughly tried. They have just done that with the nitric oxide stuff. Two out of the last four cases where they got a child into a nursery, the child bled in its head. The only thing that changed was their pharmacology treatment of the patient." A nurse also discussed some complications resulting from early attempts to use nitric oxide: "You know the preterm labor issue is a big deal. We have actually started using nitric oxide, which is a very unusual thing. They almost killed somebody because they gave her the wrong suspension. But once we figured it all out, it turns out intraoperatively to be a really good drug for preterm labor."

Future reproductive potential, defined as the ability of the woman to successfully carry subsequent pregnancies, is another issue of concern in all accounts of maternal risk—and likely of great interest to women making a decision about fetal surgery. Minimal adverse effects have been claimed regarding future reproductive potential, although women who experience fetal surgery are committed to cesarean section for all future pregnancies. In one study of eighteen human patients, seven had subsequent pregnancies and delivered by cesarean section with "good outcomes" (Harrison and Adzick 1991). The other women were still too close to their operative dates to assess subsequent fertility, making follow-up more difficult. To date, no *long-term* outcome studies have been published in which women who have undergone fetal surgery are assessed for subsequent reproductive potential or for other health problems that might stem from the surgeries and postoperative care. Possible consequences related to reproductive potential include multiple cesarean sections, back problems due to abdominal weakness, the possibility of uterine rupture, urinary impairment from sustained catheterization and/or injury, circulatory problems, unknown long-term effects of tocolytic agents, muscle loss due to immobility, and a range of other problems that have not been adequately investigated in humans.

One informant at Capital Hospital was especially deeply concerned about the risk to women's reproductive potential. She told me,

> The other big dilemma for me are these young moms. It's one thing when you're thirty-six and you've been trying for fifteen years to be pregnant, and this is your last shot. . . . But when you're seventeen years old, or eighteen or nineteen, you have a long future of fertility ahead of you. And what we're doing is putting these people at risk for complications, and at the very least for the necessity of having cesarean sections later. Is that reasonable? At some point we need to look at an age cutoff. Which women are we in good conscience putting at risk here?

Similar concerns were raised by the IRB (discussed in chapter 5), which demanded an explanation from fetal surgeons as to why one of the women operated on was seventeen years old and six others were under twenty years of age. The IRB raised two important questions for the fetal surgery team that were not adequately addressed in subsequent correspondence: Would the team consider any minimum age appropriate? Why not limit the procedures to women near the end of their reproductive phase? It is difficult to avoid the conclusion that young, healthy women may make particularly good research materials in the fetal surgery enterprise. Ironically, surgeons may be putting at most risk precisely those young women with the greatest potential for future reproduction.

Risk is contested in other ways at Capital Hospital. One surgeon told me, "The overriding number one concern is to maintain mother's health. That is, without question, number one in everybody's mind. All the friction comes about *how* to obtain that." Another surgeon described the women as "willing to risk it all in the most complex operation that's currently being undertaken." In describing the early successes and failures of the program at Capital Hospital, this informant, like others, was quick to point out that "no moms have ever been injured, though we had some fetal deaths." Other medical workers had a somewhat different construction of maternal risk in fetal surgery. One informant, a nurse, told me, "I wasn't as concerned about the mothers dying because I've come to realize that we know enough about maternal care here and we just won't let them die. But we almost lost a patient, a woman who I got to know very well. We held her baby when it died [postoperatively]. It was a very tumultuous and difficult case." In describing risk, she stated, "Even if the surgery is perfect, all of the things we have to do to keep a baby inside a mother who's postoperative and in preterm labor complicates the course for the mom and her baby." And this may certainly complicate relations among medical workers in the Fetal Treatment Unit.

Accepting a certain degree of risk on behalf of their fetuses renders the pregnant women "heroes" in the eyes of some medical workers. But observers outside the medical domain have also identified risks in fetal surgery and question the viability of treatments focused on the fetal patient. Their emphasis is often quite different from that of fetal surgeons. For example, the director of Community Services for a local chapter of the March of Dimes Birth Defects Foundation, introduced in chapter 1, told me that fetal surgery is especially challenging with respect to maternal risk and safety. Drawing on her background in public and community health, this informant shared her own concerns about what she sees as an experimental practice with "questionable benefit to fetuses and clear risks to maternal health and well-being." Given that the mission of the March of Dimes is to improve the health of babies, fetal surgery is considered worthy of financial support and is a frequent recipient of foundation grants. But because it poses significant risks to pregnant women, it becomes problematic from an epidemiological perspective and may well be considered, in this informant's words, "a serious public health issue."

In sum, fetal surgery merits fresh consideration of *maternal* risk and safety issues. As a medical practice geared toward the fetal patient, pregnant women's participation is often seen as peripheral despite the centrality of their bodies. But assuming a huge risk is hardly consistent with a "conflict" perspective that tends to erase women. For some pregnant women, who benefit (albeit indirectly) from fetal surgery with the possibility of a reasonably healthy baby, a high degree of risk is obviously worth assuming. The women who talked about fetal surgery as "worth the effort" made their own complex analyses. They may well *not* have considered "costs" and "benefits" in the traditional ethical or biomedical framing of those terms. For their part, fetal surgeons and obstetricians attempt to minimize maternal risk and prevent pregnant women's deaths. For fetal surgeons, this has to do not only with concern for "moms" and fetuses, but also with ensuring successful operations and with the continued viability of this new specialty. Thus, for surgeons "minimizing risk" has a double meaning; it may take place both in practice and in claimsmaking about fetal surgery. For obstetricians, nurses, and other informants, minimizing risk is related to their professional concern with maternal health and is often presented in opposition to the aims of the fetal surgery team. As previously discussed, because most fetal surgery has up until recently been experimental and because pregnant women participate only on behalf of their fetuses, "losing a mom" would pose a serious threat to the continuance of fetal surgery. It is for these reasons, among others, that pregnant women are carefully managed in fetal surgery.

"Optimizing Mom to Save Her Fetus": Managing the Maternal Environment

Glenn Griener (1988, 3) has written that "in the past, the only way to affect the fetus' condition was by treating the mother. Now she can be bypassed." But as fetal surgeons discovered when they attempted to access the unborn patient, the "merely geographic" barrier posed by the uterus blossomed into a living, breathing participant who talked back (and who was deemed to need human subjects protection as a patient, as we saw in Chapter 5). A fetal surgeon summed up the dilemma: "You basically have a mother who's healthy and a fetus who's sick. In order to get at the fetus, you have to go through the mother, which presents potential for harm to the mother. So we need to develop safe ways of getting to the fetus." The necessity of having to "go through" women meant that surgeons had to recognize that "there's an additional player involved, and that's the mom," as another surgeon phrased it. Taking "mom" into account means that medical workers alternate between working *with* women and working *on* women to ensure healthy fetuses. Toward that end, pregnant women have been the focus of a variety of management strategies designed to foster the making of the unborn patient.

Fetal surgery is pervaded by metaphors and practices of maternal management. Extraordinary measures are often taken to ensure that a "successful" operation, one in which the fetus lives, is followed by a successful postoperative period with continued fetal and maternal survival. A fetal surgeon claims that "the advantage [of fetal surgery] is that the mom's brought in and, under controlled circumstances, the baby is cared for." In this framing, the woman becomes a passive part of the clinical circumstances (she is "brought in") and thus can be controlled in order to focus on the recovery needs of the fetus. Another surgeon echoed this strategy: "Mom deserves the very best on our part to try to save the fetus. In order to do that we have to optimize mom." In short, surgeons attempt to control as many aspects of fetal surgery as possible, including managing pregnant women both in and out of the operating room. Management is a means of transforming women's bodies into work objects or technologies of fetal care through processes that erase women's agency and reduce them to maternal environments. The women become *technomoms* in the service of the fetal patient.

In clinical practice, medical workers are especially frustrated with the dilemmas of postoperative care. One fetal surgeon told me, "We don't lose fetuses during an operation. Now we're dealing with perioperative mortality." Practitioners' concerns stem from what happens to fetuses when they are replaced in the uterus and thus removed from surgeons' direct purview. Many fetuses that die do so in the postoperative period, even after a so-called successful surgery. A fetal surgeon reported that at one point the team had "a bunch of deaths in the first twenty-four hours, what we call mysterious deaths." This prompted renewed consideration of management issues. Another surgeon lamented that "it's very frustrating to do your best work and then lose the baby post-op. It makes one wonder if it's okay post-op to put the baby back in and assume that mom will take care of things." A similar comment was made by another surgeon in describing how the fetal surgery team evaluated a particular case after the fetus died. He stated, "We learned the value of an intensive care setting, that we had to optimize mom in order to make sure that it wasn't mom causing this fetus to die."

These comments are telling, for they illustrate cultural conceptions of the maternal environment. Not only do surgeons appear to mistrust pregnant women's bodies, but they are constrained by the material realities of pregnancy to relying on an unstable course of postoperative management. Having done their "best work" during surgery, fetal surgeons are reluctant to relinquish control of their precious and vulnerable fetal work objects back into what they are now constructing as a potentially dangerous environment. Yet they must do so because the uterus is recognized as a better (and cheaper) "recovery room" than the Neonatal Intensive Care Unit (NICU), particularly for very young fetuses that are not yet viable. Reproductive politics are clearly at work here in the ways in which pregnant women's bodies and actions are defined. But this framing is likely as much about medical work as it is about gender politics. Surgeons may be reluctant to release the unborn patient into *any* environment that they cannot control, whether women's bodies or the NICU, as we saw in chapter 4.

Surgeons' comments also reveal a discourse of blame and shifting accountability for postoperative problems—in this case, to the women who "cause" their fetuses to die. The issue is one of who will control the postoperative period, and it is clearly not "mom." Here we see surgeons staking a claim to the crucial fetal recovery period. But they do not distinguish between the bodily activities that women can control after surgery and those they cannot, for example, as we saw earlier, some women can monitor their own tocolysis postoperatively. Women certainly cannot control any of the physiological consequences of having their wombs surgically opened, nor can they control the fate of their fragile fetus. How, then, are failures accounted for in fetal surgery? Who is responsible when fetuses die? Surgeons believe that if they can control the maternal environment they might achieve better outcomes—and this may pit them against obstetricians as well as against the pregnant women whom they reduce to technomoms.

Unsurprisingly, discussions of management often occur alongside evaluations of success or failure in fetal surgery. Management issues become especially acute after fetal deaths or when there are significant problems with a case. For example, at Capital Hospital a special meeting on fetal management was convened after several consecutive fetal deaths occurred in the postoperative period. Specifically, participants wanted to discuss monitoring as a crucial aspect of management. In suggesting that I attend this meeting, one of the nurses told me that I might not understand everything that was being said, but "the politics should be interesting." During the meeting, a fetal surgeon referred to the diverse group of specialists in the room—including obstetricians, sonographers, physiologists, nurses, and others—as "a special working group to address the problems of post-op management." He remarked that mortality statistics are "so far two out of three," and "what is needed is a strategy for increasing management." Discussion during this meeting focused on ways of achieving this goal, and thus from the outset clearly linked the potential for successful procedures to enhanced management.

One case in particular illustrated some of the problems that the fetal surgery team faced regarding maternal management. A fetus with a right-sided diaphragmatic hernia survived surgery at twenty-six weeks but then died postoperatively. A fetal surgeon claimed that "the bottom line is that the operation was perfect and there was no identifiable cause of death." Another surgeon concurred, stating emphatically that this was "the first mother that was satisfactorily monitored during surgery." (It is discursively interesting, but not surprising, that the mother here is referred to as "that" rather than "who.") Yet the surgeon went on to say that during the operation the woman had experienced three uterine contractions on the operating table, causing surgeons to worry about "the effects on the fetus of controlling her." This suggests that the operation was less perfect than fetal surgeons claimed. In summing up lessons learned from this case, one of the surgeons emphasized that "we need to increase management of mom." He called for additional monitoring, particularly in the postoperative period, stating that "the issue is to monitor the uterus post-op where the kid's inside. We're not very good at it." Here, the pregnant woman becomes simply "the uterus," a container for "the kid." Obstetricians in the room reacted negatively to the surgeon's statement, expressing concerns about encroachment on "their" territory—the postoperative period. The surgeon attempted to placate them by saying "there is a terrible balance between care of the fetus and concern for the mother. But we don't monitor very well; we put the fetus back in and need to monitor more closely." As articulated by these surgeons, better management can only be accomplished through intensified control of the pregnant woman, and perhaps of obstetricians as well.

By monitoring, medical workers were referring to a range of technologies that are designed to provide crucial information about fetuses but that are used in and on pregnant women. Also discussed at the meeting were some examples of "better" monitoring techniques already in use, such as ultrasound both during and after surgery and a radio telemetric device that keeps track of the fetal heart rate during surgery. A clinician whose primary responsibility in the laboratory is to develop monitoring technologies described a new technique that embodies some of the tensions in fetal surgery between fetal care and maternal management. Not yet used for humans at the time of my research, the technique was tried first in sheep and monkeys. It works by penetrating the placental vessel with a twenty-two-gauge catheter that, according to the surgeon, "comes out and gets hooked into the mother's body under the abdominal skin. If you want to access the fetus, you put a needle into the catheter through the woman's abdomen." Because the catheter is designed to remain in place in the woman's body, it provides an easy, accessible, semipermanent channel through which to diagnose, monitor, and even treat the fetus.[14] This is an excellent example of how women are technologically transformed by the practices of fetal surgery. Another fetal surgeon described the technique as "the wave of the future," but asked others at the meeting "if it is worth the risk right now." Risk, in this case, was to the mother, and not all participants agreed that the innovation was worth the risk.

Women in fetal surgery are also subject to nonclinical management, where surveillance strategies are more refined and subtle. For the most part, the fetal surgery team at Capital Hospital—including surgeons, nurses, social workers, and administrative support personnel—is fully responsible for managing nonmedical aspects of pregnant women's participation in fetal surgery. From the moment pregnant women agree to fetal surgery and begin reorganizing their lives to accommodate this major disruption, they and their partners are closely managed and directed through the fetal surgery process. As an obstetrician remarked, "——— [a fetal surgery nurse] is running those patients and their lives." During and immediately following surgery, the women are hospitalized where they can be closely monitored clinically. After surgery, most patients are asked to remain near Capital Hospital for the remainder of their pregnancies. For those who cannot afford a hotel, there is a nearby guest house funded by the March of Dimes that can accommodate up to five patient families. It is located near the hospital and provides both lodging and support. Comments at a fetal treatment meeting are fairly typical of how patients are managed: "April is being put up at a guest house until the baby is born. Rather than sending her back to [her home state], it made more sense to keep her here so that we can better monitor her and the fetus's condition."

Examining management issues highlights another important aspect of fetal surgery. Where the term *management* is used positively to describe strategies for achieving success, the term *mismanagement* is used in this setting in a derogatory way. Conflicts occur among different specialists over how best to manage "moms," and medical workers often accuse each other of putting patients at risk. Obstetricians, somewhat inexplicably, are accused by fetal surgeons of not understanding maternal physiology and its relationship to patient management. One fetal surgeon claimed that "the obstetricians grossly mismanaged [a patient] in the perioperative period. And in fact almost cost the pregnancy." He went on to say, "That won't happen in the future. We took the time to place mom in an intensive setting, to monitor mom very carefully. I personally stayed at her bedside for forty-eight hours straight, examining her constantly, doing ultrasound measurements and recording, and just going over everything." Another fetal surgeon told me that "some of the obstetricians and OB nurses are not used to doing big operations and having patients in the ICU. They view the postoperative problem as the preterm labor problem. But it was clear that patient management went far beyond just management of preterm labor, and we couldn't not be responsible outside of monitoring. That led to friction."

The postoperative period is particularly contested because, as we have seen, preterm labor poses a grave threat and fetal surgeons have not yet developed effective management strategies. In evaluating a fetal death, one fetal surgeon remarked,

> Had it not been for some mismanagement of the mom, the fetus probably wouldn't have had any problems. No matter how much data we could give [the obstetricians] telling them they were grossly wrong, they would do what their experience told them was the right thing to do. They don't even want to look at [our data]. Any data we give them they just flat-out don't trust, because they've never had that data before and they don't know how to interpret it. In essence, they're out of their league. They've left obstetrics, where they understand what they're doing, and entered the realm of perioperative surgery, physiology they clearly have no handle on. And interestingly enough, are absolutely close-minded and unwilling to learn or to be taught.

In accusing obstetricians of being "out of their league," this surgeon is making a hierarchical rather than geographical claim. For their part, obstetricians are as adamant as fetal surgeons in accusing the other group of mismanagement of pregnant women. An obstetrician told me that "fetal surgeons just shunt patients off. They don't take care of the woman afterward. The perinatal group has now taken over the maternal management." And a perinatologist told me that "fetal surgeons tend to lose sight of the forest for the trees. A live fetus is not the only measure of success. My role is to take care of the mother." Ironically, both fetal surgeons and obstetricians accuse each other of mismanagement in relation to the pregnant women, suggesting that "moms" are key sites of professional struggles.

In sum, a variety of clinical management strategies have been used in the making of the unborn patient. Because pregnant women and their fetuses exist in one body, maternal management is seen as essential to improved fetal outcomes. Unlike fetuses, pregnant women are not always defined as patients, yet they are certainly treated as work objects and "optimized" in numerous ways. Various forms of clinical and non-clinical care are provided to the pregnant women with the aim of controlling the circumstances of fetal treatment and recovery, suggesting that a different kind of "managed care" is at work in fetal surgery. To a large degree, management strategies can be seen as attempts to create a hospitable maternal environment, one in which the fetus will survive and recover successfully. The surgical team attempts to reconfigure the pregnant women as technomoms in line with their clinical goals. But not all specialists in this domain agree with fetal surgeons' management strategies, leading to fractious turf battles and imputations of mismanagement. Nor are the women themselves merely passive environments to be shaped and prodded by technicians focused on the fetus. Women may assert their own interests and needs as they struggle for a modicum of control in the face of intensified medical management.

"We're Not So Sure We Like Them Anymore": Differences in Lay and Professional Perspectives

Not only is fetal surgery a site of contestation among professionals, it is also a site of differences between professionals and laypersons. Pregnant women and their families bring their own unique knowledge, meanings, and interpretations to the fetal surgery experience, and these may differ considerably from the "expert" perspectives claimed by fetal surgeons and other medical workers. Along a number of dimensions, ranging from evaluations of success and failure to selecting a treatment option, pregnant women's decisions and expertise are often challenged or simply ignored in fetal surgery. Once initial consent for fetal surgery is obtained, respect for women's authority as spokespersons for their fetuses seems to diminish considerably. This is not to suggest that the fetal surgery team is insidiously "out to get" pregnant women. Nor does it mean that the women passively accede to physicians' requests like the sheep that preceded them in the fetal surgery enterprise. The reality, as is often the case, is more complicated, contingent, and subtle, reflecting the many social and cultural factors that come together to shape pregnant women's experiences in a specific clinical setting.

One important difference concerns how fetal surgery is defined and evaluated by its participants. In identifying a particular operation as successful or not, fetal surgeons and patients often use varying criteria. Pregnant women choose fetal surgery with the hope that they will have a healthy baby in the end. These patients are, according to a social worker, "people who have waited a long time to have a baby" and who "are very committed." Their goals are to "save" their fetuses however possible, a goal certainly shared by fetal surgeons. Yet their reactions to success or failure may be very different from those of fetal surgeons. Susan Davis, whose surgery was successful, described the operation as an unqualified success and her daughter as "a miracle baby." For Susan, the success of the surgery extended beyond the operation and into the fabric of her family's lives. Four years after surgery, when I visited the Davises, Elizabeth was still considered a very special baby. Wendy, another patient, qualified success in a slightly different way: "It was worth the effort. Even if it had not been successful, we would have known that we'd at least tried and he might have had a slim chance. I feel sure that if we had not done anything, he wouldn't have survived the pregnancy." In Wendy's case, a live baby was a mark of success: not even making the effort to undergo the operation would have been considered a failure.

Fetal surgeons are far more interested in the *immediate* clinical success of fetal operations, with definitions of success and failure often limited to survival of the operation by the fetus. One fetal surgeon told me that "the nature of fetal surgery is that once you opt to run the race, the goal is to win." When I asked another surgeon how he defined success and failure in fetal surgery, he replied, "Surgeries are kind of a unique therapy. You do a specific invasive intervention with lots of different risks and hope to obtain a specific goal, usually cure or palliation. Ideally, you'd like to get somebody to a point of comfortable, functional living." He also defined a failed surgery: "Obviously, if you aren't able to cure somebody then that would be some degree of failure if that was your intention. But even if you can't cure somebody, in the process you can palliate their pain or disability. A miserable failure would be to make them worse off than they were before you operated and an even more miserable failure would be to make them worse off than the natural history of the disease would make them. And that should be foreseeable pre-operatively most of the time." Yet in certain cases, babies might very well be worse off after fetal surgery, chronically impaired in innumerable ways or potentially brain damaged as we saw with a sacrococcygeal teratoma case in chapter 5.

Fetal surgeons at Capital Hospital have other criteria for success: criteria that reflect both their dual position as clinical researchers and the status of fetal surgery as an "innovative" procedure. If something useful can be learned from a specific case, even if the fetus dies, the surgeons may consider the procedure a success. But some surgeons are deeply troubled by the costs of gaining biomedical knowledge in this uncertain fashion. For example, one surgeon recalled some of his earlier doubts about the value of fetal surgery:

We finally know what the hell we're doing in some small way. And we will succeed. It's very obvious to me now. It was not a year ago. I was very frustrated; I thought, we're working on all these kids. Why? What are we learning? What are we doing? We're just murdering babies. It's just a fancy, expensive way to kill kids. But now that we're taking measurements, we're doing the right thing. We're understanding, and we'll succeed. There's no doubt that we'll succeed.

In addition to invoking reproductive politics—fetal surgery and abortion both may be defined as means for killing fetuses—this surgeon clearly links success to better methods, increased knowledge gained through experience, and fetal survival.

For fetal surgeons, success may also refer to the broader enterprise of fetal surgery and not just individual clinical cases, although these too are important. Another fetal surgeon offered this response when asked about success and failure: "If you're going to go 80 percent of the way, you've got to finish the race. You've got to go the whole way. Because if you fail not having gone the whole way, did you really fail? Did you fail for the stupidity of not going the whole way or did you fail because it was truly the wrong thing to do?" He then went on to link the success of fetal surgery generally to the work at Capital Hospital: "You haven't answered the question if you don't do it right. So we have to do it right. And we're the only people in the world who can do this. We're the only people in the world who can *ask* the questions and we're the only people in the world who can *answer* the question. We have to do it right. We're under the world's spotlight." Thus, for the surgeons it appears that success and failure are intimately tied to the viability of operating on unborn babies, the survival of fetal surgery as a medical specialty, and the institutional standing of Capital Hospital as a leader in the field.[15] Certainly pregnant women desperate to save their babies do not give so much thought to the future of the fetal surgery enterprise or Capital Hospital, although they, too, may worry about the implications of excessive fetal deaths.

Another way in which differences between medical workers and pregnant women are manifest is in constructions of pregnant women as "problem" patients. To some degree, this reflects professionals' attempts to control the circumstances of fetal surgery through the maternal management strategies described above. Medical workers have a strong sense that they invest a great deal in pregnant women, and they become very disappointed when the women do not behave in expected or hoped-for ways. One social worker remarked, "We feel incredibly indebted to the patients for taking a risk like this, as long as they're cooperating. As soon as they tell us they have to get home, we're not so sure we like them any more. These patients become difficult compliance problems, and they do a lot of acting out around these lines. You really need people who understand the consequences of this, and who are responsible in their lives." There is a judgment here about women's commitment to fetal surgery. Women are expected to invest all of themselves in the making of the unborn patient and, if they do not, they are deemed irresponsible.

When pregnant women cannot be managed by the medical workers, they are often defined as "noncompliant," a punitive term that stigmatizes patients for behaving in ways outside of those prescribed by the medical model (Hunt et al. 1989). Yet such expectations of compliance, like other maternal management strategies, may be unreasonable in light of just how difficult the postoperative period is for pregnant women. One patient remarked, "Once I started coming off of morphine and they increased the two drugs, magnesium sulfate and terbutaline, that really punched me out. That really knocked me out. I mean, it was the worst time, the third or fourth day after surgery." An obstetrician who works with patients in the postoperative period stated, "They wake up out of general anesthesia like a truck has run over them," and a nurse described the women as "wet dishrags." The women's physical condition in the postoperative period may magnify differences between lay and professional perspectives. Surely the professional notion of "noncompliance" fails to recognize the many factors that may constrain a pregnant woman's ability or willingness to fully participate in fetal surgery.

This dynamic is apparent in the clinical literature as well. In discussing maternal complications resulting from unsuccessful surgery, Harrison and Adzick (1991, 289) write, "[P]oor patient compliance occurred in one case—the mother stopped her oral tocolytics and promptly went into labor and delivered vaginally." The fetus in this case survived, a point *not* emphasized by the authors. Clearly, the information they most wish to convey is that the patient subverted standard operating procedure in which cesarean section deliveries are expected of *all* women following fetal surgery. This is an important issue, as surgeons are reliant in the postoperative period on pregnant women following their orders. The educational video discussed in previous chapters illustrates how the fetal surgery team attempted to teach compliance *before* the operations took place. The narrator states, "Before you leave the hospital, we will teach you how to monitor your contractions and deliver medication to control preterm labor. Remember, you'll have to be on almost continuous bed rest during the rest of your pregnancy." Ironically, the fact that the woman in the above case delivered vaginally without complications contradicts surgeons' insistence on the threat of fetal demise resulting from vaginal birth.

Differences also surface around treatment decisions and what should be appropriate criteria for pursuing different therapeutic trajectories. Fetal surgeons, obstetricians, and other specialists tend to approach problems from a clinical perspective, often opting for more rather than less intervention. Pregnant women, on the other hand, tend to approach problems within the broader framework of their health and lives. One case in particular, presented by an obstetrician during a staff meeting, illustrates this sometimes tense dynamic.

Kelly, a young woman carrying twin fetuses at about twenty weeks' gestation, was referred to Capital Hospital because one of her fetuses was "stuck" (i.e., not growing) and the other, healthier fetus was already twice as large. She had been counseled by her regular physician to abort the smaller fetus, but she wanted a second opinion. One of Capital's obstetricians told her that she had four options: terminate the pregnancy (both fetuses), abort the smaller fetus, undergo fetal surgery to remove the smaller twin, or undergo fetal surgery to tie off the cord to the smaller fetus, thus allowing it to die in utero. All options presented significant problems and risks, including the questionable survival of the remaining fetus. Kelly and her partner told the obstetrician that an open surgical procedure was "not acceptable" *and* that they were "not willing to risk the birth of an abnormal fetus." In relaying this case to his colleagues, the obstetrician outlined a number of problems associated with it and complained that this couple had "put boundaries on what they're willing to do." Other medical staff at the meeting grumbled about this, with one doctor remarking on Kelly's "irrational boundaries." The obstetrician's preferred treatment plan was to "wait a few weeks and do noth ing to see if nature resolves the problem; [Kelly and her partner] would feel better and we'd feel better."

This case was discussed again at the next fetal treatment meeting, one month later. After leaving Capital Hospital, Kelly had decided to pursue termination of the stuck fetus at another hospital. She underwent "aggressive amniocentesis" that, according to one of the obstetricians at Capital, "apparently didn't work very well." Kelly again presented at Capital Hospital, with an even sicker stuck fetus. The obstetrician said that Kelly and her partner saw the situation as "totally unacceptable," and did not want either twin if the smaller one would have a problem. Having initially wanted to postpone treating or removing the smaller fetus, he now agreed to operate on the smaller fetus. He used a technique in which a coil is wrapped tightly around the umbilical cord, thereby shutting off the blood and oxygen supply from the placenta. The goal is to kill the stuck fetus before the healthier fetus is affected by the procedure. Yet the procedure was only partially successful; within twenty-four hours, flow was reestablished to the larger fetus and within forty-eight hours to the smaller fetus. Kelly and her partner "were adamant that they did not want to deliver an abnormal fetus," and they became dismayed when the procedure did not work. Yet a few days later, the smaller fetus died and the remaining fetus was growing. However, the obstetrician was worried because the surviving fetus may have already been damaged by its stuck twin. He remarked, "Now it's a wait-and-see game, but Kelly has achieved what she wanted. The smaller fetus is dead." His tone indicated that he clearly disagreed with Kelly's decision, despite his participation in her treatment. What is unclear is whether Kelly understood the much-increased likelihood of problems in the surviving fetus.

Kelly's story points to an important difference in the level of bio-medical knowledge that women and doctors have. The experience of repeated diagnoses, treatments, and meetings with physicians was probably harrowing for Kelly. With no medical training, her situation must at times have seemed incomprehensible; she certainly needed a physician she could trust. Yet, like Kelly, the majority of fetal surgery patients have no clinical training. For them, the world of fetal surgery, like most medicine, is complex, foreign, and confusing. Susan Davis described similar experiences for me, relaying the story as if she were a traveler in a foreign land where nobody spoke English and the signs were undecipherable. She told me that she often felt that the medical personnel "talked down" to her. Although she found the fetal surgeons supportive, their arcane language created barriers between doctor and patient. Susan and her husband, Jim, developed a close, friendly relationship with one fetal surgeon, but found other surgeons less accessible "because they were so busy." For example, she spoke of the chief surgeon with a sort of respectful awe, a noticeable contrast to the affectionate tone she used when talking about her favorite, more readily available surgeon.

Because Susan felt uncomfortable not sharing the knowledge that surgeons and other medical staff brought to their work, she decided to do something about it. She clearly wanted to seize some measure of autonomy and control for herself, and so began reading as much as she could find about fetal surgery.[16] I found Susan to be as knowledgeable as many of the clinical staff. She was well versed in the history of fetal surgery, morbidity and mortality statistics, maternal risks and complications, different types of operations, and published outcomes. She stated proudly, "I know more about fetal surgery than most of the nurses and social workers." This was a telling statement, as Susan had complained to me that she had had several uncomfortable encounters with nurses and social workers. She found one social worker, in particular, to be very unsupportive and judgmental (which, she implied, had something to do with abortion politics). Knowing more than her caretakers brought Susan great satisfaction, and also enabled her to talk to the surgeons with at least some semblance of expertise.

Kelly's and Susan's experiences, while not representative of all fetal surgery patients, illustrate some of the key differences between lay and professional perspectives. In contrast to the women's own experiential frameworks, clinical staff may appear to be "talking down" to women as they articulate their own professional perspectives. Even nurses and social workers, who usually consider themselves advocates for the pregnant women, may be positioned on the other side of the lay/professional boundary. This dichotomy was obvious in some informants' blunt comments about what is expected of the pregnant women both clinically and emotionally. Medical staff behave as if pregnant women are noncompliant "problem patients" who must be carefully managed. But within the institutional setting of fetal surgery, women's knowledge and perspectives may diverge from that of medical workers, despite their shared goal of saving babies. From the women's perspectives, medical workers may even be considered "noncompliant." In short, women and medical professionals may have fundamentally different definitions of the situation (Thomas and Thomas 1970; Thomas 1978). Both sets of actors participate in the making of the unborn patient, but the ways in which they do so may differ considerably.

Reframing Fetal Surgery as a Women's Health Issue

I began this chapter with a discussion of the maternal-fetal conflict paradigm, in which pregnant women and their fetuses are seen and represented as distinct entities. I suggested that a focus on maternal practices, or the engaged work that women do on behalf of their fetuses, provides one avenue for challenging this perspective. This chapter has presented some of the existing tensions in experimental fetal surgery between practices that reinforce the maternal-fetal conflict paradigm and those that challenge it. When women are emphasized as active participants in fetal surgery, assumptions that they are merely passive technologies in support of the fetal patient are rendered invalid. If anything, pregnant women in fetal surgery are *simultaneously* engaged and implicated actors, working subjects and work objects, part of meaningful maternal-fetal connections and enmeshed in discourses of maternal-fetal conflict. These tensions, woven into fetal surgery, have much to do with the material aspects of a practice in which pregnant women are the vehicles through which surgeons must access the fetal patient. The women are very much in the clinical frame of fetal surgery, whether or not medical workers choose to define them as such.

Within medicine and popular culture, as we have seen in previous chapters, fetal surgery is conceptualized largely as a pediatric issue. Fetuses have been transformed into unborn patients, and most work in this emergent specialty is organized around fetal health problems and biomedical needs. Fetal surgeons are trained as pediatric surgeons and not as obstetricians, illustrating that fetal surgery is viewed as pediatric surgery but "with a difference." (It is also pediatric surgery with an attitude.) Framing fetal surgery as a pediatric issue renders pregnant women barriers to be breached, bodies to be manipulated, and constraints to be managed—if they are made visible at all. However, reframing fetal surgery as a women's health issue challenges this approach and allows us to critically analyze women's complicated participation in this domain, as I have done here. A basic assumption of a women's health approach is that "women's experience in the health care system is not an isolated phenomenon, but one which is influenced by and in turn influences wider societal themes" (Olesen and Lewin 1985, 3). Thus, a major theme in this chapter has been to call attention to pregnant women's experiences in fetal surgery, including specific health issues and the wider context of reproductive and gender politics in which they exist.

In linking pregnant women's experiences to their broader social worlds, this chapter has focused on the work women do in attempting to cope with the "unimagined horror" of a defective fetus, as one informant phrased it. Pregnant women who choose fetal surgery must profoundly reorganize their lives, often traveling great distances, spending considerable sums of money, and leaving other family members behind. Contrary to the pervasive maternal-fetal conflict paradigm, in which women's interests are thought to be quite different from their fetuses', women's actual work illustrates just how committed these women are to the concept of the fetal patient. Examining women's engaged participation in the making of *their* unborn patient goes far in debunking the maternal-fetal conflict paradigm in favor of a different approach, one that recognizes that maternal-fetal relationships are both social and embodied. The specific ways in which these relationships form may vary for different women, but they are firmly grounded in lived experiences and actions taken in relation to fetuses. In this framework, it would be impossible to think of fetal surgery as just a pediatric issue.

Yet, while recognizing women's engaged complicity in the emergence of fetal surgery, a women's health perspective also encourages us to address how this practice affects women's morbidity and mortality. Although surgeons are justifiably proud that they "haven't lost a mom yet," we have seen that women's health may be severely compromised in fetal surgery. Almost all aspects of fetal surgery, from prenatal diagnosis to postoperative care, may impair women's health. As participants in fetal surgery, pregnant women are at great risk from surgical manipulations, tocolytic agents, and the like. As the patients quoted above illustrate, the intensive regimen of surgery, delivery by cesarean section, and postoperative care takes a considerable toll on pregnant women's bodies, and the long-term consequences for the women as well as the surviving fetuses remain to be studied. A women's health framework brings into sharp focus the implications for women of risk and safety issues, maternal management strategies, and struggles for control in clinical decision making such as those profiled here. An important component of reframing fetal surgery as a women's health issue is recognizing that making fetuses into unborn patients has significant implications for women's health, bodies, and lives.

In sum, this chapter has highlighted some of the many ways in which pregnant women's lives may be shaped by fetal surgery. Their decisions to undergo fetal surgery are influenced by previous experiences, by the availability of prenatal diagnostic technologies, by what their physicians tell them, and by their own political beliefs. A women's health framework enables a critical understanding of how reproductive politics imbue and mold fetal surgery, and how fetal surgery fits into the extant structure of women's emotional and political lives, including work and family circumstances. Not only do abortion politics resonate within fetal surgery, they are amplified by fetal surgery's location as a politicized reproductive practice. Although ostensibly focused only on fetuses, fetal surgery is firmly situated within the wider field of maternal-fetal medicine in which women's reproductive health is central. Thus, not only does a women's health framework challenge fetal surgery's identification as a pediatric issue, it also redefines it as a practice of great consequence for women's reproductive and postreproductive experiences in the health care system. Assessments of the value of fetal surgery must move beyond fetal survival to these broader implications.

Chapter 7

Beyond the
Operating Room

For three decades, the work of operating on fetuses—and, by extension, on pregnant women—has been central to a transformation in the social organization of reproductive medicine. Medical work in various forms has intersected with the cultural politics of reproduction in the development and consolidation of a new specialty called fetal surgery. This risky but increasingly "routine" procedure has become a major building block in the expansion of fetal medicine, itself the focus of numerous clinical, economic, and cultural resources aimed at salvaging (some) ailing, defective fetuses that might otherwise die. As we have seen, fetal surgery is unique among new medical procedures for the corporeal terrain on and within which it operates: the gravid womb. Prior to the new breed of surgical explorers who treat the fetus, few had ventured directly into the uterus for the sake of the tiny entity nestled within. As the dazzling specialty of fetal surgery has grown up within medicine, fetuses have correspondingly been reconfigured as unborn patients and persons, while women have increasingly been relegated to the status of maternal environments (albeit, active ones with their own interests and needs). For these and other reasons, fetal surgery is a sociologically rich topic.

I began this story of fetal surgery with a discussion of "fetal matters" in reproductive medicine and politics. As we have seen, certain groups of people care deeply about the fetus and have participated in the making of the unborn patient. Acting out of diverse commitments to healthier babies, medical workers and pregnant women for thirty years have collectively built fetal surgery into a vital if not yet fully legitimate medical specialty. But fetal surgery serves only a small number of women and their fetuses, at least at present. Although almost all pregnant women with access to health care face decisions about ubiquitous prenatal diagnoseis, most pregnancies are normal and only a minority of women are confronted with a severely ill fetus requiring treatment. Thus, fetal surgery will not directly touch the lives of most women in the near future, despite its rapid routinization at Capital Hospital. Rather, their encounters with fetal surgery will likely take place through a provocative excerpt on some television program or an article in a women's magazine. Given the limited nature of fetal surgery, then, does it really matter what happens to a select group of women and their fragile fetuses in a few operating rooms around the world? Why should we care?

I contend that we should care a great deal indeed about the making of the unborn patient both inside and beyond the operating room. As we have seen, fetal surgery serves as a lens through which to view medical work, health care priorities, and reproductive politics, including the cultural appeal of fetuses and ongoing confusion about women's place in the reproductive arena and in broader social life. Not only does fetal patienthood have major clinical consequences for medicine itself and for pregnant women's health and autonomy; as a new clinical, social, and cultural entity the unborn patient has journeyed out of the operating room and entered into other spheres of life. Despite fetal surgery's promise and its generally positive reception by the media, it poses a number of social dangers. The fate of the unborn patient and of fetal surgery highlights the significance of biomedicine, including its capacity to intervene in and transform human lives and to reshape relations. In focusing on the social and political consequences of the making of the unborn patient, I suggest that we need also to consider the possible *unmaking* of the unborn patient.[1] That is, we need to "ask the hard questions," to paraphrase a fetal surgeon, about the specialty itself and its role in reshaping subjectivity, medicine, reproduction, and politics. The purpose of this chapter is to raise some of those questions.

Whither Fetal Surgery?

A short time ago, one of the fetal surgeons I interviewed was recognized by *Life* magazine as among the one hundred most influential people for the twenty-first century. At around the same time, a video produced by a group of fetal surgeons was awarded top honors in a film competition sponsored by the American Medical Association (AMA). The winning video was designed to educate the public about the value of space science in contributing to solutions for medical problems. Its subject was how the monitoring of astronaut health on shuttle missions can also be applied to human fetuses. The surgeons featured in the video had worked closely with a division of NASA to develop improved monitoring devices for use in fetal treatment. Not too long after I learned of the *Life* story and the AMA award, researchers at Harvard University reported that they had used tissue harvested from sheep fetuses to grow replacement organs with which to repair congenital defects in the same animals after birth. Their efforts were lauded by fetal surgeons from coast to coast, who immediately grasped the potential impact of the experiments.

All of these events got me thinking about the future of fetal surgery, and they reminded me yet again of the connections between the promises of science fiction and the actual work of today's biomedical scientists. As we have seen, there is considerable contention surrounding the viability of fetal surgery (and of fetuses) both within and outside of medicine. According to one participant at a conference on fetal research and treatment sponsored by the Institute of Medicine (1994, 38), "Although a good deal has been learned about fetal conditions that are more or less amenable to open surgery and there have been some successful outcomes, it does not seem likely that the existing technology offers an approach that will save large numbers of endangered fetuses." Because its fate is still uncertain, fetal surgery offers a kind of cultural Etch-a-Sketch upon which participants can and often do inscribe various possible futures. Here, I offer a brief preview of the future of fetal surgery as described in the clinical literature and by many of my informants. Proponents of fetal surgery extol its virtues and envision a useful future for the specialty, while critics decry its excesses and failures and consign it to the biomedical waste bin. Regardless of his or her particular vision, each informant's prediction embodies many of the themes present throughout this book, including the significance of fetal patienthood.

Before proceeding, a couple of definitions are necessary. In place of open fetal surgery, practitioners often tout the promise of embryoscopy and fetoscopy, techniques that do not typically require surgically opening the uterus (Quintero et al. 1993). With these procedures, clinicians create small incisions in a pregnant woman's abdomen and uterus through which fiberoptic instruments and tools (such as endoscopes) are introduced for fetal diagnosis and treatment. Embryoscopy and fetoscopy are generally considered to be safer and easier to perform than open fetal surgery.[2] Some fetal surgeons refer to these techniques as "Fetendo," invoking the popular video game Nintendo (Adzick and Harrison 1994). Indeed, one fetal surgeon told me that "the best fetal surgeons of the future will be kids who are really good at video and computer games. Newer techniques will require micro-manipulations." Embryoscopy and fetoscopy lend themselves well to another major wave of the future: prenatal gene therapy, in which the actual genetic makeup of a fetus is altered. Prenatal gene therapy could potentially be used in conjunction with scopic techniques. Practitioners hope that they will be able to intervene at ever earlier stages to prevent defects and diseases from developing in the first place. One researcher remarked, "When I dare to dream, I think of intervening before the immune system has time to mature, allowing for advances that could be used in organ transplantation to replacement of genetic deficiencies" (quoted in Klass 1996, 119). As we shall see, all of these techniques have captured clinical imaginations.

In 1966, Karliss Adamsons (1966, 204) outlined the perceived major benefits of the nascent specialty of fetal surgery. The most significant advantage, he claimed, was "direct exposure of the fetus after hysterotomy." He went on to praise experimental clinical work in New Zealand and Puerto Rico, including his own contributions, that had established important precedents in fetal surgery. Yet, despite its promise, Adamsons was not entirely convinced that fetal surgery had a broad future. He (1966, 205) wrote:

> It appears unlikely that even in the distant future, fetal surgery will become a field of major concern to the clinician since most abnormalities requiring surgical correction can be dealt with after birth. . . . For the present, the sole use of fetal surgery is in the treatment of erythroblastosis fetalis [Rh disease], and even here its value is still open to debate. Nevertheless, the acceptance of the concept that diagnosis and even surgical treatment can be extended to prenatal life is an important advance. It paves the way to a more complete understanding of the environment that will ensure optimal prenatal development.

Thus, even if fetal surgery itself did not have a broad future, Adamsons was convinced at the time that the idea of the fetus as a patient would endure.

J. H. Louw (1974) was more optimistic about the specialty, framing his discussion around the future of pediatric surgery more broadly. He predicted that fetal surgery would have a place in the future as a treatment for a range of congenital defects, including that most vexing of conditions, diaphragmatic hernia. He called for intensified efforts in fetal treatment and perceived the surgical approach as an opportunity with great promise. He argued that pediatric surgery "should not stop at neonatal nor fetal anomalies, but maybe start tampering with embryos, removing a gene here and implanting one there . . . forever striving to improve the quality of life" (1974, 1597). With these words, he presaged one of the major trends occupying the contemporary group of fetal surgeons: prenatal gene therapy.

Like Adamsons and Louw before him, Pringle (1986) too reflected on the past, present, and future of fetal surgery. He described the historical efforts of the 1960s in New Zealand and Puerto Rico, pointing to all that had been learned from these activities. He argued that fetal surgery might have become more prevalent in the 1960s had Liley's group not been so successful with closed operative techniques for fetal exchange transfusions. Detailing some of its problems and achievements, Pringle forecast the future of fetal surgery in optimistic but cautious terms. He (1986, 25) wrote, "At present, fetal surgery is limited in its scope but very widespread in its application. . . . The results of these procedures are variable but fetal salvage may not have been greatly increased." For improved outcomes, he predicted the development of better tocolytic agents and methods for diagnosing which fetuses to treat. He (1986, 29) closed his predictive account with these words: "Fetal surgery has a proud history, an exciting present and a promising future. The aim of pediatric surgeons should, indeed, be to 'improve the quality of life.' . . . Fetal surgery will be just one of the means at the disposal of the medical profession to do just that."

Almost thirty years after his initial predictions when I met him in Puerto Rico, Karliss Adamsons had retained his enthusiasm for the promise of fetal surgery. His eyes sparkled throughout our interview and he showed a lively interest in the development of the specialty. He expressed admiration for the fetal surgeons at Capital Hospital who, in his view, "have managed to remain excited about their work despite very high mortality and morbidity." He wanted to know, for example, how the fetal surgeons in my study viewed their contributions to the field, and he framed his own views in moral and economic terms. He remarked,

> In the U.S., we're willing to invest lots of money, time, and resources to save one life. [Fetal surgery] is showing that we can salvage an organism that would otherwise die. It is not unethical to be changing nature in the interests of Homo sapiens. Many societies would consider fetal surgery excessive, but we're a wealthy society. Resources are misused in many ways already, so why not pursue something like fetal surgery?

What is interesting to note here is Adamsons's subtle inference that fetal surgery may be a misuse of resources, or at the very least an untested use of resources. Yet he also suggested that fetal surgery is worthwhile because it "teaches us about basic mechanisms and not just technological innovation. What fetal surgery has contributed to is a breakdown of the belief that the uterus is sacrosanct. It has basically helped the construction of the field of fetal medicine."

Vincent Freda was also optimistic about the future of fetal surgery when I spoke with him, predicting that surgeons "will probably do more cases. It will become more common." He feels that "if people go back and read what I wrote, they'll realize what can be done," believing that the field will expand to include cardiac surgery and prenatal gene therapy. He, too, asked me about Capital Hospital. When I told him in general terms about conflict among different specialists (described in chapter 4), he described who should be involved in fetal surgery at the present time:

> The pediatrician should be the surgeon for the fetus. The obstetrician should open the mother and take over after fetal surgery. There should be collaboration. Frankly, the obstetrician doesn't know his ass from his elbow about doing surgery on a fetus. So the OBs should only open the abdomen and put the baby outside, and then the pediatric surgeons should take over and do the rest. But the OBs should then close up the mother.

Obviously, as we saw in chapter 4, this is *not* the division of labor in fetal surgery today, where obstetricians have been increasingly marginalized by fetal surgeons.

Graham Liggins, who worked closely with Liley in New Zealand, was somewhat guarded about the future of fetal surgery. He told me,

> It's highly controversial, for one. In my view, fetal surgery is not going to be generally useful until we have a better understanding of the mechanism of the control of labor. To that extent, the work at Capital Hospital and my work are, you might say, intertwined. But we've still got quite some time to go before we'll be in a position to successfully control factors such as preterm labor and hormones. In general terms, though, I could see the future of fetal surgery being in endoscopic techniques, where you have direct vision into the uterus through a fiberoptic scope.

Liggins's comment raises the provocative possibility that fiberoptic techniques might well be considered the hope of the future precisely *because* they are not so controversial as open fetal surgery.

Predictions were also made by informants at Capital Hospital in the course of my interviews with them. For example, one fetal surgeon told me:

> We've done amazingly well just to have gotten this far. Now we're understanding the effects of surgery on physiology, and the ultimate outcome will be that we're able to improve everything. It's going to happen shortly. The fetal surgery enterprise will not die because there are a number of other groups starting it now. And they're starting it after discussions with all of us and incorporating a physiologic point of view. It will continue and it will grow; it's just going to take time.

This surgeon, echoing Liggins, also remarked that "endoscopic surgery *is* the wave of the future. It's less interventive because it's done using needles and thus does not require open surgery. Also, it could potentially be used in the future for nonterminal fetal conditions."

Another fetal surgeon was very enthusiastic about the future of his specialty, but told me that he hopes that it will "grow slowly." He felt that fetal surgery "could have been immensely controversial rather than just somewhat controversial." But because the initial participants "laid low and didn't go public right away, fetal surgeons were never crucified the way cardiac transplant surgeons were." They "never wanted fetal surgery to be a circus, and were very careful about not saying things publicly until they had been peer-reviewed and published." He foresees a time when fetal surgery will be used for all kinds of fetal defects, including routine diaphragmatic hernias. Yet the "Achilles' heel" of fetal surgery, preterm labor, will continue to haunt the field. Like his predecessors, this surgeon predicted that fetoscopy and endoscopic surgery will "take off." He also raised the possibility of fetus-to-fetus transplantation and prenatal gene therapy as important techniques for the future.

Yet another fetal surgeon described the future of the specialty, and of the unborn patient, in terms of early reactions to his work:

> I distinctly recall a major pediatric surgery meeting where I presented the natural history of congenital cystic adenomatoid malformation. This was in 1984. I suggested that one consideration might be to treat *before* birth. And there was like no discussion, absolute silence. And so, you just keep working away. Then last week I chaired a course in fetal diagnosis and therapy, and there were about two hundred folks there just to watch and learn. It was an interesting contrast. It was *almost* like being legitimate. The upshot is, no one knows ten years from now whether we'll be doing much open fetal surgery. I don't know. But the enterprise of the fetus as a patient, treating the fetus as a patient, is here to stay. No question about it, whether it's gene therapy in the future or whatever. It's here to stay.

Like Adamsons before him, this surgeon points to the longevity of the fetal patient despite his uncertainty about the future of the specialty as a whole. He also clearly links his predictions to changes in the legitimacy of the specialty, contrasting earlier perceptions of his work as illegitimate with current interest in the procedures.

A fetal physiologist was much more optimistic, suggesting that not just the fetal patient but "fetal surgery itself is here to stay." She told me,

> Certainly, until such time as we are able to avoid all these defects. But I think there are many aspects of this that are important. I think you have to get into the issue of *why* you would want to operate on a fetus. It's not because the lesion the fetus has is necessarily life-threatening during fetal life. Some of them are, but others are not. In a number of lesions, the presence of one defect results in secondary changes in other parts of the body. If one could correct the lesion before birth, one could avoid that development. This is the reason why there is the appeal of going to fetal surgery.

When I asked her about the success of fetal surgery, she remarked, "I think that they're getting closer to the goal, but it's quite a ways before they solve all the problems. One of the problems we have to face up to is the fact that they have operated on babies relatively late in gestation. I think what we have to aim for is to diagnose these things earlier and to consider doing something earlier as well." This informant, too, raised the prospect of endoscopic and prenatal genetic therapies.

Another informant, a sonographer, was also enthusiastic about fetal surgery:

> I think we should continue to push on with it. I'm not sure of the direction we should push, but we should clearly continue to push. Untreated cases have a very dismal outcome. We're seeing about sixty percent of these fetuses die as newborns. You can say, well, that's the name of the game and we're just going to have to accept that fetal surgery is not going to be as successful as we'd like it to be. Maybe that's true. I would very much like to say I know the answer to that question, sitting here today. But I'll tell you, if the answer turns out to be no, fetal surgery can't do it, then we have to accept something that I find to be sad.

He also placed his opinion of the fate of the specialty in historical context, remarking, "Who would have ever thought to operate on a fetus to fix up an abnormality? It seems perfectly logical to do so now." And, as with other commentators, this informant commented that endoscopic techniques represent great promise to the field.

A surgical resident was equally optimistic about the specialty, drawing an analogy with the space program and scientific research in general. He stated,

> The ultimate goal was to put somebody on the moon, which we did. But there were a bunch of incredible things that came out of it just by looking at related topics. In fetal surgery, the discovery of scarless healing is a major benefit. Even if the ultimate end of fetal surgery is no fetuses ever get operated on, I think that the process of the research is going to have beneficial effects for health care as a whole. But I do think that there will be a prominent place for fetal surgery in the future.

Yet this surgeon also felt that open surgical techniques would be replaced by prenatal gene therapy. He told me,

> I think gene therapy is the wave of the future. It's amazing. It's perfect. There is very little intervention to both the fetus and the mother, and the benefits are incredible. A lot of these big terrible diseases are just missing one amino acid, or change in one amino acid, or missing one gene sequence. And you end up with a whole cascade of abnormalities. If you can just replace that in

utero, you know it's something that will be easy, safe, and inexpensive. I think that's what will happen.

Ironically, this informant's rather glowing predictions about gene therapy as "perfect" mirror some early reactions to fetal surgery in the 1960s. Now gene therapy is framed as revolutionary just as fetal surgery was three decades ago.

One of the nurses I interviewed was less optimistic and more critical about the future of fetal surgery. She told me:

The womb is the last frontier in medicine. I'm not sure there are other frontiers, maybe the genes. But in terms of human anatomy, I think that there's really no other area that's been sacrosanct like the womb and the developing fetus has been. And I think ultimately they'll probably conquer it. As for fetal surgery, I think there will be some continuation of the C-CAM stuff, but I have my doubts about the other stuff.

This informant's comments are interesting for the degree to which she frames fetal surgery as a conquest. If the specialty has a future, she seems to be saying, then it will be shaped by surgeons' desires to go where no one has gone before.

An obstetrician was likewise not very optimistic about the future success of fetal surgery. She remarked,

Mortality data based on thirty cases, with only four surviving fetuses, is not good. I don't think any of us would consider this to be a great success. With the success, or lack of, with these procedures, you can't really counsel a woman to have surgery. There are very few fetuses for which this will be appropriate, and very few indications where this will be useful because you can't get there early enough. Whereas this is very sexy, it's not very practical. I don't think we're going to save many fetuses.

Yet the future of nonsurgical fetal treatment, according to this informant, appears to be rosy: she predicted that prenatal gene therapy would eventually be widely used.

What are we to make of these diverse opinions about the future of fetal surgery? Do they represent merely an extension of the specialty differences discussed in chapter 4? For fetal surgeons and those who preceded them historically, the future certainly seems bright. Some other informants are more cautious and critical, pointing to high fetal mortality rates and the degree of invasiveness as limiting the success of the surgical approach to fetal treatment. Preterm labor is still, thirty years after Liley's pioneering efforts, the most significant obstacle to successful open fetal surgery. As such, many specialists advocate a 180-degree turn back to closed techniques, such as endoscopy, fetoscopy, and prenatal gene therapy, in which the womb remains intact. The tools of the future for treating fetuses may well be fiberoptic scopes and genes, manipulated by a generation of surgeons trained on video and computer games. Ironically, then, the future of fetal treatment may *not* involve surgically breaching the womb after all. Having been ushered into the world through open fetal surgery, the unborn patient can now be legitimately treated through Fetendo and other innovative techniques. And if the fetal patient is here to stay, so too are its broader social implications.

The Unborn Patient Writ Large

As the above quotes demonstrate, the unborn patient has become taken for granted, a seemingly permanent feature of the clinical landscape. Consequently, this book has been as much about the emergence of a new subject—the fetal patient—as it has the growth and consolidation of a new medical specialty. As we have seen, the specialty and its precious work object are the joint outcomes of intertwined processes involving medical work activities, health care resource allocation, the intersection of various political fields (e.g., abortion, disability, professional politics), and cultural investments in fetuses. Each chapter, focused on some aspect of the work that has gone into the making of the unborn patient, has illustrated that fetal patienthood is not a natural status. Rather, the fetus-as-patient is the product of an array of activities embedded in the social organization of medicine, including medicine's reach into many aspects of a woman's reproductive life. As a social category, fetal patienthood is relational and is given shape and form by the clinicians and pregnant women who care about fetuses. But what are some of the implications that flow from fetal patienthood? What does it *mean*?

Patienthood is a unique social status related to one's involvement with health care systems and activities; it often tells us something about who counts (or who does not) in specific medical practices. To be a patient usually means to seek from health care providers some kind of palliation or treatment for pain, discomfort, disease, or distressing symptoms. Patienthood applied to the unborn means that sick fetuses are amenable to diagnosis and treatment; they may be operated on, given drugs, and monitored. The unborn patient has its own team of doctors and surgeons, and its condition may be defined clinically as healthy, ill, disabled, treatable, hopeless, and so on. Fetuses may die before, during, or after treatment, and their demise may be hastened by intervention itself. Occasionally, an unborn patient is saved by surgery, and this fuels interest in and commitment to fetal patienthood despite overall poor outcomes. Medical textbooks concern themselves with the fate of fetal patients far more regularly than ever before, and insurance companies increasingly recognize fetal patients in their reimbursement policies. Fetal patienthood, as we have seen, is also written up with some glee and fascination in popular cultural accounts. The unborn patient, it seems, is indeed here to stay as a general concept although many individual fetuses may follow a different trajectory (e.g., no treatment, abortion, postnatal treatment).

But fetuses are a unique and limited kind of patient, and fetal surgery is a rather singular kind of medical practice. Fetuses are prime *work objects* in medicine; they are challenging bodies that do not challenge clinicians socially. That is, fetuses cannot ask questions about their own illness or prognosis, nor can they disagree with a doctor's recommendation. They can be considered neither compliant nor noncompliant, for their actions, if any, are not sentient. In its transformation to the status of patient, a fetus does not have to miss work, leave its family behind, worry about how to pay for health care, navigate the social hierarchy of the doctor-patient relationship, or engage in any of the social and cultural dimensions of patienthood. For these reasons, fetal patients may well be considered the "best" patients by medical workers.

Another actor is present in fetal surgery to do precisely the kind of social work that fetuses cannot do. Pregnant women, as we have seen, inhabit the status of patients on behalf of their fetuses. They must negotiate with clinicians, assume clinical risks, ingest antilabor drugs, participate in follow-up activities, worry about insurance, miss work, leave their families behind, and deal with the emotional consequences of fetal outcomes. What is striking in the above quotes in which leading practitioners in the field reaffirm the permanence of fetal patienthood is that not a single one mentioned the women. But as we saw in chapter 6, the making of the unborn patient is also about the making and unmaking of pregnant women. Maternal patienthood makes fetal patienthood possible, although clinical and popular cultural accounts of fetal surgery often fail to recognize this. Ironically, although pregnant women are the de facto patients, fetal surgery is *not* organized around their needs, nor is it celebrated for transforming maternal identity. Patienthood, then, is a rather ambiguous concept in fetal surgery.

Despite the limited social sense in which a fetus is actually a patient, the status of fetal *patienthood* is used in attributions of fetal *personhood* both within and beyond medicine. Because they can be treated (e.g., saved, rescued, etc.), fetuses are routinely constructed within medical practices as persons. For example, throughout this story informants have referred to fetuses in humanizing (and gendered) terms: Junior, Fred, he, baby, kid, person. Fetal surgery, as we saw in the epigraph, makes fetuses into "one of us." This is significant because personhood, like patienthood, confers a set of rights as well as attributions of social worth. It is on the question of an individual's worthiness to be considered a full member of the human community that several crucial debates hinge. Abortion, disability rights, feminism, social and economic justice, anti-racism, human rights—all engage in contestation over definitions of personhood and humanity and their contingent social and political benefits. Fetal personhood is especially significant because it often leads to a diminution of women's personhood. The more fetuses are defined as people, the greater the threats to women's reproductive autonomy including abortion rights, decision making in health care settings, and everyday behavior during pregnancy. I now briefly discuss two arenas in which fetal patienthood has come to matter in terms of defining and perpetuating fetal personhood: ethics and law.

Most bioethicists accept that medicine has fundamentally transformed the relationship between a pregnant woman and her fetus by identifying and promising to serve the distinct needs of the fetal patient. Indeed, one of the most striking aspects of moral discourse about fetal treatment is the almost universal acceptance of the unborn patient. For example, Evans et al. (1990) suggest that recent technological advances have made fetuses accessible visually and surgically; as such, they have contributed to ethical constructions of fetuses as separate individuals clinically and morally. Within this framework, the question is not *whether* the fetus should be considered a patient, for that is taken for granted. Rather, it involves a determination of the moral relationship between a pregnant woman and her fetus (or, in some fetocentric framings, between a fetus and its host). This brings us back to notions of maternal-fetal conflict, as ethicists assume that any medical focus on the fetus is likely to be *in opposition to* women's needs and interests. Clinical and moral decision making centers on how to resolve these specific tensions and not on the ethics of the overall enterprise of fetal treatment.

Bioethicists who construct fetuses as moral beings, individuals, or persons tend to emphasize clinical solutions that optimize fetal well-being and health, often at the expense of pregnant women's autonomy (e.g., Chervenak and McCullough 1991). Other ethicists point to possible threats to reproductive freedom inherent in such approaches and argue instead that such conflicts should be resolved in favor of pregnant women's autonomy and bodily integrity (e.g., Nelson and Milliken 1990). Still others attempt to formulate a "middle ground" that takes into account both maternal autonomy and fetal interests—but without questioning the clinical practices themselves (e.g., Elkins 1990). Unsurprisingly, strategies for resolving maternal-fetal conflict often diverge along specialty lines (e.g., Grodin 1990). Obstetricians, for example, tend to favor bioethical proposals that respect pregnant women's autonomy, while pediatricians and fetal surgeons tend to support solutions that incorporate fetal interests. Despite these quite different perspectives, all rest on an absolute assumption that fetuses are indeed patients and thus must be at least potential persons if not full persons.

Legal perspectives share similar assumptions with ethical perspectives and are characterized by the emergence and expansion of the fetal rights framework. Fetal rights are those that are attributed to fetuses in and of themselves; such rights are distinct from, and often in opposition to, those of pregnant women (Knopoff 1991). Significantly, the fetal rights framework has been fueled by constructions of the fetus as a patient. Lenow (1983, 17; emphasis added) argues that *"with the treatment of the fetal patient a reality,* the physician may now possess independent responsibilities for both the mother and the fetus." He goes on to state that "viability continues to be an important factor in determining the rights of the unborn. . . . In light of the changing medical interpretation of viability, our perception of the rights of the fetal patient may change in the near future" (Lenow 1983, 10). What he calls "the ultimate achievement" of the removal of a fetus from a woman's uterus parallels the dichotomization of maternal and fetal rights in legal discourse and practice. As Hubbard (1982, 32) asserts, "Now the law has joined the medical profession in viewing pregnancy as pathology, though this time with *two* patients. In this way the fetus's presumed 'rights' as a patient can be used to control pregnant women."

In law as in ethics, then, two patients equal two persons equal two sets of competing interests and rights. How do these ethical and legal issues matter both in fetal surgery and beyond? One surgeon hinted at some possible implications: "It's sort of like the whole thing that surrogate motherhood has brought into play. You know, whose rights are involved, who ultimately controls those rights? What happens if we're in the middle of this, and now we've got the fetus completely monitored, and the mother wants to stop?" What comes to mind almost immediately is the pervasive use of the fetal rights argument to compel pregnant women to undergo medical procedures, especially cesarean sections, against their wishes (Gallagher 1989; Jost 1989; Willis 1989). Courts seem increasingly willing to intervene in a pregnant woman's decision making, largely for the sake of fetal well-being and survival. In other words, judges and lawyers, like ethicists, are often persuaded by biomedical claims. When I asked fetal surgeons about the eventual possibility of compelling women to undergo fetal surgery, they were uniformly horrified and assured me that it would never happen. The same surgeon who invoked surrogacy went on to tell me,

> Right now, we feel that the parents have control over what to do. We're here to help. Who knows what the legal system will do with that? I think you have

a very difficult time when you start to legislate surgery for reasons other than health and illness. When you start saying that somebody should receive an operation for some legal issue. I'm not a lawyer you know. With search and seizure or whatever, making an incision in somebody's abdomen is a completely different magnitude than opening somebody's car trunk or searching their living room. And I definitely wouldn't agree with that. I'm not sure how you can make the argument for a court-ordered cesarean, unless it was for somebody's health. I don't know. That's like Frankenstein, sometimes technology advances before the understanding of how to use it appropriately.

But arguments for court-ordered treatment *are* already made, at least ostensibly, for somebody's health: that of the fetus. Regardless of surgeons' own reluctance to envision the possibility that fetal surgery might someday be forced on a pregnant woman, practitioners in medicine, ethics, and law continue to draw on and aggressively circulate the idea of the unborn patient. They assert notions of fetal personhood and fetal rights, while correspondingly contributing to a diminishment of pregnant women's autonomy.

Of course, fetal surgery is just one of the many sites at which fetal personhood is being constructed and contested in the United States and elsewhere (Franklin 1991; Ginsburg and Rapp 1995; Hartouni 1997; Petchesky 1987) But it is a particularly authoritative site, as medical constructions may be quite consequential. Biomedicine intervenes intimately in human bodies, contributes to crucial definitions of health and illness (with significant implications), and is a key site of social control over people's lives (Casper and Berg 1995). Certain groups in medicine, reflecting extant hierarchies, are vested with the authority to create persons through a range of reproductive, surgical, and genetic technologies and practices. For example, both fetal surgery and the Human Genome Initiative are uniquely positioned to create new subjects. But fetal patienthood and its twin fetal personhood are *not* foregone conclusions. Rather, they are *potential* outcomes of social negotiation and work both in and beyond the operating room. Not all fetuses are patients, nor are all fetuses considered persons; even the same fetus may shift between these different statuses. We need to ask who views the unborn patient as a person, under what conditions, with what consequences, why such constructions matter so much, and who resists certain versions of fetal patienthood and personhood.

As medical sociologists have long argued, patienthood itself may be stunningly dehumanizing as medicine focuses on specific diseases and body parts rather than whole beings. Human bodies on biomedical frontiers are often atomized, reduced to work objects that can be manipulated to produce data. Maynard-Moody (1995, 100) has suggested in relation to fetal treatment that "being a patient is a peculiar and limited form of personhood. Critics of modern medicine complain that patients are dehumanized, that they are treated like bodies or biochemical systems, not people." And Fletcher and Jonsen (1991, 16) argue that "the designation of the fetus as a patient (i.e., as a medically treatable being) would not seem equivalent to an attribution of personhood. The latter concept, without doubt, bears much more philosophical and theological weight than the former and requires considerably more than 'treatability' to justify its attribution to the fetus." How, then, can patienthood—especially the ambiguous patienthood produced in/by fetal surgery—lead to personhood? There is something rather ironic about the causal links drawn between fetal patienthood and fetal persons. Fetal surgery, as we saw in chapter 3, was built on a body of animal experiments, yet nobody is suggesting that we define sheep and monkeys as either patients or persons. So what, precisely, is at stake when medicine, ethics, and law define human fetuses as such and then promote these definitions as natural and inviolable?

As reproductive politics, especially struggles over abortion, continue to rend the social fabric, at least some Americans are looking to medicine for answers. As Catholic physician Elio Sgreccia (1989, 16) has written, "Civilization's battlefield and the site of its conflicts has become, if I may be allowed the expression, the woman's uterus." Given the seemingly intractable gap between "pro-life" and "pro-choice" factions, marshaling medical and scientific "truth" on one side or the other may provide an edge. As we saw in chapter 2, at the same time that clinicians were attempting to rescue fetuses from life-threatening diseases, providers such as Liley were participating in the broader arena of reproductive politics to rescue fetuses from abortion (and from "selfish" women). Recall also that Susan and Jim Davis were convinced that medical definitions of fetal patienthood would transform pro-life politics. As these examples illustrate, medical constructions of fetal personhood are deployed in the cultural politics of reproduction as well as in ethical and legal domains. It would not matter to most of us if sheep and monkeys were defined as persons, but it matters a great deal to many people how human fetuses are defined. We are passionate about fetal status because the unborn tell us something about ourselves. Fetal stories have become human stories, and those who participate in their telling are often granted our undivided attention. It is thus unsurprising that fetal patienthood has been influential in several domains where fetal personhood is a core, albeit contested, value. The unborn patient both crystallizes and fuels ongoing political debates, not only in the reproductive arena, but also in the mutable U.S. health care system. New fetal subjects matter very much indeed, for fetuses are us.

Making a Fetal Surgery for Women

Focusing on fetal patienthood as a social object, as I have done in this book, presents a number of provocative challenges to perspectives that assert fundamental or natural categories, whether patienthood or personhood. Fetal subjects—like other subjects—are produced through ongoing processes, and they are continually under construction. If the unborn patient has been actively made across three decades, then what would be involved in *unmaking* the unborn patient? For example, many clinicians have resisted notions of the unborn patient, instead pointing to some of the dangers of fetal surgery. Similarly, many women opt to deal with fetal problems in other ways, either through abortion, no treatment at all, or different kinds of intervention. Some people may not be bothered by the idea of treating individual fetuses; they might think, what could be the harm? But there is growing resistance to cultural reification of fetal patienthood and personhood. Just as pro-life groups have championed the fetal patient and its ontological siblings, other groups have begun to challenge these subjectivities.

One way of resisting particular versions and implications of the unborn patient is to recast fetal surgery in terms of a women's health agenda. As we have seen throughout this book, and especially in chapter 6, fetal surgery poses a number of serious health risks and consequences for the pregnant women who undergo it. It also rather seamlessly feeds—or is fed by committed actors—into reproductive politics as part of the broader cultural construction of fetal persons with interests distinct from those of women. Because fetal surgery can be dangerous for women, both individually as patients and collectively in terms of reproductive politics, it could certainly be described as bad medicine, or at the very least cowboy surgery. Indeed, many informants at Capital Hospital have described it as such. Thus, an obvious feminist response to fetal surgery might simply be efforts to do away with it. As one colleague wrote in response to an earlier draft of this book, "I've always felt this topic was a mixed blessing; it's great empirical data—flashy, sexy, and highly relevant. Yet fetal surgery is *so* outrageous as an enterprise that in the end, you cannot but be against it."[3] Although I have raised a number of issues and problems invoked by fetal surgery, I am not necessarily "against it." To my mind, the story of fetal surgery is far more complicated than the potentially satisfying but too simple resolution of eliminating it would suggest.

As we have seen, pregnant women themselves have been active participants in fetal surgery, selecting a range of interventions for the sake of their fetuses. What is needed is a feminist intervention or response that does not claim to know better than the women who select fetal surgery.

This means finding a way to critique fetal surgery and the social relations that sustain it without criticizing the women who choose it. It also means attending to the many contradictions in reproductive medicine of which fetal surgery is a part. Reproductive medicine both heals and harms women; it both produces and destroys fetuses; it is both palliative and iatrogenic; it both opens and closes reproductive possibilities; it is both a consumer choice and a form of social control; and it both shapes cultural meanings and is a product of culture. A good example of some of these contradictions concerns the potential of embryoscopy and fetoscopy described earlier. What if fetal surgery no longer involved breaching the womb? On the one hand, fiberoptic techniques might be better for women by offering a safer, less invasive alternative for treating fetuses. On the other hand, they might contribute to the expansion of fetal patienthood and thus to the further erasure of women. Instead of cutting pregnant women open, clinicians could simply look *through* them to the unborn patient within.

In recognition of these types of paradoxes, I offer a different kind of feminist intervention, one that is more subtle and contingent. As someone who both studies *and* participates in reproductive politics, I am dismayed at how often the binary language of "pro" and "con" excludes and silences a variety of perspectives. I suggest a move away from simple, naive arguments to a more comprehensive understanding of the complexities of women's health and reproduction. A hallmark of women's health approaches is sensitivity to and regard for the diversity of women's health and illness experiences (Ruzek et al. 1997). Related to this are reproductive rights frameworks in which all of women's varied, even competing, needs and desires are represented, including both prenatal care *and* the right to abortion, voluntary sterilization *and* access to in vitro fertilization, autonomy *and* concern for fetuses—and so on. These approaches are attentive to women's own concerns, while also deliberately avoiding the usual dichotomies of reproductive politics.

Rather than eliminating fetal surgery, then, I propose an appropriation of fetal surgery on behalf of a women's health and reproductive rights agenda. If some women want to use prenatal diagnosis and treatment to attain healthier fetuses, then a certain amount of social change is in order. What, I ask, needs to be in place—clinically, socially, culturally, economically, ethically, and legally—to enable women to undergo fetal surgery safely, effectively, and autonomously? The solutions—or, rather, the struggles—I propose below must be taken *together*. One change alone is not sufficient for reformulating fetal surgery as a women's health or reproductive rights issue. For example, making the procedure safer does not address the importance of its connections to reproductive politics. As strategies for systemic social change, some of these suggestions may seem too idealistic. However, rather than dismissing them as simplistic or unattainable, I suggest they be used to reexamine the power of medicine and science in social life. If *all* of these conditions need to be in place in order for fetal interventions to address women's health needs adequately, then why, given that so many of these conditions do *not* exist, is fetal surgery pursued with such zeal? What does it tell us about medicine, culture, politics, and gender that a procedure so risky to women on a number of levels can move forward under current social conditions?

Clinical Safety. Before fetal surgery is allowed to become a routine procedure available to all women, medical workers must ensure that it is safe. Clearly, preterm labor is an ongoing problem, as are potential threats to subsequent reproduction after surgery. All additional maternal risks should be identified and, if possible, alleviated. The solution is not intensified management of pregnant women's bodies as if they were inert technologies, but rather the search for safer, better ways (for women) to diagnose and treat fetuses. If it is not possible to perform fetal surgery without jeopardizing women's safety, then perhaps it should not be done at all. If newer techniques such as embryoscopy and fetoscopy promise enhanced safety, then they should be introduced slowly in order to allow for adequate assessment by Institutional Review Boards and by the public. Of course, ensuring clinical safety may also mean *not* intervening in situations where fetuses are at risk, instead recognizing that other techniques may be equally viable. In other words, the overall aim of fetal surgery should be the *safety* of pregnant women and their fetuses, and *not* an idealistic, heroic vision of rescuing fetuses at any cost. Nor should the burden of risk assessment fall primarily on women, many of whom are likely to disregard their own safety on behalf of their fetuses. Medical workers themselves must take responsibility for assuring that their practices safeguard women's health.

Reorganization of Medicine. As we have seen, fetal surgery is characterized by considerable conflict between and among its specialist practitioners. In addition, professional and lay perspectives often chafe against each other in a clinical setting, as "experts" are positioned above patients in medical hierarchies. These dynamics are especially pernicious given the physiological and ethical magnitude of operating on fetuses inside women's bodies. For fetal surgery to be a viable option *for women*, the specialty would have to be reorganized so that it is less competitive and non-hierarchical. Fetal surgery should not proceed as if it were a battle, with "mom docs" and "baby docs" lined up against each other. This kind of conflict—the antithesis of the much-touted teamwork at Capital Hospital—certainly does *not* serve women's needs. Resolving the conflict may mean giving women and their advocates—family members, social workers, nurses, and obstetricians—a much-expanded role in fetal surgery. Every effort should be made to incorporate the women's perspectives into treatment and postoperative plans, as well as to provide detailed and adequate informed consent whether a procedure is experimental or not. Patients in routine medicine likewise should be protected to the fullest extent possible even if they are not technically considered human subjects. Biomedicine itself needs to be refashioned such that the rewards of medicine come not from glamorous, mediagenic, capital-intensive research, but rather from patient care. There is far too much emphasis in Western biomedicine today on high-tech interventions and not nearly enough on disease prevention and health promotion.

Access to Health Services. The issue of access to health care extends far beyond access to fetal treatments; it encompasses all of medicine, particularly in the United States. If fetal surgery is to be part of the arsenal with which clinicians strive to ensure healthier babies, then it should *not* be limited to a select group of mostly white, mostly middle- to upperclass women who can afford it. *All* women should have access to *all* available health care. Poor women and women of color should have just as much opportunity to get the "best" treatment for their fetuses as white women of privilege. This will likely mean addressing class relations and broader issues of social, economic, and racial justice. Strategies for increasing health care access for all pregnant women should be part of efforts to build a national health program in general. In other words, the viabilty of experimental procedures should be made part of all discussions about health care reform. If we cannot ensure that all pregnant women who desire it will be able to obtain diagnosis and treatment of their fetuses if needed, then we must seriously reconsider the wisdom of investing public funds in research on fetal surgery and related procedures. (Other nations may well organize fetal surgery differently, although these general considerations may still be applicable.)

Redefining Ethical and Legal Frameworks. As we have seen, traditional ethical and legal perspectives emphasize fetal personhood and rights, while striving to navigate the complexities of maternal-fetal conflict issues. Rather than beginning with the fetus, feminist perspectives conceptualize fetuses as moral or legal subjects *only* in concrete relation to the pregnant women in whose bodies they live. Feminist approaches acknowledge the broader social relations of reproduction and are consequently not committed to abstract, societal obligations as determinants of pregnant women's behavior. Some feminist legal scholars, for example, criticize the concept of fetal rights on the basis of sex equality and freedom from discrimination (Johnsen 1986). Others situate fetal rights within a broader framework of social justice, arguing that such rights must be defined in relation to the moral and legal status of women

(Gallagher 1987). Still others reframe these issues by bringing women back into the picture: "Women carry fetuses in their bodies, it is true. It is equally true, however, that fetuses are part of women's bodies. . . . This means that what happens in and to those bodies can adversely affect fetuses and that the only way to get at a fetus is through the body that houses it" (Purdy 1990, 273–274). In terms of resolving maternal-fetal conflicts, feminist perspectives diverge considerably from those discussed earlier; they recommend that women's interests be given the same respect that those of a white, middle-class male would recieve. In short, within a women's health framework, fetal surgery would develop in conjunction with *feminist* ethical and legal approaches that emphasize pregnant women's autonomy and agency.

Reproductive Politics. The term *reproductive politics* refers to all of the ways in which women's reproductive experiences are embedded and contested in broader social and political relations. Fetal surgery poses several distinct threats to pregnant women's autonomy, including the reaffirmation of maternal-fetal conflict issues and the erasure of women in frameworks celebrating fetal personhood. Within a women's health agenda, a different kind of maternal-fetal relationship must be realized. As we have seen, the pregnant women in fetal surgery accept an extraordinary amount of risk on behalf of their fetuses, so much so that surgeons refer to them as "heroic moms." A fetal surgery that is part of a women's health agenda must begin with pregnant women's experiences, and *not* with the fetus. Put simply, women know best. This is not to exalt some naturalized version of motherhood, but rather to recognize that women have the most at stake in reproductive decisions. They may make such decisions in concert with health care professionals, and with their partners, but only an individual woman knows the circumstances of her own life that make some choices tenable and others not. After all, it is women's bodies and lives that will be fundamentally transformed by fetal interventions of all kinds, including treatment *and* abortion.

For fetal surgery to continue (regardless of its form), its practitioners must be accountable to women's needs. This means taking women's agency seriously (not treating them like "heart-lung machines"), respecting women's decisions in clinical settings, providing as much information as possible about a given fetal treatment trajectory, de-emphasizing fetal personhood, working to ensure greater clinical safety for women, enhancing access, and recognizing that all reproductive decisions and choices are difficult. In other words, the broader social context of "choice" matters. A variety of factors, such as a woman's economic situation or her social support network or her proximity to clinics, may impinge on her reproductive decisions. Making fetal surgery responsive to a women's health agenda may require improving the conditions of women's lives such that fetal surgery is seen as just one of many possible options (and certainly not the most significant option) for ensuring healthier babies.

Politics of Prenatal Care. The politics of prenatal care is related to access to services, but goes beyond economic issues to encompass broader social and political concerns. From a women's health perspective, it is difficult to see fetal surgery as "heroic" when infant mortality rates in the United States remain astonishingly high compared to those of other industrialized nations (in 1989, nineteen countries had lower rates) and when millions of children remain uninsured. Fetal interventions raise the profound question, What types of prenatal care should be and currently are available and to whom? Which fetuses are worth saving? Whose fetuses are valued? Until *all* women have access to *basic* prenatal care, perhaps there should be a moratorium on expensive, high-tech procedures such as fetal surgery. A narrow, reductionist focus on surgically fixing extant problems precludes comprehensive preventive strategies. It would be far more heroic for clinicians, communities, and the nation at large to work collectively to ensure that all pregnant women have access to good nutrition, regular physician or midwife visits, and clean, safe places to live. Activities could include efforts to create a national health program that does not allow poor, nonwhite citizens to fall through the cracks in coverage; the promotion of community-based health activism that recognizes the collective effort required to foster healthier mothers and babies; better attention to the health needs of women in marginalized groups and enhanced public assistance for those without economic resources; language-specific and culturally sensitive health education programs that emphasize both women's health and community health aspects of prenatal care; and limitations on high-tech procedures. Fetal surgery could be reinstituted after the U.S. infant mortality rate has dropped substantially, the number of low birthweight babies has decreased, and many pregnant women are no longer deprived of basic prenatal care.

Abortion Rights. In a reproductive rights framework, women would have access to both abortion *and* fetal surgery (and a range of other reproductive options) despite increasingly popular claims of fetal personhood. If fetal surgery proceeds in a manner that undermines women's right or access to abortion (still legal in the United States as of this writing), then it should be eliminated or reframed. Beginning with women's experiences and needs, rather than with fetal needs, will help ensure that women's autonomy will be protected. But how can we be sure that fetal interventions can and will put women first? For starters, we can take some lessons directly from the practice of fetal surgery itself. As we saw in chapter 6, Susan Davis was adamantly opposed to abortion, portraying women who choose it as "selfish." Yet she was completely comfortable, even delighted, with her own decision to undergo fetal surgery. There seems to be a rather serious contradiction in this avowed pro-life position, one that deems some choices legitimate and others illegitimate and immoral. I would argue that antiabortion activists (and some medical workers) cannot have it both ways. They cannot recognize women's agency for some decisions (e.g., fetal treatment) but not for others (e.g., abortion). Their fallacy comes from a fetocentric perspective, one that blinds them to the paradoxes of their own claims. A reproductive rights perspective, on the other hand, is consistent in its recognition of women's agency in *all* reproductive decisions—including the right *not* to have an abortion. If we accept women's capacity to choose fetal surgery, then we must also accept other choices and build that recognition directly into the social organization of reproductive health care.

Fetal Well-Being. Within a women's health framework, we should also care a great deal about what happens to fetuses that are operated on prenatally. Although fetal surgery is often touted as a rescue mission, we have seen that it may contribute to fetal disability and demise. What are both the immediate and the long-term effects on fetuses of removing a fetus from the womb before it is viable, operating on it, replacing it for continued gestation, the inevitability of preterm labor, birth by cesarean section, and then more surgery after birth? Those who practice fetal surgery should make every effort to minimize trauma to the fetus, as well as to gather as much information as possible about the fate of fetuses that survive. Data can include "objective" measures such as function, size, and disability status, as well as qualitative data obtained from parents about their children's behavior. I maintain that one does not, in fact, have to be "pro-life" (in the usual framings of that term) to care about fetal well-being and the implications of prenatal interventions. In fact, some pro-life individuals and groups advocate fetal surgery because it propagates notions of fetal personhood, as we saw with Liley in chapter 2 and Susan and Jim Davis in chapter 6. But such celebratory discourse elides some of the worst hazards of these procedures, including high fetal mortality rates and the potential for increased neonatal disability. There is instead much room in women's health and reproductive rights frameworks,—themselves "pro-life" in multiple ways—for concern about the fate of fetuses.

Disability Politics. Much of the impetus for fetal surgery stems from the desire for healthy, nondisabled babies. It is likely that many reproductive decisions, from prenatal diagnosis to abortion to fetal treatment, are made in relation to contexts in which disability matters. For example, which women have the resources necessary to raise a disabled child? What are the cultural and economic implications of bearing a disabled child? For fetal surgery to be viable in terms of women's health, we need to address these complicated politics at a societal level. This means working to minimize the stigma attached to disability, as well as broadening social support for the disabled. Currently, there is an *imperative* to do anything possible to avoid disability, and women's choices may be constrained in many ways. Changing the social relations in which such decisions are made requires a rethinking of disability and its place in social life. Some women might still choose *not* to raise a disabled child for a variety of reasons. But the decision to seek fetal treatment for or to abort a potentially defective fetus would be directly related to the specific conditions of a woman's life rather than mandated by the broader social context in which she lives.

In sum, making a fetal surgery for women would involve social and political change on several fronts. Is such change possible? Perhaps not, in which case we should seriously question the existence of fetal surgery while also imagining new and better ways to secure healthier fetuses. Collectively, however, we should at least strive toward attaining the conditions proposed here. Fetal surgery is an arena in which professional status, biomedical authority, health and disease, fetal and maternal bodies, pregnancy, motherhood, fetal subjects, politics, and cultural meanings are continually produced and reproduced, often with profound social consequences. Addressing these consequences means focusing on the social relations and practices that create them. For quite some time now, reproductive politics have been dominated by concern for fetuses, and fetocentric politics have been shaped and enacted by nonfeminist activists, doctors, bioethicists, lawyers, and others. But, I ask again, is fetal surgery the kind of medicine we want? Is it the kind of reproductive politics we want? Those of us who care about women's health need to enter this new reproductive frontier boldly and reclaim the terrain of fetal politics—both in and beyond the operating room—from those who may not have women's best interests at heart. If fetal stories are human stories, then let us rewrite the story of fetal surgery so that women are the principal authors and heroes.

Notes

Chapter 1. Fetal Matters

1. An international conference, sponsored by the Kroc Foundation and held in California in 1982, brought together a number of specialists interested in fetal medicine and fetal surgery. The conference of "fetal invaders," as they called themselves, was not widely publicized (Kolata 1990).
2. See Saltus (1981) and Cadoff (1994).
3. Fetal surgery has been attempted in the United States, the Netherlands, France, Germany, Italy, Japan, the United Kingdom, and a handful of other countries, all with mixed success.
4. Financial data on fetal surgery are not widely available. However, a financial counselor at Capital Hospital provided information on inpatient and outpatient charges and the total amount paid by patients for twelve operations during the period between July 1990 and February 1992. The least expensive operation was $4,686.30 and the most expensive was $68,884.18. Average cost per operation was $23,562.27. The amount paid by patients (including insurance reimbursement) during this period ranged from zero to $14,310.20; the average amount paid was $4,368.35. I learned from another informant, a surgeon, that for the first seventeen open fetal surgery cases at one hospital, the average cost was $10,425, with operations ranging from $5,593 to $22,315. Some of the costs were reimbursed by insurance companies, but the institution absorbed most of it. For the next twenty-three fetal surgery cases, third parties were increasingly willing to pay.
5. Data are from "Healthy California 2000: California's Experience in Achieving the National Health Promotion and Disease Prevention Objectives," California Department of Health Services, 1995, and from "Vital and Health Statistics: Prenatal Care in the United States, 1980–94," U.S. Department of Health and Human Services, July 1996.
6. See Rapp (1993a; 1993b; 1993c; 1994), Rothenberg and Thomson (1994), and Morgan (1996) for a fuller discussion of this issue.
7. One reason for a gap in the literature regarding cost is that fetal treatment is

too experimental for a large-scale analysis; there is not a large enough patient population to determine average outcomes. Korenbrot and Gardner (1991) suggest that one way to evaluate the benefits of fetal surgery is to compare it to neonatal treatment, which is also quite expensive. Benefits might be defined as avoidance of childhood disability, although fetal therapies are at too early a stage of development to assess their impact on chronic childhood diseases. They suggest that fetal treatments that improve birthweight, reduce major medical problems, or reduce the need for major surgery in infants might be cost-efficient in terms of medical expenses alone.

8. See Newman (1996) for a historical analysis of such representations.
9. Police officers in San Francisco's Haight-Ashbury district confiscated five human fetuses at various developmental stages from a man who had hoped to sell them at his garage sale for $100. The police were surprised to learn they had no legal grounds upon which to arrest the entrepreneur, but took custody of the fetuses anyway because they were concerned that children would see the fetuses and become upset.
10. See Morgan (1997) for an analysis of the fetus as a cultural icon in Ecuador.
11. This is recognized even by those who claim to speak for the fetus (Stetson 1996).

Chapter 2.   Breaching the Womb

1. The information presented here on Rh disease is taken from a variety of sources, including unpublished talks and articles found in the collected papers of William Liley as well as his and others' published work (Liley 1968; Liley n.d.-b; Liley n.d.-c; Liley n.d.-d; Liley and Boylan 1965; Zimmerman 1973).
2. Unpublished paper, "Haemolytic Disease," 1973, Postgraduate School of Obstetrics and Gynecology, University of Auckland.
3. See Koenig (1988) for an excellent historical anthropological account of the development of therapeutic plasma exchange.
4. In addition to interviews with his family and colleagues and review of his papers, information on Liley was obtained from *More Famous New Zealanders* (1972), Green (1986), and Shadbolt (1976).
5. Over time, the Lileys' 1,200 acres of rough land has been transformed into a picturesque and impressive farm with Norfolk pines and a lively assortment of animals including sheep, cattle, dogs, and cats. Dr. Margaret Liley runs the farm in partnership with her son, Bill Jr., a forestry consultant.
6. Dr. G. H. Green has prepared an unpublished overview, "The Founding of the Postgraduate School of Obstetrics and Gynecology" (1976), from which much of this material is drawn. The school was established in 1951 by a group of civic-minded women working with the Obstetrical Society who felt that New Zealand should have its own training ground for obstetrics and gynecology, rather than continuing to send physicians to England and elsewhere. Spearheaded by Dr. Doris Gordon, the campaign began in the early 1940s with fundraising and advocacy efforts. Gordon wrote to a colleague, "Even though it looks as if war is in New Zealand waters, it still requires the

old methods of public clamour to generate courage to spend among our politicians." After obtaining the requisite funding and discussing a variety of possible sites, the Postgraduate School was eventually located in what had been, during World War II, the 39th General Hospital of the U.S. Army (Green 1986).

7. Liley described Rh work as such in a 1980 presentation in Long Beach, California, entitled "Rh Hemolytic Disease: Peacekeeing on the Maternofetal Frontier." Notions of maternal-fetal conflict are built right into the title.

8. The importance of the blood bank to the organization of Rh treatment cannot be overestimated, as fresh blood was absolutely necessary for both fetal and neonatal transfusions. Liley maintained continuous correspondence with staff of the Auckland Blood Bank, as well as with blood banking personnel within National Women's Hospital.

9. The contemporary incarnation of the Rh Committee at National Women's Hospital is the Fetal Medicine Advisory Panel. This is a citywide service group composed of physicians, laboratory workers, surgeons, pathologists, and others who review cases and determine fetal treatment policy.

10. Consider the following description: "The fetal position was checked and a likely spot for puncture selected. With lateral or posterior positions this was usually a site where fetal limbs were readily palpable. . . . The site having been selected, local anesthetic was injected through the parietal peritoneum. . . . Translation of the needle showed that the tip was still in the abdominal wall while angulation indicated that the tip lay somewhere in the uterus. Violent or erratic angulation suggested fetal puncture or, more commonly, that the tip lay among fetal limbs. . . . With a rather blunt needle two distinct 'gives' were felt as the anterior and posterior rectus sheaths were penetrated. A further 'give' was felt as the needle entered the amniotic sac or intervillous space. With a very sharp needle these landmarks were often imperceptible but the puncture could be more gentle and controlled. By the same token, however, puncture of . . . the fetal thigh could meet very little resistance and indeed very little protest from the fetus" (Liley 1960; 581–582).

11. Liley and his colleagues felt that clinical signs such as radiological evidence of hydrops were insufficient, and the opportunity to help the fetus in a timely fashion would almost certainly be lost. "Only a specific test on the current fetus can provide the necessary indication and only amniocentesis fulfills this role" (Liley 1965c; 70).

12. In addition, not all ethnic groups at National Women's Hospital were equally represented among Rh patients. Ross Howie told me that approximately 14 percent of women of European descent are Rh-negative. Hemolytic disease was virtually nonexistent in Polynesian, Melanesian, and Maori populations until migration resulted in ethnic mixing. Approximately 8 percent of women in Northern India are Rh-negative, and the highest Rh-negative rate is in Basque and Latin populations.

13. Quoted in Liley (1965c).

14. The difficulty in accessing fetuses resulted in two important modifications of the initial transfusion technique. The first technical modification was the introduction of two needles, one a fine guide–needle upon which the fetus was

impaled to hold it in place and the other a catheter for transfusion. Liggins (1966a; 618, 621) wrote, "The idea of blindly impaling the fetus on a skewer as a guide to the insertion of the catheter introducer is rather repugnant. . . . The impaling technic [*sic*] offers a real prospect of salvaging the fetus otherwise destined to be hydropic by Week 25–26 of pregnancy." Note that use of the catheter was not itself repugnant; the troublesome factor was performing the procedure blindly. The second technical modification was the development of a self-retaining catheter (one that would stay in place) to make transfusions more efficacious. The self-retaining catheter allowed for selecting the optimal rate of transfusion, which "could extend the scope and safety of peritoneal transfusion, particularly in the less mature fetus prior to the thirtieth week" (Liggins 1966b, 323). As with the impaling technique, the self-retaining catheter was designed to enhance access to the fetus as a work object during transfusions. These technical modifications thus contributed to the making of the unborn patient.

15. Liley's work was reported in several U.S. publications, including *Reader's Digest* and *Redbook*, virtually guaranteeing that he would be contacted by American women at risk for Rh complications. The *Redbook* article, titled "What the Rh Factor Is—And What Can Be Done About It," was authored by Liley himself (Liley and Boylan 1965). What is striking in this piece written for a lay audience is the degree to which Liley presented experimental fetal transfusion technology as normal and routine. He (1965d, 38) wrote, "While this may sound like a dangerous or painful operation to the mother, it is simple and harmless. . . . There is no discomfort to the mother and no harm to her baby. On the contrary, the baby's life probably is saved. All these techniques designed to protect the baby's life are amazingly uncomplicated and painless. . . . [W]e must live with the knowledge that hemolytic disease is dangerous. Fortunately, medical control is now possible."

16. Quote taken from an unpublished paper in Liley's files titled "A Perspective of Rh Problems" (n.d.). The last sentence of the quote is almost surely a direct response to Zimmerman (1973).

17. Liley was perhaps the best-known physician in New Zealand, particularly after being knighted by Queen Elizabeth in 1973 for his work in fetal treatment. On one of my research trips to New Zealand, I was taking a ferry from Rangitoto, a volcanic island in Hauraki Gulf, back to Auckland after a day of hiking. On board I struck up a conversation with two middle-aged women who asked what I was doing in Auckland. No sooner had I uttered Liley's name when both women began nodding in recognition, saying things like "Of course, Sir Liley, what a wonderful man" and "Oh yes, Sir Liley, who did all that work on fetuses. His death was such a tragedy." I was both pleased and somewhat astonished that these two women knew who he was, but I soon learned that just about everyone I talked to in New Zealand knew of him. The elderly couple with whom I stayed in Hawkes Bay, a visiting couple from Wellington, the Belgian couple who ran a bed-and-breakfast in Auckland—all of them knew about Liley and his work.

18. See Gluckman et al. (1989). The significance of animal research, particularly in sheep, to the development of these practices cannot be overestimated. Lig-

gins told me, "I guess we were the first people who were able to carry out what's called chronic fetal experiments. That is, do things to a fetus and have the pregnancy continue in experimental animals. Our ability to carry out these procedures was the basis for our discovery of the mechanisms of onset of labor in sheep." These issues will be further explored in chapter 3.

19. Liggins, although formally educated as an obstetrician, was deeply interested in the intricacies of fetal physiology. Trained in New Zealand, he spent a fruitful sabbatical at the University of California, Davis, in 1966 where he investigated fetal physiology, specifically the fetus's role in onset of labor, in sheep. Geoffrey Dawes (1989, 1), considered one of the premier twentieth-century fetal physiologists, wrote about that period in a *Festschrift* in Liggins's honor: "I first met, talked of fetal physiology, and fished with Mont Liggins in California in 1966, where we were both on sabbatical leave, he in Davis and I in San Francisco. . . . In retrospect it was the start of a remarkable epoch in which, over 2–3 years, experimental perinatal physiology and medicine were given a new direction through Mont Liggins' elegant and deceptively simple results." In 1970, Liggins spent three months at Oxford with Dawes, where he developed chronic fetal sheep preparations for research on fetal breathing and lung volume.

20. In 1970, the University of Puerto Rico School of Medicine resumed control of Cayo Santiago and integrated it into what is now called the Caribbean Primate Research Center (CPRC). The addition of a veterinarian to the CPRC staff in 1977 facilitated a new focus on noninvasive biomedical research on free-ranging Rhesus monkeys (Rawlins and Kessler 1986).

21. In relating this story to me, Adamsons also subtly shifted the blame onto the woman, remarking that "the woman went into labor, *without telling us about her uterine contractions.* Even though the baby was not anemic or hydropic, it died from prematurity after a vaginal delivery" (emphasis added).

22. Title taken from McCarthy (1983), writing in New Zealand's major antiabortion newsletter, *Humanity,* on the occasion of Liley's death in 1983.

23. Dr. John Simpson, senior vice president of the Queensland Right to Life Association, introduced Liley as keynote speaker at the University of Queensland, July 15, 1980.

24. This article was subsequently reprinted in the inaugural issue of *Fetal Therapy* with the following introductory note from the editors (Michejda and Pringle 1986b, 8): "Sir William Liley was one of the fathers of fetal therapy. . . . His untimely death in 1983 robbed the field of fetal therapy of a mentor of incredible experience, breadth of vision and wisdom. This paper was based upon an invited paper delivered to the Eighth Annual Congress of the Australian and New Zealand College of Psychiatry in October, 1971. A wide variety of facts about fetal physiology are reviewed, exploding the myth of the fetus as a passenger carried to term, and pointing out that the fetus is an active, developing individual responding to his environment in ways designed to improve his comfort. Liley's humor and tremendous breadth of knowledge are both amply illustrated in this article. He is sorely missed."

25. This was a particularly troublesome issue for Liley, who with his wife, Margaret, had adopted a girl with Down's Syndrome in 1976. Liley was a passion-

ate advocate for the rights of the disabled and mentally handicapped and often remarked that "the morally handicapped cause far more misery and suffering in the world than the mentally or physically handicapped ever do"
(Liley 1971a:3).

26. Margaret Liley (Liley and Day 1966, xii–xiii) described this work in her first
book: "In our hospital in Auckland, New Zealand, [we put] infants with their
mothers as soon after the birth as the mother's condition would permit, so
that the mother would know the baby, and know how to care for him when
she took him home. . . . We found, however, that most young mothers were
not equipped to receive their infants. The majority had never held a baby. . . .
Many mothers were frankly fearful of the tiny strangers they had produced.
. . . It was at this time that we created an ante-natal program designed to
teach mothers about their babies—both unborn and newborn."

27. Pat McCarthy told me, "[Margaret] was very highly qualified in her field, and
I think that perhaps she felt that she was overshadowed by Bill."

28. Pat McCarthy, Ross Howie, Florence Fraser, and Peggy Lawsom of SPUC provided background information on abortion law in New Zealand.

29. The current situation, according to McCarthy, is in theory like that in the
United States: "If there's anyone who wants an abortion, they can likely get
one." But also like the United States, questions of access remain central especially as New Zealand moves toward managed care.

30. Dunn was a retired obstetrician who still served as a consultant to National
Women's Hospital at that time and Manning was a local businessman. Liley
served as SPUC's first president, and all three men became active campaign-
ers on behalf of the organization.

31. Among its publications are pamphlets on the psychological and physical effects of abortion and on fetal development, illustrated by graphic images of
fetal body parts.

32. McCarthy told me that SPUC membership in 1994 was around 20,000, although I was unable to verify either of these figures. He lamented that SPUC
has not made much of a national impact since the 1970s, as "abortion figures
have gone up from about 3,000 per year during the Royal Commission. An of-
ficial report from 1992 states it is 11,460. That's still low by comparison to the
U.S., but very high compared to what the abortion rate in New Zealand used
to be."

33. Presented at hearings of U.S. Senate Judiciary Subcommittee on Constitutional Amendments, May 7, 1974.

34. From "The Humanity of the Unborn," which appeared in an antiabortion
newsletter in New Zealand.

35. Liley killed himself by drinking a glass of cyanide at his home in Auckland.
His wife, Margaret, was home at the time and found his body shortly thereafter. When I spoke with them in 1994, Liley's family and colleagues remained
profoundly affected by the circumstances of his death. Margaret Liley confirmed that her husband had been gravely depressed for months before
killing himself, causing his superior at National Women's Hospital to suggest
he step down. The hospital was experiencing a number of difficulties, including a scandal involving Herb Green's work on cervical screening (see Coney

1988) that affected Liley's own work. As Margaret told me, being asked to leave work "was about the worst thing that could have happened to a workaholic like him." A number of people also indicated that Liley was very concerned about the direction of abortion politics and devastated by the use of his techniques in terminating fetal life.

36. Liley's obituary was carried in newspapers across New Zealand, as well as internationally. In one article, the parents of Liley's first successfully transfused baby, Grant Liley McLeod, remarked, "We were really dumbfounded. He was too young to die, and he had too much to offer."

37. I found this among the papers that Pat McCarthy shared with me. The quote was taken from an unpublished, undated transcript.

38. The antiabortion newspaper *Humanity* (July 1983, 1) reported on Liley's funeral: "On June 18, a bleak mid-winter's day, grieving prolifers joined representatives of the Government and Opposition, university and hospital staff, and colleagues and friends of Sir William as they crowded into the Anglican Holy Trinity Cathedral in Auckland with members of his family for a memorial service. 'You and I are mesmerized by this tragic loss,' said Dean John Rymer, a SPUC patron, who conducted the service. . . . In his panegyric, Dr. Herbert Green, a colleague and friend, spoke of Sir William's prowess as a great scientist and great teacher, his human qualities and his concern for the unborn. . . . The Anglican Archbishop of New Zealand, Archbishop Paul Reeves, presided and the administrator of the Catholic diocese of Auckland, Bishop John Rodgers, was present. Sir William is survived by his wife and scientific co-worker Margaret, Lady Liley, and by their six children."

Chapter 3.   A Hybrid Practice

1. According to one fetal physiologist, "this is an area which still requires a great deal of exploration as to what is removed from the fetus and newborn when the placenta is removed." This seems to imply that scientists might want to re-create some of these maternal physiological processes in order to sustain life outside of a woman's uterus via construction of a *techno-uterus*. Indeed, there have been attempts in the biological sciences to create artificial wombs, placentas, and uteri, none of which have proved successful in practice (Borrell 1989; Hartouni 1991).

2. Ironically, this is precisely what obstetricians had done to midwives using the speculum and forceps in the nineteenth century (Arney 1982; Donegan 1978; Leavitt 1986).

3. Historically, there has been a surprising lack of application of physiology in clinical practice. For links between physiological research and clinical practice, especially legitimacy issues, see Geison (1979; 1987).

4. Amniocentesis is increasingly being recommended for women under age thirty-five, although there is no scientific evidence that amniocentesis benefits younger women.

5. Gilbert (1993) provides a rare frank discussion of risk in prenatal diagnosis.

6. See Associated Press (1991) and Institute of Medicine (1990).

7. Susan Kelly, "Stalking the Rare Fetal Cell: Social and Ethical Issues in

Emerging Prenatal Diagnostic Technologies." Talk presented at the Stanford University Center for Biomedical Ethics, Stanford, California, January 7, 1997.

8. Ibid. Kelly reports that many obstetricians she interviewed "will not take the technology seriously in their own clinical practices until another break-through of the magnitude of polymerase chain reaction (PCR) occurs." But this caution has not prevented at least one biotechnology company from planning for the future. Applied Imaging Corporation in Santa Clara, California, is developing a blood test for diagnosing chromosome-based disorders in fetuses. The company's goal is to obtain the accuracy of amniocentesis or CVS while offering the safety of maternal blood screenings; it had spent about $15 million on the project as of 1997.

9. A newer type of ultrasound technology may eventually supersede today's ul-trasound, as reported in *Fortune* magazine (Kupfer 1993). Called 3-D fetal imaging, the new technique is designed to improve on the grainy, two-dimen-sional images currently produced by ultrasound. "Invading the *real* inner sanctum to create three-dimensional images of the developing fetus quickly and easily" (Kupfer 1993, 87), the 3-D imaging system requires considerably less scanning time and does not expose the fetus to radiation. It works by pro-ducing several slices of two-dimensional images that are then combined by a computer into a solid model. The model can be examined in whole, or doctors can study the various cross-sections from any angle. According to Kupfer (1993, 87), "[P]arents will be able to take home a videotape showing a series of cross-sections that give solid form to their child, and get a head start on bond-ing with their baby."

10. A study reported at the height of the U.S. health care debates found that rou-tine use of prenatal ultrasound screening did not significantly improve out-comes for low-risk women (Leary 1993). The study claimed to demonstrate that if screening were limited to high-risk women, or about 40 percent of all women, savings of $500 million could be achieved. One physician, Richard Berkowitz, was quoted as saying that if the test is not offered to all women, "physicians will have to be extremely vigilant in searching for the many prob-lems or conditions that are indications for obtaining a scan" (Leary 1993, A16). In my own study, a sonographer addressed this issue: "Ultrasound should not be a regular part of prenatal care. The patient should have a rea-son to have a sonogram, and there are lots of reasons. The only thing that is not on the list of reasons to have sonography is a perfectly normal, healthy mother with a planned pregnancy who knows when she got pregnant and [whose] size matches her dates. [Such women] could have their babies com-pletely on their own without any technological help of any type, so they do not need the sonogram. Right now, approximately 60–70 percent of these pa-tients have one of the reasons to have a sonogram. The real question is, by adding the last 30–40 percent, how much do you really accomplish? And now we have a very good study showing that you do not add that much."

11. In 1991, as debates about "family values" raged nationwide, an entire episode of the situation comedy *Murphy Brown* featured Murphy's first look at her fe-

tus. Everyone in the room gazed in wonder at the image as the unmarried Murphy referred to it as "my baby."

12. An oft-quoted saying among antiabortion activists is that if pregnant women's abdomens were transparent, there would be no abortions. Taking these pro-life dreams of ultrasound to their (il)logical limit, such an anatomical feature would certainly make fetal diagnosis and treatment much easier.

13. A recent report of the Tufts University Center for Animals and Public Policy announced that the number of animals used in research has declined by more than 50 percent since 1968 (Hilts 1994). The report also claimed that the amount of pain experienced by animals in research was understated by universities and overstated by animal rights activists. It cited a study from the Netherlands, the only country that has collected data on animal pain and distress caused by research, which contends to show that about one-quarter of animals experienced "severe" discomfort, one-quarter "moderate" discomfort, and about half "minor" discomfort. See also Rader (1995).

14. On April 14, 1967, Liley wrote to the director of the Animal Health Division in Wellington, New Zealand: "For some time we have been interested in the 9 banded armadillo of Texas as an experimental animal for work in fetal physiology. Some months ago I enquired of Mr. Wood, Director of Auckland Zoological Gardens about the possibility of obtaining and caring for armadillos. This American enthusiasm and generosity catches us on the wrong foot and I would therefore appreciate your advice as to whether these animals, presumably captured in the wilds, could be air freighted to New Zealand and quarantined here or whether quarantine is essential in a Zoo in the U.S." After receiving a reply from the animal health officer, on April 28, Liley wrote to J. Gregory Miller, his source in Texas: "I have now heard from the Director of Animal Health Division, Department of Agriculture, and unfortunately they will only permit importation of armadillos into New Zealand on a zoo to zoo basis. If these animals you have so kindly captured could be held in the Houston or some other registered zoo for the required 6 month quarantine period we would have no difficulty getting the necessary import permits, but if this is at all inconvenient for you to bother with I guess the simplest thing would be to let them go."

15. For example, Martin and Murata (1988, 276) argue that "each species is unique, and sometimes surprising differences in physiology turn up between even fairly closely related species. . . . One should not assume that the laboratory primate is a superior surrogate for experimental observations on the human fetus simply because they are closer to humans on the phylogenetic tree."

16. Chairing refers to the process by which primates are restrained during and after operative procedures. They are strapped into chairlike apparatuses and are unable to move about or use their arms and hands. The basic purpose of chairing is to prevent the animal from disrupting the experiment by removing instruments, dislocating stitches, and so on. Because chairing seems to cause emotional distress in many animals, prechairing is used to acclimate the animal before surgery takes place. Murata et al. (1988, 233) state, "although

prechairing for one day to ten days before the operation appeared to help individual monkeys to adjust themselves to the restraining chair more easily after the operation, retrospective statistical analysis failed to demonstrate
significant effects of prechairing either on success rate or on duration of the
preparations. Moreover Chez reported an increased incidence of spontaneous
abortion in the animals that were prechaired in early gestation."

17. Flake et al. (1988, 251) state, "The initial goal of our studies was to develop
surgical, pharmacologic, and anesthetic techniques that could be successfully
applied to fetal surgery in the human."

18. Given the scope of scarring and fibrosis in medicine, it is possible that fetal
wound healing researchers would find many supporters within medicine for
their work. For example, plastic surgeries, transplantation, amputations,
prosthetics, and other areas would likely be transformed by fetal wound healing applications, suggesting multiple possibilities for enrollment of allies, a
key element in the formation of stable scientific and technological endeavors
(Latour 1987). On the other hand, fetal wound healing knowledge could provide yet another lever with which fetal surgeons attempt to gain control over
other medical specialties. Support might come from outside medicine, as
well; it is not difficult to imagine that fetal wound healing would be of great
interest to the cosmetics industry.

Chapter 4. Working on (and around) the Unborn Patient

1. The new technology was called a Rocket catheter and is still used widely in fetal treatment practices.

Chapter 5. Clinical Trials in Fetal Surgery

1. I investigated documents related to the human subjects approval process at
Capital Hospital for the period 1990–1994. Documents included research protocols, multiple versions of informed consent forms, correspondence between the IRB and the fetal surgery team, correspondence between the IRB
and the Oversight Committee, statistical reports, and copies of publications
and papers given at conferences by fetal researchers. The fetal surgery team
refused my initial request to view these documents. But because Capital Hospital receives public funding, I was able to invoke the Freedom of Information Act (FOIA) to access the records. This action provided me with ample
data upon which to base this chapter, but added to my notoriety at Capital
Hospital where only one other person had invoked FOIA over a ten-year period.

2. An administrator told me that the IRB at Capital Hospital sees fifteen to
twenty new protocols each week.

3. But see Kaufmann (1988) for an important challenge to these perspectives.

4. Beginning in 1932, low-income, illiterate, African-American men with
syphilis were misinformed of their diagnoses and denied treatment by the

U.S. Public Health Service researching the disease. According to Jones (1993, 275), "The Tuskegee Study had nothing to do with treatment. No new drugs were tested; neither was any effort made to establish the efficacy of old forms of treatment. It was a nontherapeutic experiment, aimed at compiling data on the effects of the spontaneous evolution of syphilis on black males."

5. More recently, disturbing reports revealed that American medical researchers injected hospital patients with radioactive plutonium during World War II without their explicit knowledge or informed consent (Kaufman 1997). As with the reports of the 1960s, public outrage and a federal response ensued. As Kaufman (1997, 160) argues, "the urgency and secrecy of war-time human experimentation did not justify a departure from prevailing standards either about the use of human beings in medical research or about the voluntary consent of subjects."

6. Data for this section come from the *Belmont Report* (1979), and from DHHS (1991). There is considerable overlap between these two documents.

7. Application also includes the selection of subjects, which I do not discuss at length here because it is less relevant to fetal surgery where enrollment is both limited and nonrandom. The Belmont Report (1979, 7) states that "social justice requires that distinction be drawn between classes of subjects that ought, and ought not, to participate in any particular kind of research. . . . Injustice may appear in the selection of subjects . . . [and] unjust social patterns may nevertheless appear in the overall distribution of the burdens and benefits of research." But, the report stresses, every effort should be made to ensure that the principle of social justice is used to select human subjects fairly and equitably for participation in research.

8. Moreover, Fox (1959, 46) argued, no matter how "deeply committed" they were to the ethical principles, the metabolic researchers "often subordinated their clinical desire to serve the immediate interests of the particular patients involved in such experiments, and gave priority to the more long-range, impersonal research task of acquiring information that might be of general value to medical science."

9. Such views depend, to some degree, on what kind of medicine a physician practices. Carole Joffe (1995, 179) quotes an obstetrician and abortion provider whose primary allegiance is to the pregnant woman: "It comes down to who is the patient. Is the woman the patient, or is the fetus the patient? One or the other is the patient. I've never heard a fetus talk to me. I've heard thousands and thousands of women share their pain, their desperation, and their hopelessness[.]"

10. In certain cases, the drug approval process has been relaxed. Epstein (1996) has written about activists who sought and achieved faster approval for promising drug treatments for HIV/AIDS and greater accountability from drug companies. Breast cancer activists have taken note, and are beginning to push at the boundaries of the drug approval process for innovative breast cancer treatments.

11. Thanks to Barbara Koenig for this insight.

12. The procedures covered by the documents I studied included open fetal surgery for congenital cystic adenomatoid malformation of the lung, congenital diaphragmatic hernia, and sacrococcygeal teratoma, as well as temporary trachael obstruction (PLUG) for congenital diaphragmatic hernia.

13. I attempted to clarify these statistics but was unable to obtain the relevant data despite repeated attempts.

14. The "healthy" eight-year-old requires assistance with urination twice daily. The seven-month-old underwent surgery on the abdomen for aesthetic purposes (abdominoplasty), surgical treatment of an undescended testicle (orchioplexy), and an additional operation on the urinary tract.

15. Personal correspondence, July 10, 1997.

Chapter 6.   Heroic Moms and Maternal Environments

1. Cost of treatment was covered by Susan and Jim Davis and also by the hospital itself.

2. What Charis Cussins (1998) has argued with respect to infertility clinics applies also to fetal surgery: "[T]he patient undergoes significant ontological change. . . . It is the genius of the setting—its techniques—that it allows these ontological variations to be realized and then to multiply." In other words, women's very "nature" is defined through these practices.

3. Merriam Webster's *Collegiate Dictionary* (1985) defines *engaged* as "involved in activity; greatly interested; committed." All of these definitions apply to women's participation in experimental fetal surgery.

4. This chapter is indebted to perspectives in feminist technoscience studies (e.g., Clarke 1998; Haraway 1989; Hubbard 1990) that have striven to show how science and medicine have had a significant role in the making of women, gender, and reproduction while also arguing for the centrality of women's agency and humanity.

5. The quote is from Kolata (1990, 92).

6. For a contemporary cultural analysis of maternal-infant bonding, see Eyer (1992).

7. Fraser told me that when she started at National Women's Hospital, the fetal survival rate for transfusions was around 45 percent and had risen to about 60–70 percent by the time she left. She attributed some of this improvement to women's activities. See chapter 2 for a more detailed discussion.

8. Because of the difficulties I described in chapter 1, I was only able to interview one family formally before losing my research access. I completed my analysis using secondary sources, including a videotape produced by the Fetal Treatment Unit featuring several patients, media coverage of patients discussing fetal surgery, medical workers' "hearsay" discussions of pregnant women, and other data sources. See Casper (1997) for a fuller examination of these access issues.

9. I am profoundly grateful to Rayna Rapp (personal correspondence, July 16, 1996) for reminding me of the complexity of these issues. Her own work on

prenatal diagnosis is a shining example of how to account for the many contradictions embedded in women's use of reproductive technologies.

10. Terbutaline is a tocolytic agent used to prevent preterm labor; it may be administered intravenously or subcutaneously from a pump attached to a woman's body (Scheerer and Katz 1991).

11. Not all of these drugs were in use in fetal surgery at the time of this writing.

12. In 1997, the National Women's Health Network became involved in a "SLAPP" (strategic lawsuit against public participation) related to the use of the terbutaline infusion pump (National Women's Health Network, Membership Appeal, May 8, 1997). Despite having never been approved by the FDA, a major medical technology company marketed the pump to women and doctors. While the company claimed that pregnant women could use the pump in their homes for weeks to prevent premature birth, the drug has not been proved to work for more than a few days. According to FDA reports, at least two women have died while using the terbutaline infusion pump. Yet this has not prevented the use of the terbutaline pump in women after undergoing fetal surgery.

13. Nitrous oxide is laughing gas, and would likely cause quite different reactions in the operating room.

14. This is similar to the semipermanent catheters, such as Swan-Ganz lines, used in cancer patients to introduce chemotherapy and other fluids into the bloodstream. These lines are often inserted in the chest and remain in place during treatment regimens, providing a stable channel while offsetting the need to gain intravenous access over and over again.

15. Ironically, it is precisely these evaluative criteria that are contested by obstetricians and other medical workers. One obstetrician told me, "The reason that [maternal] complications are unacceptable is you have to look at what the benefit is. The same cost would be acceptable if the benefit is fine. We've learned a lot, but that doesn't mean a fetus should have a marsupialization of the bladder today or a CDH." He pointed to high fetal mortality rates as indicative of fetal surgery's limited success, while simultaneously recognizing that important clinical and scientific "discoveries" have been made through pursuing fetal surgery. A sonographer who shares these views remarked, "The bad news is that we've had failure. The good news is that we're a long way from being out of ideas." For both these clinicians, success and failure are linked to issues beyond just saving babies. Obstetricians are aware of threats to maternal risk associated with fetal surgery, and both groups are concerned about the long-term viability of the specialty.

16. Epstein (1995) has written about autodidacts in the HIV/AIDS arena, focusing on how the acquisition of knowledge can be a powerful tool in dealing with clinicians and biomedical institutions.

Chapter 7.   Beyond the Operating Room

1. Many thanks to Lynn Morgan for suggesting this concept.

2. In 1994, surgeons at Wayne State University in Detroit, Michigan, used "tiny

needles and a miniature camera" to separate a fetus from its headless twin. According to the doctors who performed the operation, "such surgery represents a 'new frontier in fetal medicine' and could provide a new weapon against a variety of abnormalities" (Neergaard 1994, A11).

3. Marc Berg, personal correspondence, November 22, 1996.

Glossary

abdominoplasty. Surgery on the abdominal wall, usually for aesthetic purposes. In fetal surgery, such an operation may be done to repair either congenital defects or damage to the abdomen caused by treating other diseases, such as diaphragmatic hernia.

amniocentesis. A procedure for prenatal diagnosis in which a small sample of fluid is drawn from the amniotic sac (the sac surrounding the fetus) during the second trimester of pregnancy. The fluid is used to determine the sex of a fetus and genetic abnormalities.

anemia. A deficiency in the component of the blood responsible for carrying oxygen. Anemia can lead to fatigue and other symptoms.

antibody. A protein produced in the blood as an immune response to a specific antigen. Antibodies are an important way that human bodies fight disease and infection.

anti-D immunoprophylaxis. The so-called Rh vaccine used to treat hemolytic disease.

antigen. Any substance that stimulates the production of antibodies when introduced into the body. Antigens may include toxins, bacteria, or foreign cells, and they are sometimes referred to as *allergens* or *immunogens*.

ascites. The accumulation of serous or watery fluids in the peritoneal cavity (the space between the lining of the abdominal cavity and the abdominal organs). Ascites is often related to hydrops induced by Rh incompatibility.

cardiac arrhythmia. An irregularity or defect in the rhythm or force of the heartbeat.

chorioamnionitis. An infection or inflammation in the amniotic sac, often resulting from premature rupture of the membranes. This condition often leads to neonatal infection.

chorionic villus sampling (CVS). A procedure for prenatal diagnosis in which cells are collected from the chorion, the outermost layer of the fetal membrane that eventually becomes the placenta. CVS is typically done between the ninth and twelfth weeks of pregnancy.

chylothorax. A condition in which there is an accumulation of milky fluid in the membrane enveloping the lungs. It usually causes severe respiratory problems.

congenital diaphragmatic hernia (CDH). A condition in which there is a hole in the diaphragm, causing fetal organs to migrate upward into the chest cavity and impair lung development. Fetal surgery for CDH is designed to repair the diaphragm in utero and reposition the organs in the fetal abdominal cavity, thereby making room for subsequent lung development. Many fetuses with CDH die at birth; those who live and undergo surgery after birth generally have respiratory and other problems for the rest of their lives.

congenital cystic adenomatoid malformation (C-CAM). A tumor in the connective tissue surrounding the urinary bladder and gallbladder. This condition can cause severe kidney damage and/or renal failure.

corticosteroids. A steroid or hormone produced by the adrenal cortex. The adrenal glands are two small endocrine glands located above the kidneys, and the cortex is the outer layer.

embryoscopy. The use of a fiberoptic instrument to view and possibly diagnose and treat an embryo.

endometrium. The mucous membrane comprising the inner layer of the uterine wall.

enterocolitis. Inflammation of the intestinal membranes.

erythroblast. A partly formed red blood cell that is a precursor to an erythrocyte.

erythroblastosis fetalis. A blood disease of a fetus or newborn that usually results from the development in a pregnant woman of an antibody response to the Rh factor in the fetal blood. *See also* **Rh disease** or **hemolytic disease**.

erythrocyte. A normal, mature red blood cell.

fetal blood sampling. An experimental prenatal diagnostic procedure in which a blood sample is taken from a pregnant woman and then filtered using molecular biological techniques in order to locate and analyze the fetal blood cells contained within it.

fetal encephaly. Inflammation or disease of the brain in a fetus.

fetoscopy. The use of a fiberoptic instrument to view the fetus and placenta, to collect fetal blood, and possibly to treat the fetus.

hemolytic disease. Any disease that is destructive to blood cells. *See also* **Rh disease** and **erythroblastosis fetalis**.

hemoperitoneum. The presence of blood in the peritoneal cavity.

hyaluronic acid. A substance that forms a gelatinous material in the tissue spaces of bodies; also an intercellular cement substance throughout the body. It is relevant to fetal wound healing processes.

hydronephrosis. An excess buildup of fluid in the kidneys caused by an obstruction to the flow of urine. Untreated, it generally results in renal failure and death.

hydrops. An excessive accumulation of fluid in any of the tissues or cavities of the body. In the fetus, hydrops refers to the abnormal accumulation of serous fluid in fetal tissues and signifies the terminal phase of hemolytic disease.

hyperplacentation syndrome. Overattachment of the placenta.

hypertension. Abnormally high blood pressure.

hypotension. Abnormally low blood pressure.

hysterotomy. An incision in the uterus, typically lower than a cesarean section.

iatrogenic. An unfavorable condition or response caused by the therapeutic effort itself; doctor-induced.

intrauterine transfusion. Transfusion of a living fetus directly through the uterus.

jaundice. Yellowish discoloration of the eyes and tissues caused by an increase in bile; often indicative of disease.

myocardial ischemia. Constricted blood flow in the heart.

neonate. A newborn infant.

neonatology. A specialty concerned with disorders in the newborn.

oligohydramnios. A condition characterized by an insufficient amount of amniotic fluid.

orchiopexy. Surgical treatment of an undescended testicle in which it is freed and implanted in the scrotum.

parabiosis. The surgical joining of the vascular systems of two organisms.

percutaneous umbilical blood sampling (PUBS). A method of entering the bloodstream of the fetus through the umbilical vein. Also called *cordocentesis*.

perinatology. A subspecialty of obstetrics concerned with the care of a woman and her fetus during pregnancy, labor, and delivery. Perinatologists are involved especially when the woman or her fetus is ill or at risk of becoming ill.

peritoneal cavity. The space between the lining of the abdominal cavity and the abdominal organs.

placenta. A membranous vascular organ that develops in mammals during pregnancy. It lines the uterine wall and partially envelops the fetus, to which it is attached via the umbilical cord. The placental membrane is thin enough to permit the absorption of nutritive materials, oxygen, and some harmful substances (e.g., viruses) into the fetal blood. It also allows the release of carbon dioxide and nitrogenous waste from the fetus.

PLUG. "Plug the Lung Until It Grows." A type of treatment for diaphragmatic hernia in which the fetal trachea is obstructed in utero.

polyhydramnios. A condition characterized by an excessive amount of amniotic fluid.

preeclampsia. The development of hypertension with proteinuria (an abnormal concentration of urinary protein) or edema (accumulation of serous fluids), or both, due to pregnancy. Preeclampsia is dangerous if let untreated.

prenatal gene therapy. A means of treating or correcting genetic disorders in utero by introducing a normal or functioning gene into the cells of fetuses that lack the normal gene.

pulmonary edema. The accumulation of fluid in the lungs.

Rh disease. A condition brought on by immune system incompatibilities between a woman and her fetus, based on the presence or absence of a specific protein on blood cells (the Rh factor). The woman's immune system attacks the fetal blood cells, which it recognizes as foreign because of their different Rh factor. *See also* **hemolytic disease** or **erythroblastosis fetalis**.

sacrococcygeal teratoma (SCT). A tumor located on both the sacrum (the part of the vertebrae directly connected to the pelvis) and the coccyx (the end of the spinal column).

teratology. The branch of embryology concerned with the production, development, anatomy, and classification of malformed embryos and fetuses.

tocolytic. Any agent, typically a drug, that arrests or forestalls uterine contractions. In fetal surgery, tocolytics are used to prevent preterm labor.

tocolysis. The process of arresting uterine contractions or preventing preterm labor.

trophoblast. A thin layer of tissue forming the outer surface of the placenta and separating a pregnant woman's bloodstream from that of her fetus.

ultrasound. A prenatal diagnostic tool that uses sound waves to create moving images of the fetus.

urinary tract obstruction. A condition caused by any number of factors that generally results in an excess buildup of fluid in the kidneys, leading to severe kidney damage and/or renal failure.

Bibliography

AAP Committee on Bioethics. 1990. "Fetal Therapy: Ethical Considerations."
Women's Health Issues 1:16–17.

Abramovich, D. R., and K. R. Page. 1989. "Fetal Control of Amniotic Fluid Volume in the Human." Pp. 9–14 in *Fetal Physiology and Pathology*, edited by P. Belfort, J. A. Pinotti, and T.K.A.B. Eskes. Carnforth, Lancaster, U.K.: Parthenon.

ACOG Committee on Ethics. 1990. "Patient Choice: Maternal-Fetal Conflict."
Women's Health Issues 1:13–15.

Adamsons, Karliss, Jr. 1966. "Fetal Surgery." *New England Journal of Medicine* 275:204–206.

Adamsons, Karliss, Jr., Vincent J. Freda, L. S. James, and M. E. Towell. 1965. "Prenatal Treatment of Erythroblastosis Fetalis Following Hysterotomy." *Pediatrics* 35:848–855.

Adzick, N. Scott. 1992. "Fetal Animal and Wound Implant Models." Pp. 71–82 in *Fetal Wound Healing*, edited by N. Scott Adzick and Michael T. Longaker. New York: Elsevier Science Publishing Co.

Adzick, N. Scott, and Michael R. Harrison. 1992. "The Fetal Surgery Experience." Pp. 1–23 in *Fetal Wound Healing*, edited by N. Scott Adzick and Michael T. Longaker. New York: Elsevier.

———. 1994. "Fetal Surgical Therapy." *Lancet* 343:897–902.

Adzick, N. Scott, and Michael T. Longaker. 1992a. "Characteristics of Fetal Tissue Repair." Pp. 53–70 in *Fetal Wound Healing*, edited by N. Scott Adzick and Michael T. Longaker. New York: Elsevier.

———. 1992b. "Preface." Pp. xi in *Fetal Wound Healing*, edited by N. Scott Adzick and Michael T. Longaker. New York: Elsevier.

Alexander, Leo. 1949. "Medical Science Under Dictatorship." *New England Journal of Medicine* 241:39–47.

Anspach, Renée R. 1993. *Deciding Who Lives: Fateful Choices in the Intensive-Care Nursery*. Berkeley and Los Angeles: University of California Press.

Arney, William Ray. 1982. *Power and the Profession of Obstetrics.* Chicago: University of Chicago Press.

Aronson, Naomi. 1984. "Science as a Claims-Making Activity: Implications for Social Problems Research." Pp. 1–30 in *Studies in the Sociology of Social Problems,* edited by Joseph W. Schneider and John I. Kitsuse. Norwood, N.J.: Ablex.

Asensio, Stanley H., Juan G. Figueroa-Longo, and Ivan A. Pelegrina. 1966. "Intrauterine Exchange Transfusion." *American Journal of Obstetrics and Gynecology* 95:1129–1133.

Associated Press. 1991. "Experimental Maternal Blood Test for Fetal Ills." *New York Times,* October 9, B6.

Associated Press. 1994. "Gap Seen in Infant Mortality." *New York Times,* May 3, B7.

"Baby Makes Headlines Over World: Case a Tribute to Doctors." 1963. N.p.: n.p.

Backman, Carl B. 1982. "Institutional History." Unpublished dissertation chapter.

Bassin, Donna, Margaret Honey, and Meryle Mahrer Kaplan. 1994. "Introduction." Pp. 1–25 in *Representations of Motherhood,* edited by Donna Bassin, Margaret Honey, and Meryle Mahrer Kaplan. New Haven, Conn.: Yale University Press.

Becker, Howard. 1986. *Doing Things Together.* Evanston, Ill.: Northwestern University Press.

Beecher, Henry K. 1966. "Ethics and Clinical Research." *New England Journal of Medicine* 274:1354–1360.

The Belmont Report: Ethical Principles and Guidelines for the Protection of Human Subjects in Research. 1979. Washington, D.C.: GPO, April 18.

Berg, Marc. 1992. "The Construction of Medical Disposals: Medical Sociology and Medical Problem Solving in Clinical Practice." *Sociology of Health and Illness* 14:151–180.

Bevis, David C. A. 1952. "The Antenatal Prediction of Hemolytic Disease." *Lancet* 1:395.

———. 1956. "Blood Pigments in Hemolytic Disease of the Newborn." *Journal of Obstetrics and Gynecology, British Empire* 63:68.

Blum, Deborah. 1994. *The Monkey Wars.* New York: Oxford University Press.

Borrell, Merriley. 1989. *Album of Science: The Biological Sciences in the Twentieth Century.* New York: Scribners.

Bosk, Charles L. 1979. *Forgive and Remember: Managing Medical Failure.* Chicago: University of Chicago Press.

———. 1992. *All God's Mistakes: Genetic Counseling in a Pediatric Hospital.* Chicago: University of Chicago Press.

Bowes, Watson A., Jr., and Brad Selgestad. 1981. "Fetal Versus Maternal Rights: Medical and Legal Perspectives." *Obstetrics and Gynecology* 58:209–214.

Boyd, R.D.H., and C. P. Sibley. 1989. "Potential for Control of Placental Transfer of Osmotically Important Small Molecules." Pp. 3–8 in *Fetal Physiology and Pathology,* edited by P. Belfort, J. A. Pinotti, and T.K.A.B. Eskes. Carnforth, Lancaster, U.K.: Parthenon.

Braidotti, Rosi. 1996. "Signs of Wonder and Traces of Doubt: On Teratology and Embodied Differences." Pp. 135–152 in *Between Monsters, Goddesses, and*

Cyborgs: Feminist Confrontations with Science, Medicine, and Cyberspace, edited by Nina Lykke and Rosi Braidotti. Atlantic Highlands, N.J: Zed.

Brans, Yves W., and Thomas J. Kuehl (eds.). 1988. *Nonhuman Primates in Perinatal Research.* New York: Wiley.

Bucher, Rue. 1962. "Pathology: A Study of Social Movements within a Profession." *Social Problems* 10:40–51.

Bucher, Rue, and Anselm Strauss. 1961. "Professions in Process." *American Journal of Sociology* 66:325–334. [Reprinted in Anselm L. Strauss. 1991. *Creating Sociological Awareness.* New Brunswick, NJ: Transaction, 245–262.]

Burd, D. Andrew R., Michael T. Longaker, and N. Scott Adzick. 1992. "In Vitro Fetal Wound Healing Models." Pp. 255–264 in *Fetal Wound Healing,* edited by N. Scott Adzick and Michael T. Longaker. New York: Elsevier.

Cadoff, Jennifer. 1994. "Miracle Babies: Fetal Surgery's Lifesaving Results." *Parents,* June, 53–55.

Camosy, Pamela. 1995. "Fetal Medicine: Treating the Unborn Patient." *American Family Physician* 52:1385–1392.

Canguilhem, Georges. 1977. *On the Normal and the Pathological.* Dordrecht: Reidel.

Cartwright, Lisa. 1995. *Screening the Body: Tracing Medicine's Visual Culture.* Minneapolis: University of Minnesota Press.

Casper, Monica J. 1992. "Anatomy of a Scientific Controversy: The Politics of Fetal Tissue Research." Unpublished paper, Department of Social and Behavioral Sciences, University of California, San Francisco.

———. 1994a. "At the Margins of Humanity: Fetal Positions in Science and Medicine." *Science, Technology, and Human Values* 19:307–323.

———. 1994b. "Reframing and Grounding 'Non-Human' Agency: What Makes a Fetus an Agent?" *American Behavioral Scientist* 37(6):839–856.

———. 1997. "Feminist Politics and Fetal Surgery: Adventures of a Research Cowgirl on the Reproductive Frontier." *Feminist Studies* 23(2):233–262.

———. Forthcoming. "Operation to the Rescue: Feminist Encounters with Fetal Surgery." in *The Fetal Imperative: Feminist Perspectives,* edited by Lynn M. Morgan and Meredith Michaels. Philadelphia: University of Pennsylvania Press.

Casper, Monica J., and Marc Berg. 1995. "Introduction: Constructivist Perspectives on Medical Work: Medical Practices and Science and Technology Studies." *Science, Technology, and Human Values* 20(4):395–407.

Chavkin, Wendy. 1992. "Women and the Fetus: The Social Construction of Conflict." Pp. 193–202 in *The Criminalization of a Woman's Body,* edited by Clarice Feinman. New York: Haworth.

Chervenak, Frank A., and Laurence B. McCullough. 1985. "Perinatal Ethics: A Practical Method of Analysis of Obligations to Mother and Fetus." *Obstetrics and Gynecology* 66:442–446.

———., and Laurence B. McCullough. 1991. "The Fetus as Patient: Implications for Directive Versus Nondirective Counseling for Fetal Benefit." *Fetal Diagnosis and Therapy* 6:93–100.

Clarke, Adele E. 1987. "Research Materials and Reproductive Science in the

United States, 1910–1940." Pp. 323–350 in *Physiology in the American Context, 1845–1940*, edited by Gerald L. Geison. Bethesda, Md.: American Physiological Society.

———. 1990. "Controversy and the Development of Reproductive Sciences." *Social Problems* 37:18–37.

———. 1998. *Disciplining Reproduction: Modernity, American Life Sciences, and "The Problem of Sex"*. Berkeley and Los Angeles: University of California Press.

Coney, Sandra. 1988. *The Unfortunate Experiment*. Auckland, New Zealand: Penguin Books.

Creasy, Robert K., and Robert Resnick (eds.). 1994. *Maternal-Fetal Medicine: Principles and Practice*. Philadelphia: W. B. Saunders.

Cussins, Charis. 1998. "Ontological Choreography: Agency for Women Patients in an Infertility Clinic." In *Differences in Medicine:Unraveling Practices, Techniques, and Bodies*, edited by Marc Berg and Annemarie Mol. Durham N.C.: Duke University Press.

Dancis, Joseph. 1987. "Placental Physiology." Pp. 1–34 in *Prenatal and Perinatal Biology and Medicine*, edited by Norman Kretchmer, Edward J. Quilligan, and John D. Johnson. Chur: Harwood Academic.

Daniels, Cynthia R. 1993. *At Women's Expense: State Power and the Politics of Fetal Rights*. Cambridge: Harvard University Press.

Dawes, Geoffrey S. 1989. "Mont Liggins on Birth, the Fetal Lung and the Weddell Seal." Pp. 1–12 in *Advances in Fetal Physiology: Reviews in Honor of G. C. Liggins*, edited by Peter D. Gluckman, Barbara M. Johnston, and Peter W. Nathanielsz. Ithaca N.Y.: Perinatology Press.

Day, Beth, and Margaret Liley. 1968. *The Secret World of the Baby*. New York: Random House.

DHHS (Department of Health and Human Services). 1991. *Code of Federal Regulations, Title 45, Part 46—Protection of Human Subjects*. Office for Protection from Research Risks, National Institutes of Health, June 18.

Donald, Ian. 1969. "On Launching a New Diagnostic Science." *American Journal of Obstetrics and Gynecology* 1:609–628.

Donegan, Jane B. 1978. *Women and Men Midwives: Medicine, Morality, and Misogyny in Early America*. Westport, Conn.: Greenwood.

Duden, Barbara. 1993a. *Disembodying Women: Perspectives on Pregnancy and the Unborn*. Cambridge, Mass.: Harvard University Press.

———. 1993b. "Visualizing 'Life.' " *Science as Culture* 3(4):562–600.

Ehrenreich, Barbara, and Deirdre English. 1978. *For Her Own Good: 150 Years of the Experts' Advice to Women*. New York: Doubleday.

Elkins, Thomas E. 1990. "The Case for a Middle Ground." *Women's Health Issues* 1:34–36.

Epstein, Steven. 1995. "The Construction of Lay Expertise: AIDS Activism and the Forging of Credibility in the Reform of Clinical Trials." *Science, Technology, and Human Values* 20:408–437.

———. 1996. *Impure Science: AIDS, Activism, and the Politics of Knowledge*. Berkeley and Los Angeles: University of California Press.

Evans, Mark I., Mark Paul Johnson, and Wolfgang Holzgreve. 1990. "Fetal Therapy: The Next Generation." *Women's Health Issues* 1:31–33.

Eyer, Diane E. 1992. *Mother-Infant Bonding: A Scientific Fiction.* New Haven, Conn.: Yale University Press.

Filly, Roy A. 1991. "Sonographic Anatomy of the Normal Fetus." Pp. 92–124 in *The Unborn Patient: Prenatal Diagnosis and Treatment,* edited by Michael R. Harrison, Mitchell S. Golbus, and Roy A. Filly. Philadelphia: W. B. Saunders.

Fisher, Sue. 1988. *In the Patient's Best Interests: Women and the Politics of Medical Decisions.* New Brunswick: Rutgers University Press.

Flake, Alan W., Michael R. Harrison, and N. Scott Adzick. 1988. "Intrauterine Intervention: Fetal Surgery in the Nonhuman Primate." Pp. 245–262 in *Nonhuman Primates in Perinatal Research,* edited by Yves W. Brans and Thomas J. Kuehl. New York: Wiley.

Fletcher, John C., and Albert R. Jonsen. 1991. "Ethical Considerations in Fetal Treatment." Pp. 14–18 in *The Unborn Patient: Prenatal Diagnosis and Treatment,* edited by Michael R. Harrison, Mitchell S. Golbus, and Roy A. Filly. Philadelphia: W. B. Saunders.

Foucault, Michel. 1972. *The Archaeology of Knowledge.* London: Tavistock.

———. 1973. *The Birth of the Clinic: An Archaeology of Medical Perception.* New York: Vintage Books.

———. 1979. *Discipline and Punish: The Birth of the Prison.* New York: Vintage Books.

Fowden, A. L. 1989. "The Endocrine Regulation of Fetal Metabolism and Growth." Pp. 229–244 in *Advances in Fetal Physiology: Reviews in Honor of G. C. Liggins,* edited by Peter D. Gluckman, Barbara M. Johnston, and Peter W. Nathanielsz. Ithaca N.Y.: Perinatology Press.

Fox, Renée C. 1959. *Experiment Perilous: Physicians and Patients Facing the Unknown.* Philadelphia: University of Pennsylvania Press.

Fox, Renée C., and Judith P. Swazey. 1974. *The Courage to Fail: A Social View of Organ Transplants and Dialysis.* Chicago: University of Chicago Press.

Franklin, Sarah. 1991. "Fetal Fascinations: New Dimensions to the Medical-Scientific Construction of Personhood." Pp. 190–205 in *Off-Centre: Feminism and Cultural Studies,* edited by Sarah Franklin, Celia Lury, and Jackie Stacey. London: HarperCollins.

———. 1993. "Postmodern Procreation: Representing Reproductive Practice." *Science as Culture* 3:522–561.

Freda, Vincent J., and Karliss Adamsons, Jr. 1964. "Exchange Transfusion In Utero: Report of a Case." *American Journal of Obstetrics and Gynecology* 89:817–821.

Freund, Peter E. S., and Meredith B. McGuire. 1995. *Health, Illness, and the Social Body: A Critical Sociology.* Englewood Cliffs, N.J.: Prentice Hall.

Fuchs, Victor R. 1968. "The Growing Demand for Medical Care." *New England Journal of Medicine* 279:190–195.

Fujimura, Joan H. 1988. "The Molecular Biological Bandwagon in Cancer Research: Where Social Worlds Meet." *Social Problems* 35:261–283.

Gallagher, Janet. 1987. "Prenatal Invasion and Interventions: What's Wrong with Fetal Rights." *Harvard Women's Law Journal* 10:9–58.

———. 1989. "Fetus as Patient." Pp. 185–235 in *Reproductive Laws for the 1990s*, edited by Sherrill Cohen and Nadine Taub. Clifton, N.J.: Humana Press.

Geison, Gerald L. 1979. "Divided We Stand: Physiologists and Clinicians in the American Context." Pp. 67–90 in *The Therapeutic Revolution: Essays in the Social History of American Medicine*, edited by Morris J. Vogel and Charles Rosenberg. Philadelphia: University of Pennsylvania Press.

Geison, Gerald L. (ed.). 1987. *Physiology in the American Context: 1850–1940*. Bethesda, Md.: American Physiological Society.

Gilbert, Susan. 1993. "Waiting Game." *New York Times Magazine*, April 25, 70–73.

Ginsburg, Faye D., and Rayna Rapp (Eds.). 1995. *Conceiving the New World Order: The Global Politics of Reproduction*. Berkeley and Los Angeles: University of California Press.

Glaser, Barney G. and Anselm Strauss. 1967. *The Discovery of Grounded Theory*. Chicago: Aldine.

Gluckman, Peter D., Barbara M. Johnston, and Peter W. Nathanielsz (eds.). 1989. *Advances in Fetal Physiology: Reviews in Honor of G. C. Liggins*. Ithaca N.Y.: Perinatology Press.

Golbus, Mitchell S. 1991. "Selective Termination." Pp. 166–171 in *The Unborn Patient: Prenatal Diagnosis and Treatment*, edited by Michael R. Harrison, Mitchell S. Golbus, and Roy A. Filly. Philadelphia: W. B. Saunders.

Gould, Stephen Jay. 1996/1981. *The Mismeasure of Man*. Revised and expanded edition. New York: Norton.

Green, G. H. 1985. "Historic Perspective on Liley's 'Fetal Transfusion.'" *Vox Sanguinis* 48:184–187.

———. 1986. "William Liley and Fetal Transfusion: A Perspective in Fetal Medicine." *Fetal Therapy* 1:18–22.

Green, G. H., A. W. Liley, and G. C. Liggins. 1964. "The Place of Foetal Transfusion in Haemolytic Disease." Unpublished paper, Postgraduate School of Obstetrics and Gynecology, Auckland, New Zealand.

Griener, Glenn. 1988. "Introduction." Pp. 1–4 in *Biomedical Ethics and Fetal Therapy*, edited by Carl Nimrod and Glenn Griener. Waterloo, Canada: Wilfrid Laurier University Press.

Grobstein, Clifford. 1988. *Science and the Unborn: Choosing Human Futures*. New York: Basic Books.

Grodin, Michael A. 1990. "Patient Choice and Fetal Therapy." *Women's Health Issues* 1:18–20.

Haraway, Donna. 1989. *Primate Visions: Gender, Race, and Nature in the World of Modern Science*. New York: Routledge.

———. 1992. "The Promises of Monsters: A Regenerative Politics for Inappropriate/d Others." Pp. 295–337 in *Cultural Studies*, edited by Lawrence Grossberg, Cary Nelson, and Paula Treichler. New York: Routledge.

———. 1997. *Modest_Witness@Second_Millenium.FemaleMan©_Meets_OncoMouse™: Feminism and Technoscience*. New York: Routledge.

Harding, Jane E., and Valerie Charlton. 1991. "Experimental Nutritional Supplementation for Intrauterine Growth Retardation." Pp. 598–613 in *The Unborn Patient: Prenatal Diagnosis and Treatment*, edited by Michael R. Harrison, Mitchell S. Golbus, and Roy A. Filly. Philadelphia: W. B. Saunders.

Harrison, Michael R. 1982. "Unborn: Historical Perspectives of the Fetus as a Patient." *The Pharos* 45:19–24.

———. 1991a. "Professional Considerations in Fetal Treatment." Pp. 8–13 in *The Unborn Patient: Prenatal Diagnosis and Treatment*, edited by Michael R. Harrison, Mitchell S. Golbus, and Roy A. Filly. Philadelphia: W. B. Saunders.

———. 1991b. "The Fetus as a Patient: Historical Perspective." Pp. 3–7 in *The Unborn Patient: Prenatal Diagnosis and Treatment*, edited by Michael R. Harrison, Mitchell S. Golbus, and Roy A. Filly. Philadelphia: W. B. Saunders.

———. 1993. "Fetal Surgery." *Western Journal of Medicine* 159:341–349.

Harrison, Michael R., and N. Scott Adzick. 1991. "The Fetus as a Patient: Surgical Considerations." *Annals of Surgery* 213:279–291.

Harrison, Michael R., and Roy A. Filly. 1991. "The Fetus with Obstructive Uropathy: Pathophysiology, Natural History, Selection, and Treatment." Pp. 328–402 in *The Unborn Patient: Prenatal Diagnosis and Treatment*, edited by Michael R. Harrison, Mitchell S. Golbus, and Roy A. Filly. Philadelphia: W. B. Saunders.

Harrison, Michael R., Mitchell S. Golbus, and Roy A. Filly (eds.). 1991. *The Unborn Patient: Prenatal Diagnosis and Treatment*. Philadelphia: W. B. Saunders.

Harrison, Michael R., and Michael T. Longaker. 1991. "Maternal Risk and the Development of Fetal Surgery." Pp. 189–202 in *The Unborn Patient: Prenatal Diagnosis and Treatment*, edited by Michael R. Harrison, Mitchell S. Golbus, and Roy A. Filly. Philadelphia: W. B. Saunders.

Hartouni, Valerie. 1991. "Containing Women: Reproductive Discourse in the 1980s." Pp. 27–56 in *Technoculture*, edited by Constance Penley and Andrew Ross. Minneapolis: University of Minnesota Press.

———. 1992. "Fetal Exposures: Abortion Politics and the Optics of Allusion." *Camera Obscura* 29:131–149.

———. 1994. "Breached Births: Reflections on Race, Gender, and Reproductive Discourses in the 1980s." *Configurations* 2:73–88.

———. 1997. *Cultural Conceptions: On Reproductive Technologies and the Remaking of Life*. Minneapolis: University of Minnesota Press.

Hilts, Philip J. 1994. "Research Animals Used Less Often." *New York Times*, March 3, A7.

Himmelstein, David U., and Steffie Woolhandler. 1994. *The National Health Program Book: A Source Guide for Advocates*. Monroe, Maine: Common Courage.

Howell, Lori J., N. Scott Adzick, and Michael R. Harrison. 1993. "The Fetal Treatment Center." *Seminars in Pediatric Surgery* 2:143–146.

Hubbard, Ruth. 1982. "The Fetus as Patient." *Ms.*, October, 31–32.

———. 1990. *The Politics of Women's Biology*. New Brunswick, N.J.: Rutgers University Press.

Huet, Marie-Hélène. 1993. *Monstrous Imagination*. Cambridge Mass.: Harvard University Press.

Hughes, Everett C. 1971. *The Sociological Eye: Selected Papers.* New Brunswick, N.J.: Transaction.

Hunt, Linda M., Brigitte Jordan, and Carole H. Browner. 1989. "Compliance and the Patient's Perspective: Controlling Symptoms in Everyday Life." *Culture, Medicine and Psychiatry* 13:315–334.

Institute of Medicine. 1990. *Science and Babies: Private Decisions, Public Dilemmas.* Washington, D.C.: National Academy Press.

———. 1994. *Fetal Research and Applications: A Conference Summary.* Washington, D.C.: National Academy Press.

Jennings, Russell W., Thomas E. MacGillivary, and Michael R. Harrison. 1993. "Nitric Oxide Inhibits Preterm Labor in the Rhesus Monkey." *Journal of Maternal-Fetal Medicine* 2:170–175.

Joffe, Carole. 1995. *Doctors of Conscience: The Struggle to Provide Abortion Before and After* Roe v. Wade. Boston: Beacon.

Johnsen, Dawn E. 1986. "The Creation of Fetal Rights: Conflicts With Women's Constitutional Rights to Liberty, Privacy, and Equal Protection." *Yale Law Journal* 95:599–625.

Johnson, John D., and Robert E. Greenberg. 1987. "Regulation of Fetal Growth." Pp. 35–92 in *Prenatal and Perinatal Biology and Medicine,* edited by Norman Kretchmer, Edward J. Quilligan, and John D. Johnson. Chur: Harwood Academic.

Jones, James. 1993. "The Tuskegee Syphilis Experiment: 'A Moral Astigmatism.'" Pp. 275–286 in *The "Racial" Economy of Science: Toward a Democratic Future,* edited by Sandra Harding. Bloomington: Indiana University Press.

Jost, Kenneth. 1989. "Mother Versus Child." *ABA Journal* April:84–88.

Kaufert, Joseph M., and John D. O'Neil. 1990. "Biomedical Rituals and Informed Consent: Native Canadians and the Negotiation of Clinical Trust." Pp. 41–63 in *Social Science Perspectives on Medical Ethics,* edited by George Weisz. Philadelphia: University of Pennsylvania Press.

Kaufman, Sharon R. 1997. "The World War II Plutonium Experiments: Contested Stories and Their Lessons for Medical Research and Informed Consent." *Culture, Medicine and Psychiatry* 6:1–37.

Kaufmann, Caroline L. 1988. "Perfect Mothers, Perfect Babies: An Examination of the Ethics of Fetal Treatments." *Reproductive and Genetic Engineering* 1:133–139.

Klass, Perri. 1996. "The Artificial Womb Is Born." *New York Times Magazine,* September 29, 117–119.

Knopoff, Katherine A. 1991. "Can a Pregnant Woman Morally Refuse Fetal Surgery?" *California Law Review* 79:499–540.

Koenig, Barbara A. 1988. "The Technological Imperative in Medical Practice: The Social Creation of a 'Routine' Treatment." Pp. 465–496 in *Biomedicine Examined,* edited by Margaret Lock and Deborah R. Gordon. Dordrecht, Netherlands: Kluwer Academic.

Kogan, Barry A. 1991. "The Fetus with Obstructive Uropathy: Alternative Approaches." Pp. 399–402 in *The Unborn Patient: Prenatal Diagnosis and Treat-*

ment, edited by Michael R. Harrison, Mitchell S. Golbus, and Roy A. Filly. Philadelphia: W. B. Saunders.

Kolata, Gina. 1983. "Fetal Surgery for Neural Defects." *Science* 221:441.

———. 1990. *The Baby Doctors: Probing the Limits of Fetal Medicine*. New York: Delacorte.

Korenbrot, Carol C., and Laura Gardner. 1991. "Economic Considerations in Fetal Treatment." Pp. 25–35 in *The Unborn Patient: Prenatal Diagnosis and Treatment*, edited by Michael R. Harrison, Mitchell S. Golbus, and Roy A. Filly. Philadelphia: W. B. Saunders.

Kretchmer, Norman, Edward J. Quilligan, and John D. Johnson (eds.). 1987. *Prenatal and Perinatal Biology and Medicine*. Chur: Harwood Academic.

Krummel, Thomas M., and Michael T. Longaker. 1991. "Fetal Wound Healing." Pp. 526–536 in *The Unborn Patient: Prenatal Diagnosis and Treatment*, edited by Michael R. Harrison, Mitchell S. Golbus, and Roy A. Filly. Philadelphia: W. B. Saunders.

Kupfer, Andrew. 1993. "New Images of Babies Before Birth." *Fortune*, August 9, 87.

Latour, Bruno. 1987. *Science in Action: How to Follow Scientists and Engineers Through Society*. Cambridge, Mass.: Harvard University Press.

———. 1991. *We Have Never Been Modern*. Cambridge, Mass.: Harvard University Press.

Layne, Linda. 1990. "Motherhood Lost: Cultural Dimensions of Miscarriage and Stillbirth." *Women and Health* 16:75–104.

———. 1996. "How's the Baby Doing?: Struggling With Narratives of Progress in a Neonatal Intensive Care Unit." *Medical Anthropology Quarterly* 10 (4): 624–656.

Leary, Warren E. 1993. "Waste is Found in Use of Prenatal Ultrasound." *New York Times*, September 16, A16.

Leavitt, Judith Walzer. 1986. *Brought to Bed: Childbearing in America, 1750–1950*. New York: Oxford University Press.

Leigh, Wilhelmina A. 1994. "The Health Status of Women of Color." Pp. 154–196 in *The American Woman 1994–95: Where We Stand [Women and Health]*, edited by Cynthia Costello and Anne J. Stone. New York: Norton.

Lenow, Jeffrey L. 1983. "The Fetus as a Patient: Emerging Rights as a Person?" *American Journal of Law and Medicine* 9:1–29.

Lewin, Ellen, and Virginia Olesen (eds.). 1985. *Women, Health, and Healing: Toward a New Perspective*. New York: Tavistock.

Liggins, Graham C. 1966a. "Fetal Transfusion by the Impaling Technic." *Obstetrics and Gynecology* 27(5):617–621.

———. 1966b. "A Self Retaining Catheter for Fetal Peritoneal Transfusion." *Obstetrics and Gynecology* 27(3):323–326.

———. 1969. "Premature Delivery of Fetal Lambs Infused with Glucocorticoids." *Journal of Endocrinology* 45:515–523.

Liggins, Graham C., and Ross N. Howie. 1972. "A Controlled Trial of Antepartum Glucocorticoid Treatment for Prevention of the Respiratory Distress Syndrome in Premature Infants." *Pediatrics* 50:515–525.

Liley, A. W. 1960. "The Technique and Complications of Amniocentesis." *New Zealand Medical Journal* 59:581–86.

———. 1961. "Liquor Amnii Analysis in the Management of the Pregnancy Complicated by Rhesus Sensitization." *American Journal of Obstetrics and Gynecology* 82:1359–1370.

———. 1963. "Amniotic Fluid." Pp. 227–244 in *Modern Trends in Human Reproductive Physiology*, edited by H. M. Carey. London: Butterworths.

———. 1964. "The Technique of Foetal Transfusion in the Treatment of Severe Haemolytic Disease." *Australia and New Zealand Obstetrics and Gynecology* 4:145–148.

———. 1965a. "Amniocentesis." *New England Journal of Medicine* 272:731–732.

———. 1965b. "Intrauterine Transfusion." *Jewish Memorial Hospital Bulletin* 10:70–76.

———. 1965c. "The Use of Amniocentesis and Fetal Transfusion in Erythroblastosis Fetalis." *Pediatrics* 35:836–847.

———. 1968. "Diagnosis and Treatment of Erythroblastosis in the Fetus." Pp. 29–63 in *Advances in Pediatrics*, edited by S. Z. Levine. Chicago: Year Book Medical Publishers.

———. 1969. "Intrauterine Transfusion." Unpublished paper, Postgraduate School of Obstetrics and Gynecology, Auckland, New Zealand.

———. 1971a. "A Case Against Abortion." *A Liberal Studies Broadsheet*, 1–4.

———. 1971b. "The Development of the Idea of Fetal Transfusion." *American Journal of Obstetrics and Gynecology* 3:302–304.

———. 1971c. "The Rights of the Fetus." Unpublished paper, Postgraduate School of Obstetrics and Gynecology, Auckland, New Zealand.

———. 1971d. "The Unborn Child." *Health*, 12–13.

———. 1972a. "Disorders of Amniotic Fluid." Pp. 157–206 in *Pathophysiology of Gestation*. New York: Academic Press.

———. 1972b. "The Foetus as a Personality." *Australia and New Zealand Journal of Psychiatry* 6:99–105.

———. 1979. "The Medical Reality of Achieving the Pro-Life Ideal." Unpublished paper, Postgraduate School of Obstetrics and Gynecology, Auckland, New Zealand.

———. 1980. "Rh Haemolytic Disease: Peacekeeping on the Maternofetal Frontier." Unpublished paper, Postgraduate School of Obstetrics and Gynecology, Auckland, New Zealand.

———. 1982. "Medical Research in Mental Retardation." Unpublished paper, Postgraduate School of Obstetrics and Gynecology, Auckland, New Zealand.

———. 1983. "Development of Life." *Humanity*, July, 6–8.

———. 1986. "The Fetus as a Personality," [Originally published in 1972 in Australian and New Zealand Journal of Psychiatry, 6:99–105.] *Fetal Therapy* 1:8–17.

———. n.d.-a. "The Humanity of the Unborn." Unpublished paper, Postgraduate School of Obstetrics and Gynecology, Auckland, New Zealand.

———. n.d.-b. "Physiological Problems in Foetal Transfusion." Unpublished paper, Postgraduate School of Obstetrics and Gynecology, Auckland, New Zealand.

————. n.d.-c. "Prenatal Treatment of Haemolytic Disease: Sociomedical Aspects." Unpublished paper, Postgraduate School of Obstetrics and Gynecology, Auckland, New Zealand.

————. n.d.-d. "Rh Disease." Unpublished paper, Postgraduate School of Obstetrics and Gynecology, Auckland, New Zealand.

Liley, A. William, and Brian Richard Boylan. 1965. "The Expectant Mother: What the Rh Factor is and What Can Be Done About It." *Redbook,* November, 38–39.

Liley, H.M.I., and Beth Day. 1966. *Modern Motherhood: Pregnancy, Childbirth, and the Newborn Baby.* New York: Random House.

Longo, Lawrence D. 1978. "An Appreciation of Donald Henry Barron." Pp. xxvii–xxxiv in *Fetal and Newborn Cardiovascular Physiology,* edited by Lawrence D. Longo and Daniel D. Reneau. New York: Garland.

Louw, J. H. 1974. "Wither Pediatric Surgery?" *South African Medical Journal* 48:1597–1598.

Lynch, Michael. 1988. "Sacrifice and the Transformation of the Animal Body into a Scientific Object: Laboratory Culture and Ritual Practice in the Neurosciences." *Social Studies of Science* 18:265–289.

Macklin, Ruth. 1990. "Maternal-Fetal Conflict: An Ethical Analysis." *Women's Health Issues* 1:28–30.

Manning, Frank A. 1995. *Fetal Medicine: Principles and Practice.* Norwalk, Conn.: Appleton & Lange.

Martin, Chester B., Jr., and Yuji Murata. 1988. "Perspective on the Fetus." Pp. 275–280 in *Nonhuman Primates in Perinatal Research,* edited by Yves W. Brans and Thomas J. Kuehl. New York: Wiley.

Marwick, Charles. 1993. "Coming to Terms with Indications for Fetal Surgery." *Journal of the American Medical Association* 270:2025, 2029.

Mastroianni, Luigi, Jr. 1986. "Ethical Aspects of Fetal Therapy and Experimentation." Pp. 3–8 in *The Intrauterine Life: Management and Therapy,* edited by J. G. Schenker and D. Weinstein. New York: Elsevier.

Mattingly, Susan S. 1992. "The Maternal-Fetal Dyad: Exploring the Two-Patient Obstetric Model." *Hastings Center Report* January-February:13–18.

Maynard-Moody, Steven. 1995. *The Dilemma of the Fetus: Fetal Research, Medical Progress, and Moral Politics.* New York: St. Martin's.

McCarthy, Pat. 1983. "A Legacy of Life." *Humanity,* July, 5.

Mead, George Herbert. 1934. *Mind, Self, and Society, from the Standpoint of a Social Behaviorist.* Chicago: University of Chicago Press.

Michejda, Maria, and Kevin Pringle. 1986a. "Editorial." *Fetal Therapy* 1:3–7.

————. 1986b. "Note from the Editors." *Fetal Therapy* 1:8.

Moise, Kenneth, Jr. 1993. "Percutaneous Umbilical Blood Sampling." Paper presented at the Institute of Medicine Conference on Fetal Research and Applications, Irvine, California, June 20–22, 1993.

More Famous New Zealanders. 1972. Christchurch, New Zealand: Whitcombe and Tombs.

Morgan, Lynn M. 1989. "When Does Life Begin? A Cross-Cultural Perspective on the Personhood of Fetuses and Young Children." Pp. 97–114 in *Abortion Rights and Fetal Personhood*, edited by Edd Doerr and James W. Prescott. Long Beach, Calif.: Centerline.

———. 1996. "Fetal Relationality in Feminist Philosophy: An Anthropological Critique." *Hypatia* 11:47–70.

———. 1997. "Imagining the Unborn in the Ecuadoran Andes." *Feminist Studies* 23:323–350.

Morgan, Lynn M., and Meredith M. Michaels (eds.). Forthcoming. *The Fetal Imperative: Feminist Positions.* Pennsylvania: University of Pennsylvania Press.

Moore, Lisa Jean. 1996. "Producing Safer Sex: Knowledge, Latex, and Sex Workers in the Age of AIDS." Doctoral dissertation, Department of Social and Behavioral Sciences, University of California, San Francisco.

Morowitz, Harold J., and James S. Trefil. 1992. *The Facts of Life: Science and the Abortion Controversy.* New York: Oxford University Press.

Moscucci, Ornella. 1990. *The Science of Woman: Gynecology and Gender in England, 1800–1929.* Cambridge, U.K.: Cambridge University Press.

Murata, Yuji, Shunichi Fujisaki, Chikara Endo, and Chester B. Martin, Jr. 1988. "Chronic Instrumentation of the Fetal Primate." Pp. 231–243 in *Nonhuman Primates in Perinatal Research*, edited by Yves W. Brans and Thomas J. Kuehl. New York: Wiley.

Neergaard, Lauran. 1994. "Surgery by Needles Saves Periled Fetus." *San Francisco Chronicle*, February 17, A11.

Nelson, Cary, Paula A. Treichler, and Lawrence Grossberg. 1992. "Cultural Studies: An Introduction." Pp. 1–22 in *Cultural Studies*, edited by Lawrence Grossberg, Cary Nelson, and Paula Treichler. New York: Routledge.

Nelson, Lawrence J., and Nancy Milliken. 1990. "Compelled Medical Treatment of Pregnant Women: Life, Liberty, and Law in Conflict." Pp. 224–240 in *Ethical Issues in the New Reproductive Technologies*, edited by Richard T. Hull. Belmont, Calif.: Wadsworth.

Newman, Karen. 1996. *Fetal Positions: Individualism, Science, Visuality.* Stanford: Stanford University Press.

New York Academy of Sciences. 1968. "Fetology: The Smallest Patients." *Child and Family Quarterly* 8(2):159–164.

Nilsson, Lennart. 1990. *A Child Is Born.* New York: Delta-Seymour Lawrence.

Oakley, Ann. 1984. *The Captured Womb: A History of the Medical Care of Pregnant Women.* Oxford, U.K.: Basil Blackwell.

Olesen, Virginia, and Ellen Lewin. 1985. "Women, Health, and Healing: A Theoretical Introduction." Pp. 1–24 in *Women, Health, and Healing: A New Perspective*, edited by Ellen Lewin and Virginia Olesen. New York: Tavistock.

Oudshoorn, Nelly. 1994. *Beyond the Natural Body: An Archaeology of Sex Hormones.* London: Routledge.

Park, Robert Ezra. 1952. *Human Communities.* Glencoe, IL: Free Press.

Petchesky, Rosalind Pollack. 1987. "Fetal Images: The Power of Visual Culture in the Politics of Reproduction." Pp. 57–80 in *Reproductive Technologies: Gen-*

der, Motherhood, and Medicine, edited by Michelle Stanworth. Minneapolis: University of Minnesota Press.

——. 1990. *Abortion and Woman's Choice: The State, Sexuality, and Reproductive Freedom.* Revised ed. Boston: Northeastern University Press.

Pringle, Kevin C. 1986. "Fetal Surgery: It Has a Past, Has It a Future?" *Fetal Therapy* 1:23–31.

Proctor, Robert N. 1988. *Racial Hygiene: Medicine Under the Nazis.* Cambridge, Mass.: Harvard University Press.

Purdy, Laura M. 1990. "Are Pregnant Women Fetal Containers?" *Bioethics* 4:273–291.

Quintero, Ruben A., Karoline S. Puder, and David B. Cotton. 1993. "Embryoscopy and Fetoscopy." *Obstetrics and Gynecology Clinics of North America* 20:563–581.

Rader, Karen. 1995. "Making Mice: C. C. Little, the Jackson Laboratory, and the Standardization of *Mus Musculus* for Research." Unpublished paper, University of California, Berkeley.

Ramirez de Arellano, Annette B., and Conrad Seipp. 1983. *Colonialism, Catholicism, and Contraception: A History of Birth Control in Puerto Rico.* Chapel Hill: University of North Carolina Press.

Rapp, Rayna. 1987. "Moral Pioneers: Women, Men and Fetuses on a Frontier of Reproductive Technology." *Women's Health* 13:101.

——. 1990. "Constructing Amniocentesis: Maternal and Medical Discourses." Pp. 28–42 in *Uncertain Terms: Negotiating Gender in American Culture,* edited by Faye Ginsburg and Anna Lowenhaupt Tsing. Boston: Beacon.

——. 1993a. "Accounting for Amniocentesis." Pp. 55–75 in *Knowledge, Power, and Practice: The Anthropology of Medicine in Everyday Life,* edited by Shirley Lindenbaum and Margaret Lock. Berkeley and Los Angeles: University of California Press.

——. 1993b. "Amniocentesis in Sociocultural Perspective." *Journal of Genetic Counseling* 2:183–196.

——. 1993c. "Ethnocultural Diversity and Genetic Counseling Training: The Challenge of the 21st Century." *Journal of Genetic Counseling* 2:155–58.

——. 1994. "Women's Responses to Prenatal Diagnosis: A Sociocultural Perspective on Diversity." In *Women and Prenatal Testing: Facing the Challenges of Genetic Technology,* edited by Karen Rothenberg and Elizabeth Thompson. Athens: Ohio University Press.

——. 1995. "Real Time Fetus: The Role of the Sonogram in the Age of Monitored Reproduction." Paper presented at conference on Cyborgs and Citadels: Anthropological Interventions on the Borderlands of Technoscience, Santa Fe, New Mexico.

Rawlins, Richard G., and Matt J. Kessler. 1986. "The History of the Cayo Santiago Colony." Pp. 13–45 in *The Cayo Santiago Macaques: History, Behavior, and Biology,* edited by Richard G. Rawlins and Matt J. Kessler. Albany: State University of Ney York Press.

Reid, Tony. 1973. "Seeing Children As People." *New Zealand Listener,* September 10, 8.

Reiser, Stanley Joel. 1982. *Medicine and the Reign of Technology.* Cambridge, U.K.: Cambridge University Press.

Reiser, Stanley Joel, and Michael Anbar. 1986. *The Machine at the Bedside: Strategies for Using Technology in Patient Care.* Cambridge, U.K.: Cambridge University Press.

Riessman, Catherine Kohler. 1983. "Women and Medicalization: A New Perspective." *Social Policy* 14:3–18.

Roberts, Leslie. 1991. "FISHing Cuts the Angst in Amniocentesis." *Science* 254:378–379.

Rojas, Aurelio. 1994. "S.F. Police Confiscate 5 Fetuses from Haight Street Garage Sale." *San Francisco Chronicle,* January 10, A18.

Rothenberg, Karen H., and Elizabeth J. Thomson (eds.). 1994. *Women and Prenatal Testing: Facing the Challenges of Genetic Technology.* Columbus: Ohio State University Press.

Rothman, Barbara Katz. 1982. *In Labor: Women and Power in the Birthplace.* New York: Norton.

———. 1986. *The Tentative Pregnancy: Prenatal Diagnosis and the Future of Motherhood.* New York: Penguin Books.

———. 1989. *Recreating Motherhood: Ideology and Technology in a Patriarchal Society.* New York: Norton.

Rothman, David J. 1990. "Human Experimentation and the Origins of Bioethics in the United States." Pp. 185–200 in *Social Science Perspectives on Medical Ethics,* edited by George Weisz. Philadelphia: University of Pennsylvania Press.

Rouse, Joseph. 1993. "What are Cultural Studies of Scientific Knowledge?" *Configurations* 1:1–22.

Ruzek, Sheryl Burt, Virginia L. Olesen, and Adele E. Clarke. 1997. *Women's Health: Complexities and Differences.* Columbus: Ohio State University Press.

Ryan, Kenneth J. 1990. "Erosion of the Rights of Pregnant Women: In the Interest of Fetal Well-Being." *Women's Health Issues* 1:21–24.

Saltus, Richard. 1981. "Successful Surgery on Unborn Child." *San Francisco Examiner,* July 26, 1.

Sandelowski, Margarete, and Linda Corson Jones. 1996. "'Healing Fictions': Stories of Choosing in the Aftermath of the Detection of Fetal Anomalies." *Social Science and Medicine* 42:353–361.

Scheerer, Lourdes J., and Michael Katz. 1991. "Tocolysis for Fetal Intervention." Pp. 182–188 in *The Unborn Patient: Prenatal Diagnosis and Treatment,* edited by Michael R. Harrison, Mitchell S. Golbus, and Roy A. Filly. Philadelphia: W. B. Saunders.

Schulman, Joseph D., and Mark I. Evans. 1991. "The Fetus with a Biochemical Defect." Pp. 205–209 in *The Unborn Patient: Prenatal Diagnosis and Treatment,* edited by Michael R. Harrison, Mitchell S. Golbus, and Roy A. Filly. Philadelphia: W. B. Saunders.

Sgreccia, Elio. 1989. "Ethical Issues in Prenatal Diagnosis and Fetal Therapy: A Catholic Perspective." *Fetal Therapy* 4:16–27.

Shadbolt, Maurice. 1976. *Love and Legend: Some Twentieth-Century New Zealanders*. Auckland, New Zealand: Hodder and Stoughton.

Sherwin, Susan. 1992. *No Longer Patient: Feminist Ethics and Health Care*. Philadelphia: Temple University Press.

Simonds, Wendy. 1996. *Abortion At Work: Ideology and Practice in a Feminist Clinic*. New Brunswick, N.J.: Rutgers University Press.

Skerrett, P.J. 1991. "Wound Healing in the Womb." *Science* 252:1066.

Stabile, Carol. 1992. "Shooting the Mother: Fetal Photography and the Politics of Disappearance." *Camera Obscura* 28:179–206.

Stafford, Barbara Maria. 1991. *Body Criticism: Imaging the Unseen in Enlightenment Art and Medicine*. Cambridge, Mass.: MIT Press.

Star, Susan Leigh. 1986. "Triangulating Clinical and Basic Research: British Localizationists, 1870–1906." *History of Science* 24:29–48.

Starr, Paul. 1982. *The Social Transformation of American Medicine*. New York: Basic Books.

Steinbock, Bonnie. 1992. *Life Before Birth: The Moral and Legal Status of Embryos and Fetuses*. New York: Oxford University Press.

Stetson, Brad (ed.). 1996. *The Silent Subject: Reflections on the Unborn in American Culture*. Westport, Conn.: Greenwood.

Strauss, Anselm L. 1967. "Strategies for Discovering Urban Theory." in *Urban Research and Policy Planning*. Vol. 1, *Urban Affairs Annual Reviews*, edited by Leo F. Schnore and Henry Fagin. Beverly Hills, Calif.: Sage.

———. 1988. "The Articulation of Project Work: An Organizational Process." *Sociological Quarterly* 29:163–178.

———. 1993. *Continual Permutations of Action*. New York: de Gruyter.

Strauss, Anselm, Leonard Schatzman, Rue Bucher, Danuta Erlich, and Melvin Sabshin. 1964. *Psychiatric Ideologies and Institutions*. Glencoe, Ill.: Free Press.

Taylor, Janelle Sue. 1993. "The Public Fetus and the Family Car: From Abortion Politics to a Volvo Advertisement." *Science as Culture* 3:601–618.

Thomas, William I. 1978. "The Definition of the Situation." Pp. 54–57 in *Social Deviance*, edited by Ronald Farrell and Victoria Swigert. Philadelphia: Lippincott.

Thomas, William I., and Dorothy Swaine Thomas. 1970. "Situations Defined as Real are Real in Their Consequences." Pp. 154–155 in *Social Psychology Through Symbolic Interaction*, edited by Gregory Prentice Stone and Harvey A. Farberman. Waltham, Mass.: Xerox Publishers.

Thong, Y. H., and S. C. Harth. 1991. "The Social Filter Effect of Informed Consent in Clinical Research." *Pediatrics* 87:568–569.

Todd, Alexandra Dundas. 1989. *Intimate Adversaries: Cultural Conflict Between Doctors and Women Patients*. Philadelphia: University of Pennsylvania Press.

Twomey, John G., Jr. 1989. "The Ethics of In Utero Fetal Surgery: A Possible Threat to the Autonomy of Pregnant Women?" *Nursing Clinics of North America* 24:1025–1032.

van der Ploeg, Irma. 1994. "Fetal Surgery: Mending the Future, or: The Female

Body as Prosthesis." Paper presented at the Annual Meeting of the Society for Social Studies of Science, October, New Orleans, Louisiana.

Walters, LeRoy. 1986. "Ethical Issues in Intrauterine Diagnosis and Therapy." *Fetal Therapy* 1:32–37.

Weber, Max. 1949. *The Methodology of the Social Sciences*. New York: Free Press.

Weisz, George (ed.). 1990. *Social Science Perspectives on Medical Ethics*. Philadelphia: University of Pennsylvania Press.

West, Candace. 1984. *Routine Complications: Troubles with Talk Between Doctors and Patients*. Bloomington: Indiana University Press.

Willis, Ellen. 1989. "The Wrongs of Fetal Rights." *Voice*, April 11, 41–44.

Yoxen, Edward. 1987. "Seeing with Sound: A Study of the Development of Medical Images." Pp. 281–303 in *The Social Construction of Technological Sytems: New Directions in the Sociology and History of Technology*, edited by Wiebe E. Bijker, Thomas P. Hughes, and Trevor Pinch. Cambridge, Mass.: MIT Press.

Zimmerman, David R. 1973. *Rh: The Intimate History of a Disease and Its Conquest*. New York: Macmillan.

Index

About the Author

Monica J. Casper is an assistant professor of sociology at the University of California, Santa Cruz, where she teaches courses on medical sociology, science and technology studies, cultural theory, and feminist studies. She is also affiliated with the Stanford University Center for Biomedical Ethics and has served as a consultant for women's health groups. In 1996 the work on which this book is based won the Roberta G. Simmons Award for Outstanding Dissertation in Medical Sociology, given annually by the Medical Sociology Section of the American Sociological Association.

CPSIA information can be obtained
at www.ICGtesting.com
Printed in the USA
LVOW08s1250190517
534671LV00001B/1/P

9 780813 525167